Hematological Malignancies: Molecular Mechanisms and Therapy

Hematological Malignancies: Molecular Mechanisms and Therapy

Guest Editor

Stella Bouziana

MDPI

Basel • Beijing • Wuhan • Barcelona • Belgrade • Novi Sad • Cluj • Manchester

Guest Editor
Stella Bouziana
Department of Hematology
King's College Hospital
London
UK

Editorial Office
MDPI AG
Grosspeteranlage 5
4052 Basel, Switzerland

This is a reprint of the Special Issue, published open access by the journal *International Journal of Molecular Sciences* (ISSN 1422-0067), freely accessible at: https://www.mdpi.com/journal/ijms/special_issues/4CNOX7S98D.

For citation purposes, cite each article independently as indicated on the article page online and as indicated below:

Lastname, A.A.; Lastname, B.B. Article Title. *Journal Name* **Year**, *Volume Number*, Page Range.

ISBN 978-3-7258-4869-0 (Hbk)
ISBN 978-3-7258-4870-6 (PDF)
https://doi.org/10.3390/books978-3-7258-4870-6

Cover image courtesy of BReMeL
Fibrocyte intercalation pattern from a 92-day culture of normal human bone marrow. Safranin staining, (400X)

Contents

About the Editor vii

Preface ix

Stella Bouziana
Hematological Malignancies: Molecular Mechanisms and Therapy
Reprinted from: *Int. J. Mol. Sci.* **2025**, *26*, 2438, https://doi.org/10.3390/ijms26062438 1

Ana Guijarro-Hernández, Cristina Hurtado, Estibaliz Urizar-Compains, Begoña Ezcurra, Alberto Galiana-Sáenz, Enrique Baquero, et al.
Myeloproliferative Neoplasm-like Mutations of Calreticulin Induce Phenotypes Associated with Calreticulin Dysfunction in *C. elegans*
Reprinted from: *Int. J. Mol. Sci.* **2024**, *25*, 11606, https://doi.org/10.3390/ijms252111606 6

Abhay Singh, Nuria Mencia Trinchant, Rahul Mishra, Kirti Arora, Smit Mehta, Teodora Kuzmanovic, et al.
Immune Checkpoint Inhibitor Therapy and Associations with Clonal Hematopoiesis
Reprinted from: *Int. J. Mol. Sci.* **2024**, *25*, 11049, https://doi.org/10.3390/ijms252011049 25

Natalya Risinskaya, Abdulpatakh Abdulpatakhov, Yulia Chabaeva, Olga Aleshina, Maria Gladysheva, Elena Nikulina, et al.
Biallelic Loss of 7q34 (*TRB*) and 9p21.3 (*CDKN2A/2B*) in Adult Ph-Negative Acute T-Lymphoblastic Leukemia
Reprinted from: *Int. J. Mol. Sci.* **2024**, *25*, 10482, https://doi.org/10.3390/ijms251910482 36

Cameron K. Tebbi, Jiyu Yan, Eva Sahakian, Melanie Mediavilla-Varela, Javier Pinilla-Ibarz, Saumil Patel, et al.
Mycovirus-Containing *Aspergillus flavus* Alters Transcription Factors in Normal and Acute Lymphoblastic Leukemia Cells
Reprinted from: *Int. J. Mol. Sci.* **2024**, *25*, 10361, https://doi.org/10.3390/ijms251910361 47

Roberta Vadeikienė, Baltramiejus Jakštys, Danguolė Laukaitienė, Saulius Šatkauskas, Elona Juozaitytė and Rasa Ugenskienė
The Role of Mutated Calreticulin in the Pathogenesis of *BCR-ABL1*-Negative Myeloproliferative Neoplasms
Reprinted from: *Int. J. Mol. Sci.* **2024**, *25*, 9873, https://doi.org/10.3390/ijms25189873 64

Maiia Soloveva, Maksim Solovev, Natalya Risinskaya, Elena Nikulina, Igor Yakutik, Bella Biderman, et al.
Loss of Heterozygosity and Mutations in the RAS-ERK Pathway Genes in Tumor Cells of Various Loci in Multiple Myeloma
Reprinted from: *Int. J. Mol. Sci.* **2024**, *25*, 9426, https://doi.org/10.3390/ijms25179426 95

Johanna Pohl, Angela Litz, Omar El Ayoubi, Armando Rodríguez-Alfonso, Ludger Ständker, Mirja Harms, et al.
An Optimized Peptide Antagonist of CXCR4 Limits Survival of BCR–ABL1-Transformed Cells in Philadelphia-Chromosome-Positive B-Cell Acute Lymphoblastic Leukemia
Reprinted from: *Int. J. Mol. Sci.* **2024**, *25*, 8306, https://doi.org/10.3390/ijms25158306 110

Husam B. R. Alabed, Roberto Maria Pellegrino, Sandra Buratta, Anair Graciela Lema Fernandez, Roberta La Starza, Lorena Urbanelli, et al.
Metabolic Profiling as an Approach to Differentiate T-Cell Acute Lymphoblastic Leukemia Cell Lines Belonging to the Same Genetic Subgroup
Reprinted from: *Int. J. Mol. Sci.* **2024**, *25*, 3921, https://doi.org/10.3390/ijms25073921 . . . . . . **130**

Anna Marszołek, Maria Leśniak, Anna Sekunda, Aleksander Siwek, Zuzanna Skiba, Monika Lejman and Joanna Zawitkowska
Haploidentical HSCT in the Treatment of Pediatric Hematological Disorders
Reprinted from: *Int. J. Mol. Sci.* **2024**, *25*, 6380, https://doi.org/10.3390/ijms25126380 . . . . . . **149**

Stella Bouziana and Dimitrios Bouzianas
The Current Landscape of Secondary Malignancies after CAR T-Cell Therapies: How Could Malignancies Be Prevented?
Reprinted from: *Int. J. Mol. Sci.* **2024**, *25*, 9518, https://doi.org/10.3390/ijms25179518 . . . . . . **176**

Maria Teresa Bochicchio, Giovanni Marconi, Carmen Baldazzi, Lorenza Bandini, Francesca Ruggieri, Alessandro Lucchesi, et al.
ETV6::ABL1-Positive Myeloid Neoplasm: A Case of a Durable Response to Imatinib Mesylate without Additional or Previous Treatment
Reprinted from: *Int. J. Mol. Sci.* **2024**, *25*, 118, https://doi.org/10.3390/ijms25010118 . . . . **190**

About the Editor

Stella Bouziana

Stella Bouziana is a Hematologist and a Senior Clinical Research Fellow at King's College Hospital (KCH), London, UK, affiliated with King's College London. She has a specialist interest in cellular therapies and lymphoproliferative diseases. She obtained her Medical Degree and PhD from the Aristotle University of Thessaloniki, Greece, and she completed her Hematology training at the George Papanikolaou General Hospital, Thessaloniki, Greece. Dr Bouziana has been a member of the research and clinical team of the Hematology Department at KCH since 2021.

Dr Bouziana's research focuses on investigating the tumor microenvironment of lymphoma and chronic lymphocytic leukemia patients, especially those being considered or treated with cellular therapies or immune activators. This includes the spatial analysis and deep immunophenotyping of the cellular components with the aid of bioinformatics, while in parallel profiling transcriptional and molecular signatures. She has also been leading research activities in several early and late phase clinical trials in the field of cellular therapies, lymphoproliferative and plasma cell disorders.

Dr Bouziana has published extensively in peer-reviewed journals, while she serves as an editor, board member and reviewer in multiple prestigious journals. She is a member of the British Society of Hematology, the European Hematology Association (EHA), and the European Society for Blood and Marrow Transplantation. She has also served as an expert reviewer of cellular immunotherapy and gene therapy abstracts submitted at the annual congress of the EHA. Dr Bouziana currently offers advisory to a start-up biotechnological company under establishment (BreMeL) based in Greece, including the co-authorship of a European patent under preparation on a new method regarding the optimization of the cell dose in autologous CAR T-cell therapies.

Preface

The field of hematological cancers is advancing at an unprecedented pace, driven by groundbreaking discoveries and emerging research pipelines that enhance patient care and outcomes. The aim of this Reprint is to bring together the latest advancements in hematological malignancies, allowing readers to immerse themselves in the exploration of this dynamic field. Leading experts share their pioneering research with a vision to further accelerate progress in the arena of hematological cancers. Readers have the opportunity to delve into the investigation of molecular, genetic, and immunological mechanisms underlying these cancers, leveraging this knowledge to drive the development of innovative therapeutics. Featuring twelve high-quality articles, this collection spans a diverse spectrum of research, from preliminary preclinical studies to clinical cohort analyses. Addressed to researchers and clinicians passionate about deepening their understanding of hematological malignancies, we hope that this Reprint will inspire more researchers to contribute to the ongoing advancement of this exciting field.

Stella Bouziana
Guest Editor

International Journal of
Molecular Sciences

MDPI

Editorial

Hematological Malignancies: Molecular Mechanisms and Therapy

Stella Bouziana [1,2]

[1] Comprehensive Cancer Centre, School of Cancer and Pharmaceutical Medicine, King's College London, London SE5 8AF, UK; styliani.bouziana@nhs.net
[2] Department of Haematology, King's College Hospital National Health Service (NHS) Foundation Trust, London SE5 9RS, UK

Hematological malignancies comprise a wide range of relatively rare cancers with a diverse spectrum of biological and clinical presentations. Hematological malignancies can affect both children and adults, with some of them showing a preference for developing at a certain age group [1]. Over the recent decades, the advent and implementation of novel technologies, such as next-generation sequencing (NGS), have enabled deciphering the molecular and genetic signature of hematological malignancies. In addition, epigenetic, transcriptional, and translational analyses have also contributed to delineating the pathogenesis of these cancers [2,3]. Analysis at the single-cell level, including spatial immunophenotyping and multiomics, has resulted in the generation of bulk data, which have significantly contributed, with the aid of bioinformatic pipelines, to gaining a deeper understanding of disease mechanisms in terms of carcinogenesis, disease progression, and resistance to treatment modalities [4,5]. The acquisition of this emerging data has resulted in the development of novel diagnostic tools that offer an accurate and early detection of hematological cancers. In addition, the exploitation of novel technologies, imaging techniques, and the detection of circulating tumor DNA has massively streamlined disease monitoring over natural evolution and treatment of hematological malignancies while offering new predicting, preventive, and prognostic platforms [6,7].

More importantly, the unravelling of molecular pathways has resulted in unprecedented advances in establishing new therapeutic targets and developing innovative types of therapies for hematological cancers. These therapies include targeted therapies, such as bruton's tyrosine kinase, B-cell lymphoma 2, tyrosine kinase, and isocitrate dehydrogenase inhibitors; immune checkpoint inhibitors that block checkpoint proteins, such as programmed death-1 and programmed death-ligand 1; and a wide variety of immunotherapies, such as monoclonal antibodies and antibody drug conjugates. In addition, epigenetic modifiers, such as DNA methyltransferase inhibitors, have notably improved the overall prognosis of patients with myeloid neoplasms [8]. A major milestone towards curing hematological malignancies has been the advent of allogeneic hematopoietic stem cell transplantation (HSCT), the refinement of which has profoundly improved patient outcomes while minimizing treatment-related toxicities [9]. Another rapidly growing field includes bispecific antibodies, which are engineered to bind to two different targets simultaneously, enhancing the immune system's ability to attack cancer cells [10]. The landscape of treatment for hematological malignancies is rapidly evolving, with cellular and gene therapies, such as chimeric antigen receptor (CAR) T-cell therapies, constituting groundbreaking options in the treatment armamentarium [8,11]. A combinatorial approach to these novel therapies has revolutionized the field of hematooncology, offering long-term remission or even curing hematological patients, even those with highly aggressive and refractory malignancies.

However, despite this massive progress, there are still hematological malignancies that remain uncured, while there are treatment regimens that confer detrimental or even life-threatening toxicities. Aggressive and refractory types of hematological malignancies entail devastating outcomes, and their successful management to control the disease and induce remission represents a great challenge. Significant research is still needed to be undertaken in order to demystify key pathways towards developing more potent and safer treatments.

This Special Issue aims to compile the latest research advances on investigating the molecular, genetic, and immunological pathways that contribute to the pathogenesis of hematological malignancies or can serve as predictive, preventive, and prognostic disease markers. In addition, this Special Issue focused on collecting cutting-edge knowledge on novel therapeutics of hematological malignancies. Twenty-one manuscripts were submitted for consideration for this Special Issue, and all of them underwent a rigorous peer review process. Finally, eleven articles were accepted for publication and were included in this Special Issue: eight research articles, one review article, one opinion article, and one case report. An overview of the contributed articles is listed below:

1. An experimental *C. elegans* model with homozygous mutations in calreticulin similar to those found in patients with myeloproliferative neoplasms and without the influence of JAK/STAT activation explored the relationship of phenotypic characteristics with transcriptomic alterations. It was shown for the first time that phenotypes related to the alteration of the extracellular matrix, fat levels, and fertility could be a consequence of a partial loss of calreticulin function, suggesting potential targets for innovative therapies by further investigating these effects (Guijarro-Hernández, A.; Hurtado, C.; Urizar-Compains, E.; Ezcurra, B.; Galiana-Sáenz, A.; Baquero, E.; Cabello, J.; Vizmanos, J.L. Myeloproliferative Neoplasm-like Mutations of Calreticulin Induce Phenotypes Associated with Calreticulin Dysfunction in *C. elegans*. *Int. J. Mol. Sci.* 2024, 25, 11606. https://doi.org/10.3390/ijms252111606).

2. An observational cohort aimed to elucidate the impact of immune checkpoint blockade on hematopoietic myeloid clonal expansion in patients with melanoma and non-small cell lung cancer. Sequencing of a targeted panel of genes was performed on serial blood samples to identify mutations, and preliminary results revealed clonal expansion in epigenetic modifier genes, such as *DNMT3A* and *TET2*, potentially indicating a selective pressure of immune checkpoint blockade/T-cell activating therapies on hematopoietic stem cells. Further investigations could assess the predictive role of these mutations as biomarkers of response to immune checkpoint blockade or risk for developing myeloid malignancies (Singh, A.; Trinchant, N.M.; Mishra, R.; Arora, K.; Mehta, S.; Kuzmanovic, T.; Zokaei Nikoo, M.; Singh, I.; Przespolewski, A.C.; Swaminathan, M.; et al. Immune Checkpoint Inhibitor Therapy and Associations with Clonal Hematopoiesis. *Int. J. Mol. Sci.* 2024, 25, 11049. https://doi.org/10.3390/ijms252011049).

3. In patients with de novo T-cell acute lymphoblastic leukemia (ALL), biallelic deletions of genes were investigated by chromosomal microarray analysis. Biallelic loss of 7q34 (*TRB*) and 9p21.3 (*CDKN2A/2B*) was identified in a significant number of patients, while both biallelic deletions were considered to serve as favorable prognostic factors (Risinskaya, N.; Abdulpatakhov, A.; Chabaeva, Y.; Aleshina, O.; Gladysheva, M.; Nikulina, E.; Bolshakov, I.; Yushkova, A.; Dubova, O.; Vasileva, A.; et al. Biallelic Loss of 7q34 (TRB) and 9p21.3 (CDKN2A/2B) in Adult Ph-Negative Acute T-Lymphoblastic Leukemia. *Int. J. Mol. Sci.* 2024, 25, 10482. https://doi.org/10.3390/ijms251910482).

4. In vitro studies in normal and ALL cell lines assessed the impact of the products of a mycovirus-containing *Aspergillus flavus* in certain transcription factors, such as PAX5, Ikaros, and NF-κB. The results showed alterations in the cell cycle and transcription factors along with induced cell apoptosis, highlighting a potential contributing role of environmental factors in leukemogenesis (Tebbi, C.K.; Yan, J.; Sahakian, E.; Mediavilla-Varela, M.; Pinilla-Ibarz, J.; Patel, S.; Rottinghaus, G.E.; Liu, R.Y.; Dennison, C. Mycovirus-Containing Aspergillus flavus Alters Transcription Factors in Normal and Acute Lymphoblastic Leukemia Cells. *Int. J. Mol. Sci.* 2024, 25, 10361. https://doi.org/10.3390/ijms251910361).

5. The role of the *CALR* 52 bp deletion and 5 bp insertion in the pathogenesis of myeloproliferative neoplasms (MPNs) was assessed in vitro in *CALR*-mutated cells offering a deeper understanding of molecular mechanisms in *CALR*-mutated MPNs. It was found that the JAK/STAT and PI3K/Akt/mTOR pathways are activated in *CALR*-mutated cells independent of the CALR and MPL interactions, while *CALR* mutations that impair calreticulin function lead to DNA damage by reducing responses to oxidative stress. (Vadeikienė, R.; Jakštys, B.; Laukaitienė, D.; Šatkauskas, S.; Juozaitytė, E.; Ugenskienė, R. The Role of Mutated Calreticulin in the Pathogenesis of BCR-ABL1-Negative Myeloproliferative Neoplasms. *Int. J. Mol. Sci.* 2024, 25, 9873. https://doi.org/10.3390/ijms25189873).

6. Liquid biopsy studies analyzing plasma free circulating tumor DNA, bone marrow cells, and plasmacytomas for STR profiles in patients with multiple myeloma highlighted the anatomical tumor heterogeneity. In addition, rare *KRAS* or *NRAS* gene mutations were related to a variety of adverse laboratory and clinical factors, suggesting a potential role in predicting an unfavorable prognosis in high-risk multiple myeloma. (Soloveva, M.; Solovev, M.; Risinskaya, N.; Nikulina, E.; Yakutik, I.; Biderman, B.; Obukhova, T.; Chabaeva, Y.; Kulikov, S.; Sudarikov, A.; et al. Loss of Heterozygosity and Mutations in the RAS-ERK Pathway Genes in Tumor Cells of Various Loci in Multiple Myeloma. *Int. J. Mol. Sci.* 2024, 25, 9426. https://doi.org/10.3390/ijms25179426).

7. In vitro studies in Philadelphia-chromosome-positive cell models explored an array of peptide-based inhibitors of CXC chemokine receptor 4 (CXCR4), which seems crucial for the survival of BCR–ABL1-transformed mouse pre-B-cells. The results of this study showed that JM#170, an optimized derivative of EPI-X4, which is an endogenous peptide antagonist of CXCR4, induced cell death both in mouse and human cell lines by activating the intrinsic apoptotic pathway. This killing effect was stronger when Imatinib, an ABL1 kinase inhibitor, was combined with JM#170 which may represent a novel drug against Philadelphia positive B-ALL (Pohl, J.; Litz, A.; El Ayoubi, O.; Rodríguez-Alfonso, A.; Ständker, L.; Harms, M.; Münch, J.; Jumaa, H.; Datta, M. An Optimized Peptide Antagonist of CXCR4 Limits Survival of BCR–ABL1-Transformed Cells in Philadelphia-Chromosome-Positive B-Cell Acute Lymphoblastic Leukemia. *Int. J. Mol. Sci.* 2024, 25, 8306. https://doi.org/10.3390/ijms25158306).

8. Metabolic and lipidomic analysis using liquid chromatography/mass spectrometry set to differentiate four T-ALL cell lines belonging to the same TAL/LMO genetic subgroup based on metabolic profiles. Significant differences and similarities were found in metabolites across the four cell lines, while bioinformatic tools identified differences in enzymes involved in diverse pathways among the cell lines (Alabed, H.B.R.; Pellegrino, R.M.; Buratta, S.; Lema Fernandez, A.G.; La Starza, R.; Urbanelli, L.; Mecucci, C.; Emiliani, C.; Gorello, P. Metabolic Profiling as an Approach to Differentiate T-Cell Acute Lymphoblastic Leukemia Cell Lines Belonging to the Same Genetic Subgroup. *Int. J. Mol. Sci.* 2024, 25, 3921. https://doi.org/10.3390/ijms25073921).

9. The most recent advances in haploidentical allogeneic HSCT for treating pediatric hematological disorders were reviewed. Outcomes of haploidentical allogeneic HSCT have significantly improved; however, multiple challenges are still in place needing further

research to be tackled (Marszołek, A.; Leśniak, M.; Sekunda, A.; Siwek, A.; Skiba, Z.; Lejman, M.; Zawitkowska, J. Haploidentical HSCT in the Treatment of Pediatric Hematological Disorders. *Int. J. Mol. Sci.* 2024, 25, 6380. https://doi.org/10.3390/ijms25126380).

10. An opinion article presented the current landscape of secondary malignancies post CAR T-cell therapies given the new safety concern triggered by the Food and Drug Administration announcement in November 2023 on reported cases of T-cell malignancies in patients previously treated with either anti-CD19 or anti-BCMA autologous CAR T-cell therapies. A proposed strategy for future research aiming at potentially diminishing or abrogating the risk of developing secondary malignancies after CAR T-cell therapies was also presented (Bouziana, S.; Bouzianas, D. The Current Landscape of Secondary Malignancies after CAR T-Cell Therapies: How Could Malignancies Be Prevented? *Int. J. Mol. Sci.* 2024, 25, 9518. https://doi.org/10.3390/ijms25179518).

11. An interesting case report of a patient with an *ETV6::ABL1*-positive myeloid neoplasm was presented. The diagnosis was established by NGS, which identified both *ETV6::ABL1* type A and B fusion transcripts and was later confirmed by FISH, while the patient was treated with imatinib mesylate, achieving a deep, durable response lasting more than one year according to the last follow-up (Bochicchio, M.T.; Marconi, G.; Baldazzi, C.; Bandini, L.; Ruggieri, F.; Lucchesi, A.; Agostinelli, C.; Sabattini, E.; Orsatti, A.; Ferrari, A.; et al. ETV6::ABL1-Positive Myeloid Neoplasm: A Case of a Durable Response to Imatinib Mesylate without Additional or Previous Treatment. *Int. J. Mol. Sci.* 2024, 25, 118. https://doi.org/10.3390/ijms25010118).

This compilation of articles encompasses a diverse spectrum of research ranging from early stage preliminary pre-clinical studies to clinical cohorts. All of these articles tried to shed light into key molecular, genetic and cellular pathways of different hematological malignancies in an attempt to better understand the pathogenesis, discover new biomarkers and develop novel therapies. Further research is warranted to expand and validate these results in more complex in vivo models and subsequent clinical studies. This highlights the need for collaboration of researchers from a multi-disciplinary background in an effort to further accelerate advances in the field of hematological malignancies with an overall aim of translating research findings into clinical practice and improving patient outcomes. We hope that this Special Issue will serve towards this direction by attracting the scientific interest of researchers across the globe.

Conflicts of Interest: The author declares no conflicts of interest.

References

1. Siegel, R.L.; Miller, K.D.; Fuchs, H.E.; Jemal, A. Cancer statistics, 2021. *CA Cancer J. Clin.* **2021**, *71*, 7–33. [CrossRef] [PubMed]
2. Kwon, R.; Yeung, C.C. Advances in next-generation sequencing and emerging technologies for hematologic malignancies. *Haematologica* **2024**, *109*, 379–387. [CrossRef] [PubMed]
3. Cao, X.; Huber, S.; Ahari, A.J.; Traube, F.R.; Seifert, M.; Oakes, C.C.; Secheyko, P.; Vilov, S.; Scheller, I.F.; Wagner, N.; et al. Analysis of 3760 hematologic malignancies reveals rare transcriptomic aberrations of driver genes. *Genome Med.* **2024**, *16*, 70. [CrossRef] [PubMed]
4. Campillo-Marcos, I.; Alvarez-Errico, D.; Alandes, R.A.; Mereu, E.; Esteller, M. Single-cell technologies and analyses in hematopoiesis and hematological malignancies. *Exp. Hematol.* **2021**, *98*, 1–13. [CrossRef] [PubMed]
5. Larsson, L.; Frisén, J.; Lundeberg, J. Spatially resolved transcriptomics adds a new dimension to genomics. *Nat. Methods* **2021**, *18*, 15–18. [CrossRef] [PubMed]
6. Talotta, D.; Almasri, M.; Cosentino, C.; Gaidano, G.; Moia, R. Liquid biopsy in hematological malignancies: Current and future applications. *Front. Oncol.* **2023**, *13*, 1164517. [CrossRef] [PubMed]
7. Parghane, R.V.; Basu, S. Role of Novel Quantitative Imaging Techniques in Hematological Malignancies. *PET Clin.* **2024**, *19*, 543–559. [CrossRef] [PubMed]
8. Lica, J.J.; Pradhan, B.; Safi, K.; Jakóbkiewicz-Banecka, J.; Hellmann, A. Promising Therapeutic Strategies for Hematologic Malignancies: Innovations and Potential. *Molecules* **2024**, *29*, 4280. [CrossRef] [PubMed]

9. Phelan, R.; Chen, M.; Bupp, C.; Bolon, Y.-T.; Broglie, L.; Brunner-Grady, J.; Burns, L.J.; Chhabra, S.; Christianson, D.; Cusatis, R.; et al. Updated Trends in Hematopoietic Cell Transplantation in the United States with an Additional Focus on Adolescent and Young Adult Transplantation Activity and Outcomes. *Transplant. Cell. Ther.* **2022**, *28*, 409. [CrossRef] [PubMed]
10. Goebeler, M.-E.; Bargou, R.C. T cell-engaging therapies—BiTEs and beyond. *Nat. Rev. Clin. Oncol.* **2020**, *17*, 418–434. [CrossRef] [PubMed]
11. Cappell, K.M.; Kochenderfer, J.N. Long-term outcomes following CAR T cell therapy: What we know so far. *Nat. Rev. Clin. Oncol.* **2023**, *20*, 359–371. [CrossRef] [PubMed]

International Journal of
Molecular Sciences

MDPI

Article

Myeloproliferative Neoplasm-like Mutations of Calreticulin Induce Phenotypes Associated with Calreticulin Dysfunction in *C. elegans*

Ana Guijarro-Hernández [1], Cristina Hurtado [1], Estibaliz Urizar-Compains [1], Begoña Ezcurra [2], Alberto Galiana-Sáenz [1,2], Enrique Baquero [3,4], Juan Cabello [2] and José Luis Vizmanos [1,*]

[1] Department of Biochemistry and Genetics, School of Sciences, University of Navarra, 31008 Pamplona, Spain; aguijarro@alumni.unav.es (A.G.-H.); churtado@unav.es (C.H.); eurizarc@unav.es (E.U.-C.); agalianasae@alumni.unav.es (A.G.-S.)

[2] Center for Biomedical Research of La Rioja (CIBIR), 26006 Logroño, Spain; bezcurra@riojasalud.es (B.E.); juan.cabello@riojasalud.es (J.C.)

[3] Department of Environmental Biology, School of Sciences, University of Navarra, 31008 Pamplona, Spain; ebaquero@unav.es

[4] Institute for Biodiversity and Environment BIOMA, University of Navarra, 31008 Pamplona, Spain

* Correspondence: jlvizmanos@unav.es

Abstract: In previous research, we created a *C. elegans* model with homozygous mutations in calreticulin similar to those found in patients with essential thrombocythemia (ET) and primary myelofibrosis (PMF), two myeloproliferative neoplasms (MPNs). This model, lacking JAK orthologs, enabled us to examine the transcriptomic effects caused by mutant calreticulin without the influence of JAK/STAT activation, the primary pathogenic mechanism associated with calreticulin mutations known to date. Most of the gene expression changes observed seemed to be due to a partial loss of protein function, with the alteration of the extracellular matrix being particularly notable. In this study, our aim was to determine whether this model exhibited any phenotype related to these transcriptomic alterations. The results demonstrate that these strains exhibit multiple phenotypes related to the alteration of the extracellular matrix, fat levels, and fertility, which could be a possible consequence of a partial loss of calreticulin function. These phenotypes resemble some of the clinical and molecular characteristics described in patients with MPNs, but they had never before been linked to a loss of protein function in humans. Thus, these results collectively suggest that *CALR* mutations could have significant effects on MPNs due to loss of protein function. Delving deeper into these effects to develop innovative therapies for these patients offers considerable potential and interest, given that targeted therapies for these patients have not yielded very promising results so far.

Keywords: calreticulin; myeloproliferative neoplasms; loss of function; development; molting; *Caenorhabditis elegans*

1. Introduction

The nematode *Caenorhabditis elegans* has made significant contributions to our understanding of the molecular mechanisms involved in cancer development, including processes like apoptosis [1]. Likewise, this organism has helped uncover the link between hypoxia and apoptosis in tumor progression [2] and has provided important insights into the roles of autophagy, the cell cycle, and other processes involved in cancer development [3–5].

The approach to study cancer in *C. elegans* is very particular since this organism is incapable of generating malignant tumors [1]. However, this limitation can be overcome by comparative analyses of phenotypes. Orthologous phenotypes, or phenologs, are defined as the phenotypes arising from the disruption of equivalent gene orthologs in two organisms.

For example, mutations in the genes of the *him* family produce a high incidence of males in *C. elegans*, while alterations in their human orthologs (*TP53* and *BRCA1*) are implicated in several types of cancer. Thus, the identification of orthologous phenotypes results in a list of genes associated with the phenotype, from which potential molecular mechanisms involved in the disease can be identified [1,6].

In this study, we used the model organism *C. elegans* to investigate myeloproliferative neoplasms (MPNs), a group of rare blood cancers characterized by the clonal expansion of mature myeloid cells. Our work was focused on the study of essential thrombocythemia (ET) and primary myelofibrosis (PMF), two MPNs that can be caused by mutations in *CALR*, the gene encoding calreticulin.

Patients with ET may present with a broad spectrum of symptoms, ranging from asymptomatic cases to complications associated with thrombosis, bleeding, and vasomotor disturbances. PMF patients typically experience symptoms such as night sweat, fatigue, weight loss, and pruritus. Moreover, PMF is characterized by extramedullary hematopoiesis and fibrosis of the bone marrow. The gene harboring the driver mutation plays a significant role in shaping the clinical presentation. Thus, *CALR* mutations have been associated with higher platelet counts in ET patients and an increased risk of transformation to fibrosis, which is one of the main causes of mortality among individuals with ET [7].

The mechanism by which *CALR* mutations induce myeloproliferation remains unclear. It has been reported that mutant CALR binds to the extracellular domain of MPL in the endoplasmic reticulum, resulting in dimerization, transport to the cell surface, and activation of the JAK2/STAT pathway [7–9]. Additionally, a recent study has suggested that the activation of the JAK2/STAT signaling pathway in *CALR*-mutated cells may also occur in an MPL-independent manner [10]. In any case, although a role for the JAK2/STAT pathway in MPNs has been emphasized repeatedly, there are certain complexities in this relationship. The presence of an inflammatory state in MPNs may complicate the understanding of the role of the JAK2/STAT pathway in these disorders, as inflammation and cytokine production can influence the activation of the pathway in ways that are not specific to MPNs [7].

In this context, there is a growing emphasis on investigating alternative mechanisms independent of JAK2/STAT activation that may elucidate the reasons why mutations in *CALR* result in myeloproliferation. To date, several mechanisms triggered by mutant CALR that are independent of JAK2/STAT activation have been identified (reviewed in [11]). First, mutant CALR appears to cause resistance to UPR-induced apoptosis and genomic instability by downregulating OXR1 in K562 cells [12]. A recent study also demonstrated that *CALR* mutations impair calreticulin function, leading to weakened responses to oxidative stress and DNA damage [10], a result previously suggested by our *C. elegans* model with calreticulin mutations [13]. Additionally, *CALR* mutations increase protein secretion and bind to CALR receptors on antigen-presenting cells, limiting their ability to phagocytize cancer cells that express wild-type CALR and promoting immune evasion [14]. This effect is further exacerbated by decreased binding affinity for PDIA3, resulting in a loss of function in the peptide loading complex, which is responsible for loading cellular antigens onto MHC-I molecules [15,16]. It has also been reported that defective interaction between mutant CALR and the SOCE machinery triggers TPOR-independent cytosolic calcium fluxes in megakaryocytes that lead to their uncontrolled proliferation [17]. Finally, various studies suggest that *CALR* mutations promote tumorigenesis by modulating transcription through interactions with nuclear transcription factors [15,18], and other reports support their role in activating key pathways of MPNs, including Hedgehog signaling, in a JAK2/STAT-independent manner across different models [10,13].

Despite the advances made in the molecular description of the pathogenesis of *CALR*-mutated ET and PMF, so far it has not been possible to develop any targeted therapy capable of curing these diseases or reducing the mutant allele burden in these patients. Currently, the only approved targeted therapy for patients with myelofibrotic-phase ET and for non-transplanted patients with PMF is the JAK1/JAK2 inhibitor ruxolitinib, which aims to decrease the activation of the JAK2/STAT pathway [19]. However, this therapy does not appear to be more effective than other second-line treatments for ET [20] and only palliates symptoms such as splenomegaly in patients with PMF [19]. Therefore, studying JAK2/STAT-independent mechanisms derived from mutant calreticulin could be of great interest, as it could lead to the discovery of new therapeutic targets in order to develop new treatment approaches or to improve the efficacy of existing therapies based on JAK inhibitors.

In this context, *C. elegans* seems to be a suitable organism for studying the JAK2/STAT-independent pathogenic mechanisms of mutant calreticulin since it shows an ortholog of calreticulin (*crt-1*) and lacks orthologs of JAK proteins. In this way, the introduction of mutations similar to those causing myeloproliferative neoplasms in humans could allow the identification of the JAK2/STAT-independent effects of mutant calreticulin.

Expanding upon this logic, we created two strains of *C. elegans* with mutations in homozygosity in *crt-1* (*crt-1(knu378)* and *crt-1(jvp1)*) in a previous study [13]. These mutations, respectively, recreate those known as type 1 and type 2 mutations, typically found in heterozygosity in the calreticulin of patients with MPNs [13]. Transcriptomic analyses of these nematodes allowed us to elucidate some possible altered mechanisms resulting from mutant calreticulin [13]. Most of the observed expression changes appeared to correspond to a partial loss of protein function, with the alteration of the extracellular matrix being particularly notable. In the present work, we aim to study whether *crt-1(knu378)* and *crt-1(jvp1)* mutants exhibit any phenotype related to the transcriptomic alteration of the extracellular matrix (development, molting, and morphology and resistance of the cuticle), as well as other phenotypes previously associated with the loss of function of *crt-1* in *C. elegans* (fertility, response to endoplasmic reticulum (ER) stress, and regulation of lipid homeostasis) [21,22] that could be related to some of the alterations that emerged in the transcriptomic analyses. The description of these phenotypes can help to identify new mechanisms that may be key in the development or progression of *CALR*-mutated ET and PMF and point to new possible therapeutic targets for these diseases.

2. Results

2.1. *crt-1* Mutations Delay Larval Development and Affect Molting

The mutant strains in *crt-1* exhibited a temporal growth delay in length compared to the wild-type strain under both baseline conditions (20 °C) (Figure 1a) and conditions that slightly induce overexpression of *crt-1* (25 °C) [21] (Figure 1b). The growth delay was very similar between *crt-1(knu378)* and *crt-1(jvp1)* worms and lower than that observed for the *crt-1(jh101)* strain at both temperatures (Figure 1a,b). Differences between *crt-1(knu378)*/*crt-1(jvp1)* worms and the *crt-1(jh101)* strain were more pronounced between 29 and 53 h at 20 °C (Figure S1) and between 24 and 53 h at 25 °C (Figure S2).

To determine if the growth delay in terms of length was also associated with a developmental delay, the larval stage of the worms was evaluated at each of the time points studied based on their morphological characteristics. The results showed that the *crt-1* mutant strains also took longer than the wild-type strain to reach various larval stages, both under baseline conditions (20 °C) (Figure 1c) and under conditions that slightly induce the overexpression of *crt-1* (25 °C) (Figure 1d). This delay in development was similar to that observed with length and was also very similar between *crt-1(knu378)* and *crt-1(jvp1)* worms and less than that observed for the *crt-1(jh101)* strain at both temperatures (Figure 1c,d). Also, as in the case of length, the differences between *crt-1(knu378)*/*crt-1(jvp1)* worms and the *crt-1(jh101)* strain were more noticeable between 29 and 53 h at 20 °C (Figure S3) and between 24 and 53 h at 25 °C (Figure S4).

As expected, all strains grew faster at 25 °C than at 20 °C, both in length and larval development. However, at 25 °C, the differences between strains were greater (Figure 1b,d).

The analysis of molting at 20 °C confirmed that the *crt-1(knu378)* and *crt-1(jvp1)* strains exhibited a very similar larval development, and in both cases, it was intermediate to that observed in the wild-type and *crt-1(jh101)* strains (Figure 2).

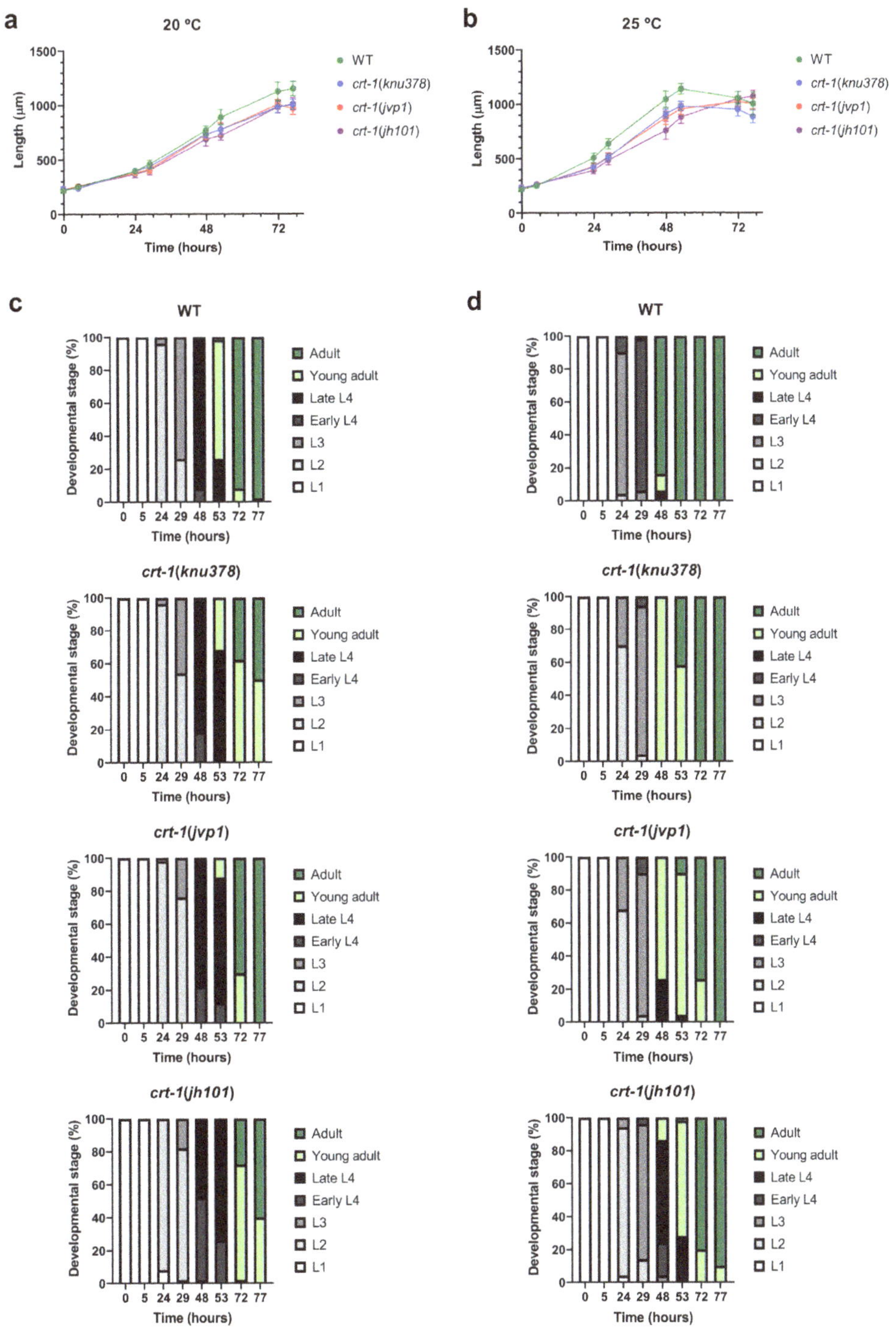

Figure 1. Larval development at 20 and 25 °C. *crt-1* mutations delay larval development at 20 and 25 °C. (**a**,**b**) Length of individuals during growth at 20 and 25 °C, respectively. The mean lengths obtained for 50 worms per strain at 0, 5, 24, 29, 48, 53, 72, and 77 h are represented, along with their

standard deviation. (**c**,**d**) Classification into larval stages of the individuals at 20 and 25 °C, respectively. The percentage of worms in each larval stage (L1, L2, L3, early L4, late L4, young adult, or adult) out of a total of 50 worms assessed per strain at 0, 5, 24, 29, 48, 53, 72, and 77 h is represented. The results of the statistical analysis conducted for these assays are detailed in Figures S1–S4.

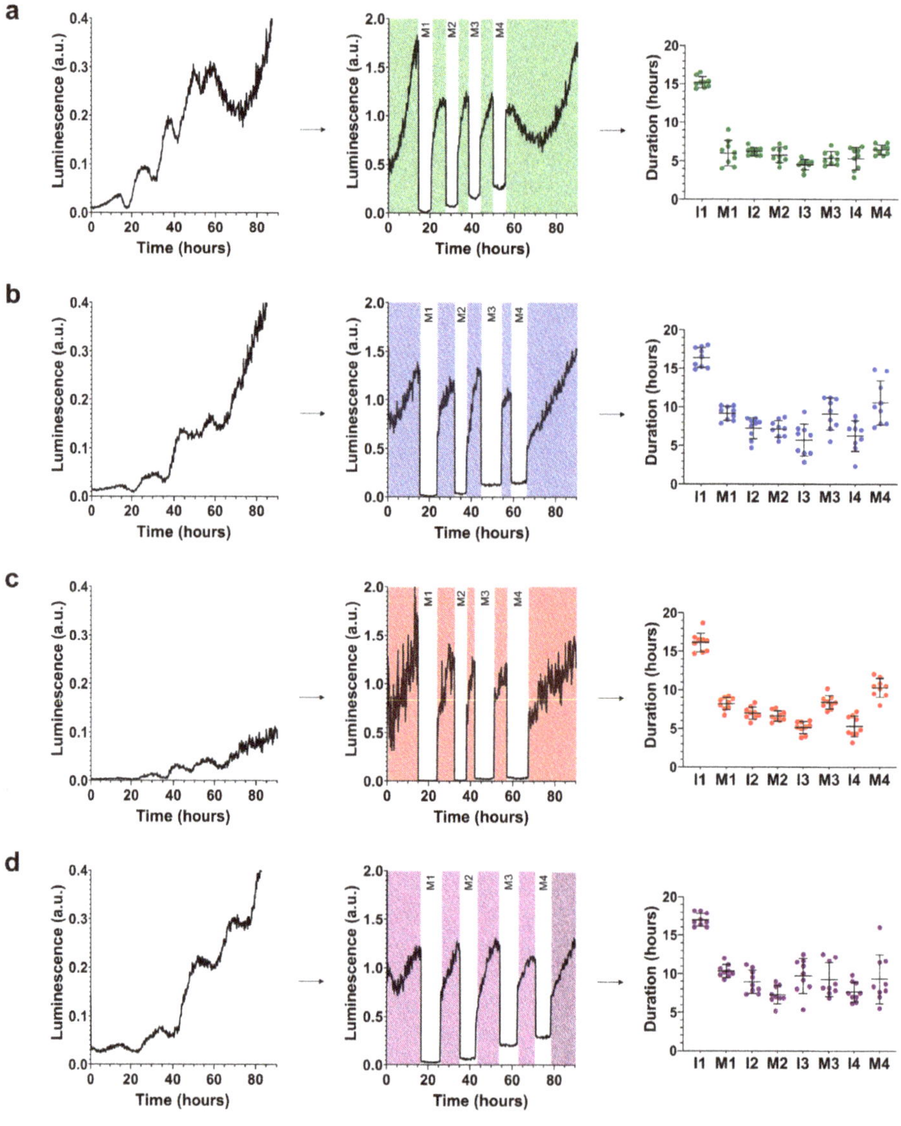

Figure 2. Molting patterns at 20 °C. *crt-1* mutants show aberrant molting patterns at 20 °C. The molting pattern of each strain was studied using bioluminescence. On the left side of each panel, the raw bioluminescence values obtained are represented. In the middle part, the corrected interphase values are represented by dividing the raw data of the interphases by the mean of each interphase while maintaining the raw bioluminescence values obtained in each molt (M; in white). On the right side, the duration values of each interphase (I) and molt (M) are represented, along with their mean and standard deviation ($n = 9$). Results corresponding to (**a**) wild-type strain, (**b**) *crt-1(knu378)*, (**c**) *crt-1(jvp1)*, and (**d**) *crt-1(jh101)*. The results of the statistical analysis conducted for this assay are detailed in Figure 3.

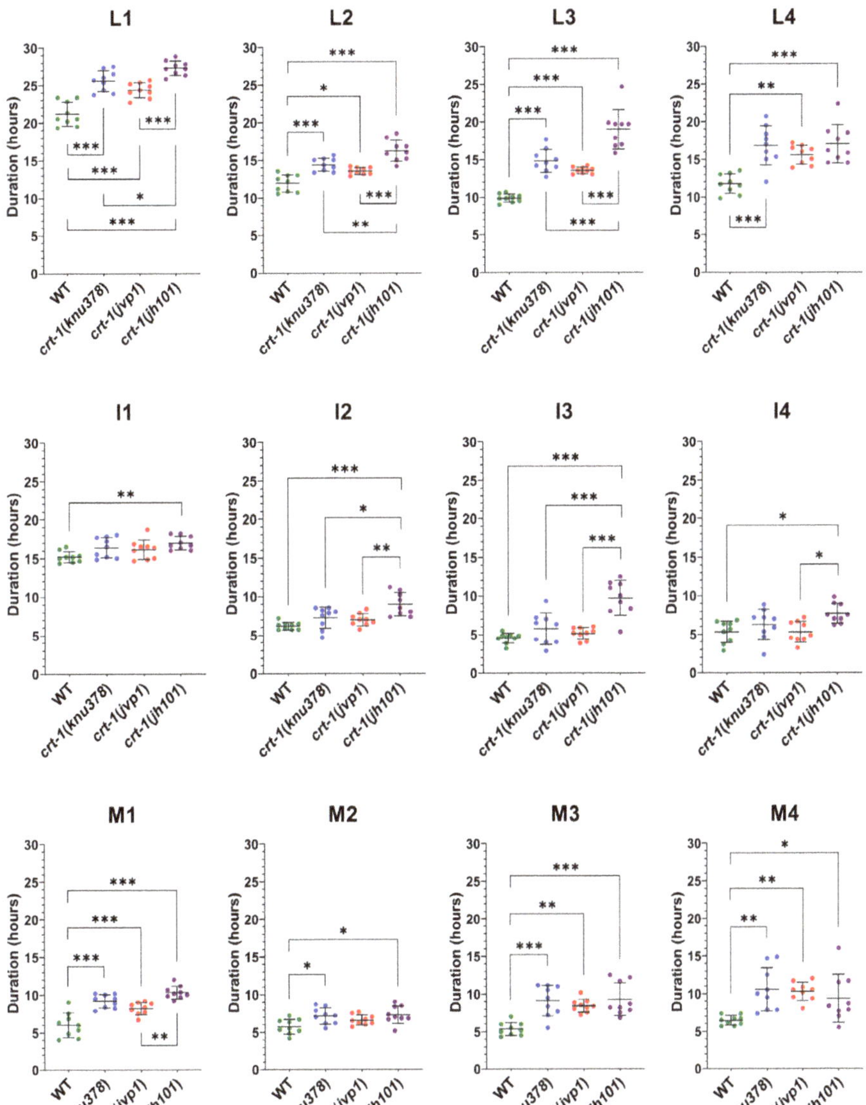

Figure 3. Molting duration at 20 °C. *crt-1* mutants exhibit longer molts than those of the wild-type strain, and the interphases of *crt-1(jh101)* worms are larger than those of *crt-1(knu378)* and *crt-1(jvp1)* mutants. The duration of the larval stage (L), interphase (I), and molt (M) at 20 °C is represented. The duration of the larval stage is the sum of the duration of the interphase and the molt. Individual data ($n = 9$), mean, and standard deviation are represented. Differences were considered significant (*) when $p < 0.05$, very significant (**) when $p < 0.01$, and highly significant (***) when $p < 0.001$.

Specifically, the duration of L1, L2, and L3 stages in *crt-1(knu378)* and *crt-1(jvp1)* worms was longer than that observed for the wild-type strain and shorter than that of the *crt-1(jh101)* strain (Figure 3). The length of the L4 stage in *crt-1(knu378)*, *crt-1(jvp1)*, and *crt-1(jh101)* worms was also longer than that of the wild-type strain, but in this case, no differences were found between the *crt-1* mutant strains (Figure 3). Worms from the mutant strains in *crt-1* exhibited molts (M1, M2, M3, and M4) that were very similar to each other and longer than those of the wild-type strain, causing the delay in the development of the L1, L2, L3, and L4 stages compared to the wild-type strain (Figure 3). In general, the *crt-1(jh101)* strain showed longer interphases than the wild-type strain and *crt-1(knu378)* and *crt-1(jvp1)* worms. In the three latter strains, the length of interphases I1, I2, I3, and I4 was very similar (Figure 3).

2.2. crt-1 Mutants Show Cuticle Defects Without Major Alterations of the Hypodermal Cell Lineage

To assess the possible function of CRT-1 during embryonic development, we performed 4D microscopy analysis of *crt-1(knu378)*, *crt-1(jvp1)*, and *crt-1(jh101)* mutant embryo development and compared them to wild-type controls. To ensure the embryos developed under the exact same conditions and that there were no experimental variations from wild-types to mutants, we recorded a mutant and a wild-type embryo side-by-side in the same preparation for each case. For each genotype, the recordings were performed in triplicate to score the penetrance of the phenotype. In all cases, we found a reproducible effect of the *ctr-1* mutation on hypodermic cells and the embryonic cuticle. Two embryos, one *crt-1(jvp1)* and one *crt-1(jh101)*, died during development due to an incomplete ventral closure of the hypodermal cells (ventral closure defect) and the subsequent extrusion of internal tissues (Figure 4). As for the rest of the embryos analyzed, three *crt-1(knu378)*, two *crt-1(jvp1)*, and two *crt-1(jh101)* developed normally but showed notable cuticle blebbing after 7–9 h of development as early as the three-fold stage. The bleb size was larger in *crt-1(jh101)* embryos than in *crt-1(knu378)* or *crt-1(jvp1)* embryos, and one of the *crt-1(jh101)* exploded after 10 h of development (Figure 4).

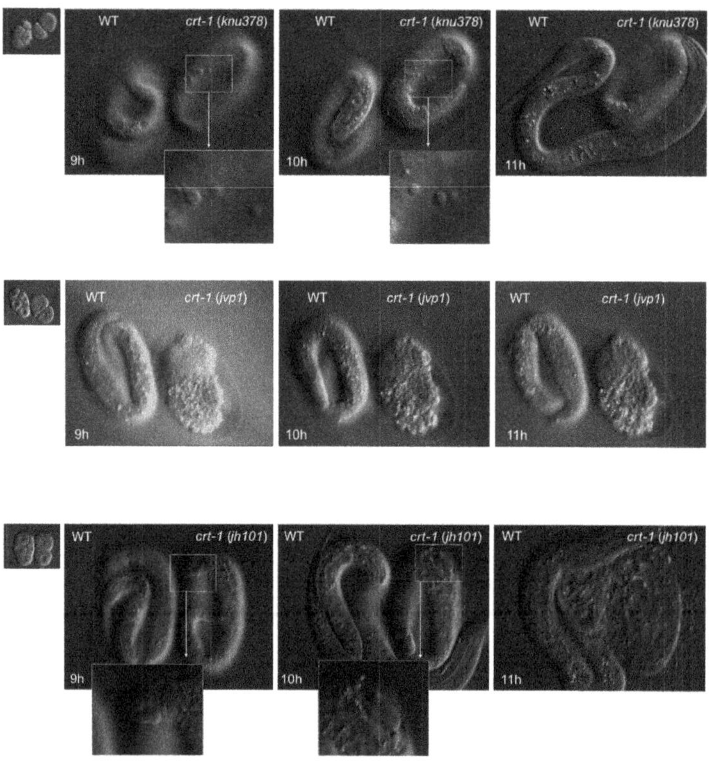

Figure 4. Embryo development. *crt-1* mutants show cuticle defects during embryo development. Differential interference contrast still images (time 0, 9 h, 10 h, and 11 h) of developing wild-type and

crt-1 mutant embryos analyzed using 4D microscopy. *crt-1(knu378)* are shown in the **top row**, *crt-1(jvp1)* in the **middle row**, and *crt-1(jh101)* in the **bottom row**. Details of cuticle blebbing are highlighted for *crt-1(knu378)* and *crt-1(jh101)*. Example of *crt-1(jvp1)* (**middle panel**) that died due to ventral enclosure defect, while other specimens also show cuticle blebbing during development.

To determine whether the cuticle blebbing and ventral closure defects of *crt-1* mutants were a consequence of an error in the fate specification of the hypodermis during development, we took advantage of the invariant *C. elegans* embryo cell lineage. We reconstructed the cell lineage of ABpra blastomere descendants fated to differentiate as hypodermal cells. Cell lineage analysis of *crt-1* mutant vs. wild-type embryos did not identify any abnormal cell division pattern beyond a slight delay in the timing of late cell division (Figure 5). This delay in late development is further supported by the fact that none of the mutants hatched during the 12 h that the recordings lasted, while the corresponding paired wild-types did.

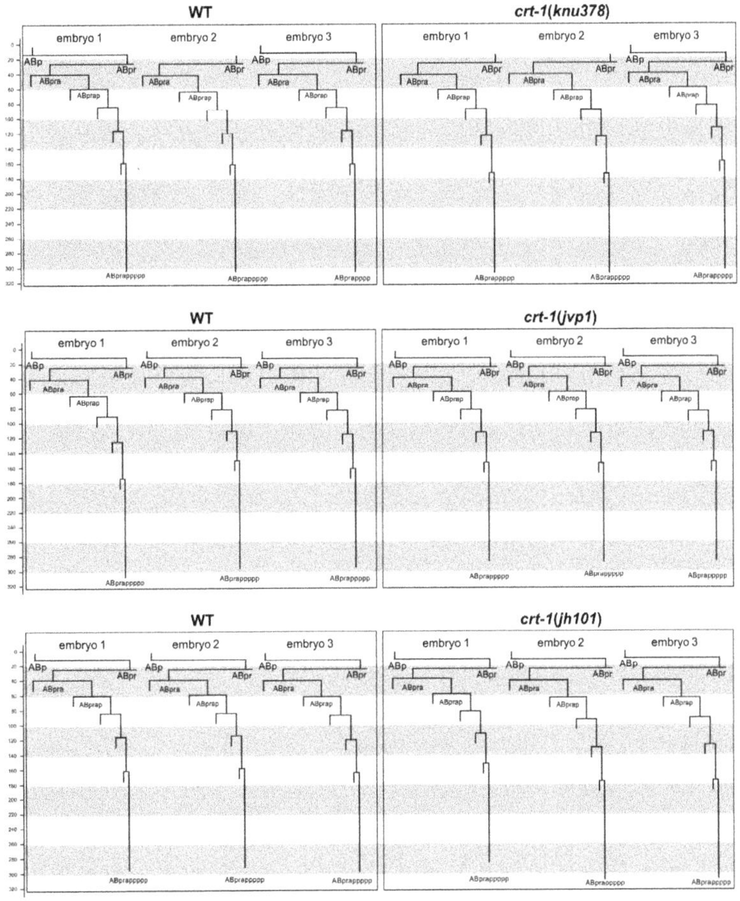

Figure 5. Embryo development. Cell lineage of a hypodermal cell (ABpra) in wild-type and *crt-1* mutant embryos. **Top panels** show the comparison between three wild-type embryos (**left**) and three *crt-1(knu378)* mutant embryos (**right**). **Middle panels** show the comparison between three wild-type embryos (**left**) and three *crt-1(jvp1)* mutant embryos (**right**). **Bottom panels** show the comparison between three wild-type embryos (**left**) and three *crt-1(jh101)* mutant embryos (**right**). Timing is shown in minutes. The cleavage pattern of wild-type hypodermis is generally conserved in *ctr-1* mutants. Cell lineage was traced up to 320 min; cells cannot be followed beyond this time due to embryo movement.

Altogether, these results highlight a function of CRT-1 in embryonic hypodermal cells (responsible for cuticle secretion) independent of fate specification. In addition, given its phenotype and that it is a true loss-of-function deletion allele, *crt-1(jh101)* might be considered the strongest allele.

Observation by FE-SEM microscopy showed that the cuticle of adult *crt-1* mutants did not show any notable defects compared to the wild-type strain in the mouth, body, or tail regions (Figure 6). The alae and annuli, key structures of the cuticle, were particularly examined, but no differences were detected between the strains. However, adults from *crt-1* mutant strains exhibited a less resistant cuticle compared to wild-type strains when exposed to sodium hypochlorite (Figure 7).

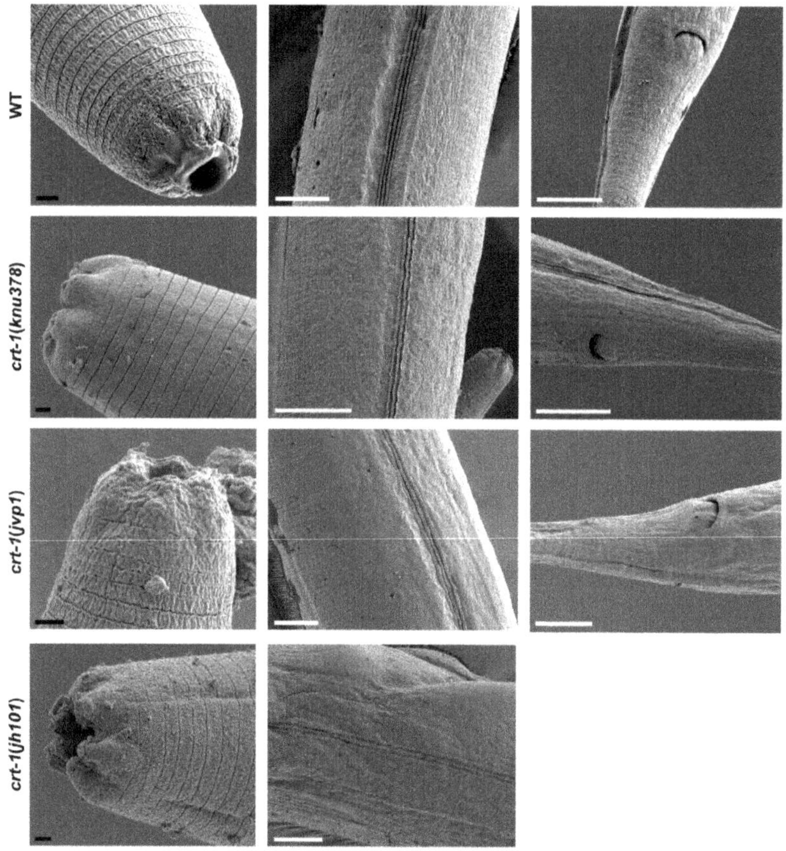

Figure 6. Images of the cuticle obtained by FE-SEM from the mouth, body, and tail regions. *crt-1* mutants do not show any morphological alteration of the cuticle in the adult stage. The images of the mouth, body, and tail are taken at magnifications of 10,000–20,000×, 4000×, and 4000–6000×, respectively. The black scale bar corresponds to 1 μm and the white scale bar to 10 μm.

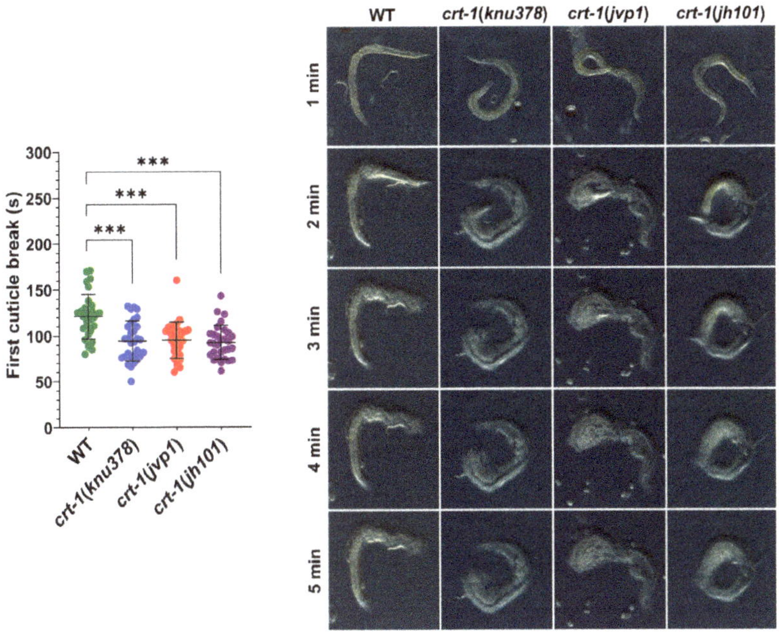

Figure 7. Cuticle resistance. *crt-1* mutants show lower resistance of the cuticle than the wild-type strain. Individual values of the first cuticle breakage after exposure to sodium hypochlorite with 6–14% active chlorine for 30 worms per strain are represented, along with the mean and standard deviation. Differences were considered highly significant (***) when $p < 0.001$. Representative images of the behavior of each of the evaluated strains taken at 13.5× magnifications after 1, 2, 3, 4, and 5 min of exposure to the chemical product are included.

2.3. crt-1(knu378) and crt-1(jvp1) Mutants Exhibit Some Phenotypes Consistent with the Loss of Function of CRT-1

Individuals from the *crt-1(jvp1)* and *crt-1(jh101)* strains exhibited a decrease in fertility compared to individuals from the wild-type strain at 25 °C. Firstly, worms from the *crt-1* mutant strains lost the ability to self-fertilize and lay eggs prior to worms from the wild-type strain (Figure 8a). Moreover, worms from the *crt-1* mutant strains laid fewer eggs throughout their fertile life compared to the wild-type strain. In this case, slight differences were observed between the *crt-1(jvp1)* strain and the *crt-1(jh101)* strain, with the number of eggs laid by individuals of the latter strain being lower (Figure 8b).

Although individuals from the wild-type, *crt-1(jvp1)*, and *crt-1(jh101)* strains were impaired in development at 25 °C after exposure to ER stress induced by 2 μg/μL tunicamycin (Figure 8c), the effects were not uniform between individuals of different strains. Regarding individual length data, a significant dispersion of the data was observed in the three strains between 48 and 53 h of growth. However, from 72 h onward, dispersion persisted only in the *crt-1(jh101)* strain (Figure S5). Regarding larval development, it was observed that most of the worms of the *crt-1(jh101)* strain were arrested between the L1 and L4 stages. In contrast, worms of the wild-type and *crt-1(jvp1)* strains mostly reached the adult stage (Figure S6). Therefore, it seems that the *crt-1(jh101)* strain is the most affected by the presence of 2 μg/μL of tunicamycin, while the *crt-1(jvp1)* strain was affected similarly to the wild-type, indicating it does not behave like a loss-of-function allele in this case.

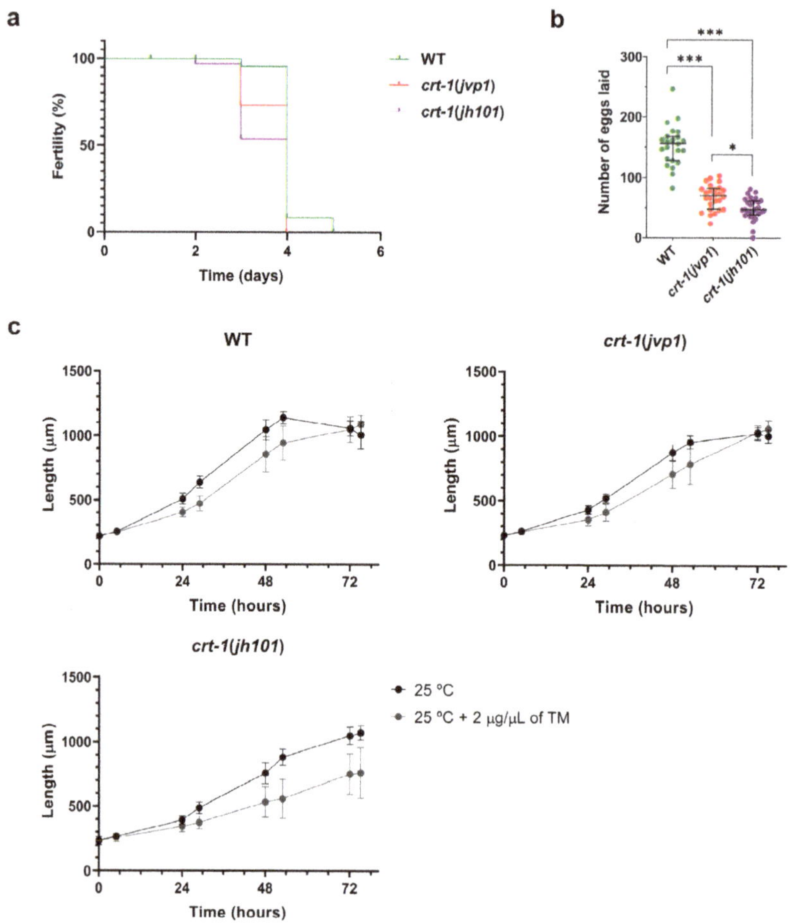

Figure 8. Fertility and resistance to ER stress. *crt-1(jvp1)* mutants have reduced fertility similar to strain *crt-1(jh101)*, but they withstand ER stress better than *crt-1(jh101)* worms. (**a**) Kaplan–Meier curve representing the day on which the strains cease to lay eggs at 25 °C (n = 36). (**b**) Number of eggs laid by each of the strains throughout their fertile lifespan (n = 36). Differences were considered significant (*) when $p < 0.05$, and highly significant (***) when $p < 0.001$. (**c**) Growth in length of *crt-1* mutants at 25 °C and 25 °C when 2 µg/µL of tunicamycin was added to the medium. In all cases, the mean lengths obtained for 50 worms per strain at 0, 5, 24, 29, 48, 53, 72, and 77 h are represented, along with their standard deviation.

Regarding fat levels, *crt-1(knu378)* worms showed no differences compared to wild-type worms at either 20 or 25 °C. However, *crt-1(jvp1)* worms showed slightly lower fat levels than those of the wild-type strain at both temperatures (Figure 9). The decrease in fat compared to the wild-type strain was most pronounced at 25 °C, a temperature at which calreticulin is slightly overexpressed. Finally, *crt-1(jh101)* worms showed lower fat levels than those of the wild-type and *crt-1(jvp1)* worms at both 20 and 25 °C (Figure 9). In this case, the decrease in fat compared to the wild-type strain remained unchanged at 25 °C.

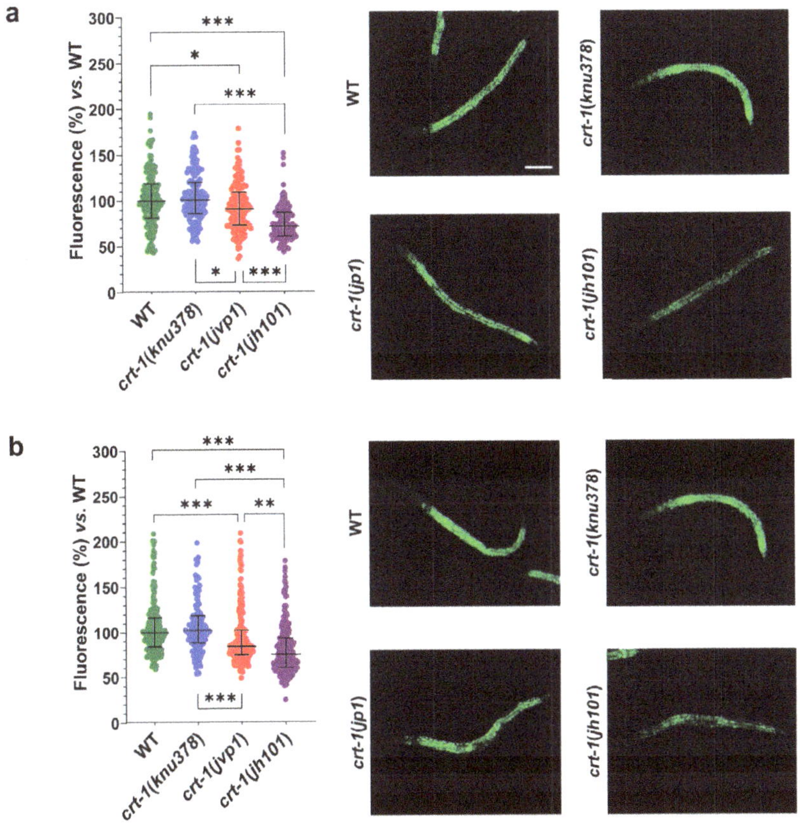

Figure 9. Fat levels with Nile Red staining. *crt-1(jvp1)* and *crt-1(jh101)* mutants exhibit lower fat levels than the wild-type strain at 20 °C and 25 °C. (**a**,**b**) Results of Nile Red staining of worms developed at 20 and 25 °C, respectively. In both cases, the (**left**) percentage of fluorescence emitted after staining of 127–214 L4 worms per strain and temperature with Nile Red is represented compared to the mean fluorescence emitted by stained wild-type worms. The statistics used are the mean and standard deviation. Differences were considered significant (*) when $p < 0.05$, very significant (**) when $p < 0.01$, and highly significant (***) when $p < 0.001$. The images on the right are representative of the fluorescence emitted by each of the strains at a 10× magnification. The scale bar corresponds to 100 μm.

3. Discussion

Mutations in *CALR* are capable of inducing ET and PMF, two MPNs characterized by the clonal expansion of mature myeloid cells. Although it is well known that calreticulin mutations activate the JAK2/STAT cascade, other mechanisms not involving JAK/STAT activation that may also contribute to these diseases have been proposed for the mutant protein. These JAK/STAT-independent mechanisms have not been extensively investigated yet and could be valuable for developing new targeted therapies, given the apparent lack of efficacy of JAK inhibitors in patients.

In this context, we developed a model in *C. elegans* with mutations in calreticulin that are orthologous to those present in patients with ET and PMF (*crt-1(knu378)* and *crt-1(jvp1)*) and lacking JAK orthologs, as established in a previous study. According to published data, transcriptomic analysis of these strains revealed some possible JAK/STAT-independent mechanisms derived from mutant calreticulin [13]. Most of the observed expression changes appeared to correspond to a partial loss of protein function, with the alteration of the extracellular matrix being particularly remarkable. In this study, our aim was to investigate whether these mutant strains in *crt-1* exhibit any phenotype related to extracellular matrix alteration (development, molting, and morphology and resistance of the cuticle), as well as to assess other phenotypes previously associated with calreticulin dysfunction (fertility, response to ER stress, and regulation of lipid homeostasis). The study of these orthologous phenotypes may be useful for identifying key mechanisms that could be relevant in the pathogenesis of the disease in humans.

Firstly, we observed that strains *crt-1(knu378)* and *crt-1(jvp1)* exhibited a developmental delay. Since the hours at which differences were found between these strains are the same when comparing both the length of growth and the larval stage throughout their development, it seems that the growth delay in the length of the strains is due to a delay in their larval development. The molting assay showed that the differences in development between *crt-1* mutant strains and the wild-type strain were due to the longer molts of M1-M4. The development of the *crt-1(jh101)* strain, used as a control for the loss of function of calreticulin, was slower than in the strains *crt-1(knu378)* and *crt-1(jvp1)* due to longer intervals between molts.

Next, we decided to investigate whether these strains also exhibited alterations in their embryonic development. An embryo from strain *crt-1(knu378)* and one from strain *crt-1(jvp1)* died during their development due to a ventral closure defect, resulting in the extrusion of their internal tissues. Ventral closure relies on actin cytoskeleton reorganization [23], but no other defects typically associated with *ced-10*/RAC1 (involved in actin polymerization) were detected. On the other hand, most embryos analyzed from strains *crt-1(knu378)* and *crt-1(jvp1)*, and all analyzed from strain *crt-1(jh101)*, developed normally but exhibited cuticle blebbing during development, with the latter strain showing a greater extent. Subsequent experiments showed that this phenotype was not due to an error in the fate specification of the hypodermis during development. Thus, the blebbing could be caused by the cuticle being detached from the hypodermis or because its structure or composition is altered. Electron microscopy results discarded any structural alterations in the cuticle of the strains, suggesting that this defect was caused by an altered composition of the cuticle, a result supported by the altered expression of multiple cuticle components in the previously published transcriptomic study [13] or because the cuticle was detached from the hypodermis. Both hypotheses are consistent with the finding that the cuticle of *crt-1* mutant strains exhibits lower resistance to external stress than the wild-type strain.

In all the phenotypes observed, strains *crt-1(knu378)* and *crt-1(jvp1)* behaved in an intermediate manner between the wild-type strain and the strain *crt-1(jh101)*. In *C. elegans*, development, molting, cuticle morphology, and cuticle resistance are intricately connected to the extracellular matrix. Specifically, the extracellular matrix plays a fundamental role during development by providing structural support and signaling cues that guide the differentiation and organization of tissues. Additionally, studies on molting, morphology, and resistance aim to investigate various aspects of the cuticle, which serves as a primary form of extracellular matrix in this nematode. Thus, these findings imply that all three *crt-1* mutant strains exhibit an alteration in their extracellular matrix, suggesting that this is due to a loss of function of the CRT-1 protein. This result is particularly noteworthy because patients with PMF present an alteration of the extracellular matrix in the bone marrow, which leads to fibrosis [24], and also because alterations in the centrosome have been repeatedly associated with MPNs [25]. Therefore, the disruption of the extracellular matrix in patients with PMF may be caused by the mechanisms that lead to the aforementioned phenotypic alterations in the *C. elegans* model.

Furthermore, our results support the idea that in addition to the well-known oncogenic function of mutant calreticulin in patients with ET and PMF by activating JAK/STAT signaling through its binding to the thrombopoietin receptor, there would also be a loss of function that may lead to major alterations [26]. This also suggests that the changes observed in the extracellular matrix of these patients could be a consequence of this loss of function. In fact, an important role has been described for the non-mutated version of calreticulin in the extracellular matrix and in the secretion and processing of collagen [27].

Regarding the study of other phenotypes related to the loss of function of calreticulin, the results confirmed that the strain *crt-1(jh101)* does not exhibit defects in the ER stress, but it does have them in fertility and lipid metabolism.

Thus, the study of ER stress at 25 °C demonstrated that the strain *crt-1(jh101)* is more affected by the presence of 2 µg/µL tunicamycin than the wild-type strain. On the contrary, worms from the strain *crt-1(jvp1)* were affected similarly to individuals from the wild-type strain. This indicates that, while calreticulin plays a role in the response to ER stress in the worm, the introduced mutations (in this case, type 2) do not seem to affect this function. These results also appear to be consistent with a recent publication indicating that while some calreticulin mutations seem to activate the IRE1α/XBP1 pathway of the Unfolded Protein Response to drive MPNs, the type 2 mutations that have been recreated in the mutant strain *crt-1(jvp1)* do not seem to have this effect [28].

In the fertility assay, the strain *crt-1(jvp1)* exhibited fertility defects similar to those of *crt-1(jh101)* animals. Specifically, these strains lost the ability to self-fertilize and lay eggs earlier than the wild-type strain, in addition to decreasing the number of eggs laid during their fertile lifespan. In the latter case, minor differences were observed between both strains, which again would be compatible with a partial loss of function of the mutant calreticulin. Previously, it has been reported that calreticulin may be important for the proper development of sperm and oocytes in *C. elegans* [21], so the *crt-1(jvp1)* animals could have a defect in the development of both, leading to reduced fertility. Regarding this assay, we find it inappropriate to establish an orthologous phenotype in humans because the mutations in patients are somatic and, therefore, do not affect the germline or gonads. Thus, this result simply verifies that the introduction of mutations similar to those found in MPN patients leads to a loss-of-function effect; therefore, the mutations in humans could also have corresponding effects related to a loss of function of the protein.

Finally, the study of fat levels revealed that strain *crt-1(knu378)* behaves similarly to the wild-type strain, while *crt-1(jvp1)* and *crt-1(jh101)* animals exhibit lower fat levels than wild types. Fat levels in *crt-1(jh101)* mutants were lower than those in *crt-1(jvp1)* worms, again suggesting a partial loss of function of calreticulin in *crt-1(jvp1)*. In support of our findings, it has been recently described that the loss of calreticulin regulates lipid homeostasis by altering the Ca^{2+} levels in the ER in mice. However, this article describes that the loss of calreticulin results in an increase in neutral lipid levels in both mice and *C. elegans* [22]. The differences in the results obtained in the present study could be due to intrinsic differences between the capacities of dyes to stain fat stores in live and fixed worms [29]. It is well known that lipid metabolism is important in hematopoiesis and, more specifically, in myeloproliferative neoplasms. In fact, it has been described that hematopoietic cells with defective cholesterol efflux in a hypercholesterolemic environment are noted to phenocopy MPNs [30]. Therefore, it does not seem unreasonable to think that lipid alterations in *CALR*-mutated patients with MPNs may be due, at least in part, to a loss of function of the mutant calreticulin.

As mentioned earlier, some of the phenotypes observed in this study have also been found in patients, but for many of them, it had not been previously proposed that the mechanism by which they are triggered could be a loss of function of calreticulin. This may have occurred because the majority of studies have been conducted in mice, which could have posed a limitation for the analysis of loss-of-function effects since calreticulin deficiency is lethal [31], unlike in *C. elegans*. Although it has been described that these mice overcome embryonic lethality and survive to term through the expression of calcineurin in the heart [32], this model remains suboptimal for studying JAK/STAT-independent mechanisms of mutant calreticulin due to the presence of JAK orthologs, contrary to what occurs in *C. elegans*. The *C. elegans* model employed in this study not only allows mutations to be homozygous without being lethal but also enables the clear observation of loss-of-function effects, which are undoubtedly independent of JAK/STAT activation, as there are no JAK orthologs. Thus, the use of *C. elegans* in this study has allowed for verification that many of the phenotypes triggered by type 1 and type 2 mutations of calreticulin could be due to a loss of function because they behave similarly to the calreticulin-deficient strain.

This finding presents an opportunity to explore calreticulin loss of function as a potential therapeutic target for MPN patients, either as a standalone approach or in combination with existing JAK inhibitors. A logical initial strategy could involve delivering a functional copy of the *CALR* gene to the patient's cells. Although gene therapy has shown promise in treating other diseases, its application in MPNs has not yet been developed. Additionally, providing a non-mutated version of calreticulin directly is currently not a feasible option due to the challenges associated with protein delivery, intracellular localization, and ensuring proper functionality. In the near term, it may be more practical to explore therapies that target extracellular matrix components or antifibrotic agents, as well as treatments aimed at mitigating ER stress and oxidative stress resulting from calreticulin loss of function.

4. Materials and Methods

4.1. C. elegans Strains and Maintenance

To evaluate the effects of patient-like calreticulin mutations, the strains COP1358 (*crt-1(knu378)*) and JLV544 (*crt-1(jvp1)*) were used. Both were obtained using CRISPR/Cas9 technology in a previous study [13] and recreate type 1 and type 2 mutations, respectively. Additionally, the wild-type strain *Bristol* N2 and the *crt-1* null mutant strain KJ216 (*crt-1(jh101)*) were used as controls of the normal function of calreticulin and the complete loss of function of the protein, respectively. Both strains were obtained from the *Caenorhabditis* Genetics Center (CGC, University of Minnesota, Minneapolis, MN, USA). All nematodes were maintained at 20 °C on NGM agar plates seeded with ampicillin-resistant *E. coli* OP50 according to standard protocols.

4.2. Larval Development

The larval development assay was conducted on synchronized L1 worms until they reached the adult stage using an SMZ18 stereomicroscope equipped with a DS-Fi2 camera (Nikon Instruments Inc., Tokyo, Japan) as previously described [13]. Briefly, approximately 400 synchronized L1 worms were transferred onto a total of four NGM-OP50 plates per strain, resulting in approximately 100 worms per plate. Two of the plates were incubated at 20 °C, while the remaining two were incubated at 25 °C for a duration of four days. At 0, 5, 24, 29, 48, 53, 72, and 77 h after transferring the worms, photographs of 50 worms per strain (25 per plate) were taken using a Nikon SMZ18 stereomicroscope equipped with a DS-Fi2 camera (Nikon Instruments Inc., Tokyo, Japan). The length of each worm was measured using Nis Elements Documentation software version 4.00 (Nikon Instruments Inc., Tokyo, Japan). Subsequently, an estimation of the developmental stage of each worm at each time point (L1, L2, L3, early L4, late L4, young adult, or adult) was made based on its length and morphological characteristics.

4.3. Molting

Molting was studied in a conventional luminometer using the bioluminescence-based method previously published by our laboratory [33]. For this experiment, the strains COP1358 (*crt-1(knu378)*), JLV544 (*crt-1(jvp1)*), and KJ216 (*crt-1(jh101)*) were crossed with the reporter strain PE255 (*feIs5[sur-5p::luciferase::GFP + rol-6(su1006)]* X) until a homozygous strain for the *crt-1* mutations and the reporter construction was obtained.

4.4. Embryonic Cell Lineage Analysis

Embryonic cell lineage analysis was carried out by 4D microscopy (multi-focal time-lapse microscopy) as described in [34,35]. Briefly, gravid hermaphrodites were dissected, and 2- to 4-cell stage embryos were mounted on 4% agar pads in water and sealed with vaseline. Images on 30 focal planes (1 micron/section) were taken every 30 s for 12 h at 25 °C on a Leica DM6000 microscope fitted with DIC optics (Leica Microsystems GmbH,

Wetzlar, Germany). The use of DIC optics allows cell tracing without using any dye or fluorescent markers that might alter cell cycle progression. The microscope was controlled with Time to Live software version 11_2010, and embryo lineages were analyzed with SIMI® BioCell software version 4.0.149 (www.simi.com [36]).

4.5. Field Emission Scanning Electron Microscopy (FE-SEM)

To evaluate the effects of *crt-1* mutations on the cuticle morphology of *C. elegans* strains, worms at different larval stages were examined using Field Emission Scanning Electron Microscopy (FE-SEM).

Sample preparation followed the protocols described [37,38] with minor modifications. Briefly, worms from various larval stages grown at 20 °C on an NGM-OP50 plate were collected and washed with PBST. The worm pellets were then fixed by adding 20 µL of 2% glutaraldehyde and incubated overnight at room temperature (RT) with gentle agitation. After this period, the worms were washed again in PBST, and 1 mL of 1% osmium tetroxide dissolved in PBST was added to the tube in a chemical fume hood. After incubating for 30 min at RT, the tube was centrifuged, and the supernatant was removed using a micropipette. Finally, the samples were dehydrated in a series of ethanol solutions of increasing concentration to gradually displace the water from the sample. For this, 1 mL of a 35% ethanol solution diluted in PBST was added, and it was incubated at 4 °C for 30 min with gentle agitation. After this, the tube was centrifuged, and the liquid content was aspirated as much as possible. To the sediment, 1 mL of 50% ethanol was added. This process was repeated with a solution of 100% ethanol. Subsequently, the samples were dried by critical point drying with liquid carbon dioxide at 50 atm pressure and then mounted on aluminum SEM stubs and shadowed by cathodic sputtering with 16 nm gold. Samples were visualized using the Zeiss Sigma 300 VP scanning electron microscope (Carl Zeiss Industrielle Messtechnik GmbH, Oberkochen, Germany), obtaining images of the cuticle in the mouth, body, and tail regions.

4.6. Cuticle Resistance

The cuticle resistance was evaluated using the protocol described in [39] with minor modifications. Briefly, worms were grown at 20 °C on an NGM-OP50 plate. Subsequently, 5 µL of a sodium hypochlorite solution with 6–14% active chlorine (Sigma-Aldrich Co., St. Louis, MO, USA) were pipetted onto ten adults from each strain. Using a Nikon SMZ18 stereoscopic microscope equipped with a DS-Fi2 camera (Nikon Instruments Inc., Tokyo, Japan), the moment of the first cuticle rupture was recorded, and photos were taken after 1, 2, 3, 4, and 5 min of exposure to bleach.

4.7. Fertility

Gravid worms were synchronized with bleach and incubated for 48 h at 20 °C in M9. After this time, 200 L1 larvae were seeded on an NGM-OP50 plate and incubated at 20 °C until reaching the L4 stage. Once in this stage, 36 worms per strain were individually transferred to each of the wells of a 12-well plate with NGM (2 mL per well) and ampicillin-resistant *E. coli* OP50 (25 µL per well), and they were incubated at 25 °C until individuals from each strain stopped laying eggs. Every 24 h, each worm was transferred to a new well, and the number of eggs laid by the same worm on the previous day was counted. This assay allowed us to evaluate both the total number of eggs laid by each worm during its fertile life and the point at which the worms stopped laying eggs.

4.8. Resistance to Endoplasmic Reticulum (ER) Stress

The ER stress assay was carried out following the same procedure used in the larval development assay, but in this case, synchronized L1 worms were exposed to 25 °C on NGM-OP50 plates containing 2 µg/mL tunicamycin.

4.9. Fat Levels with Nile Red Staining

The levels of fat in *C. elegans* strains were quantified using Nile Red staining. To carry out this assay, gravid worms were synchronized and incubated at 20 °C and 25 °C on NGM-OP50 plates. Once the worms reached the L4 stage, they were collected and washed twice with PBST. Tubes were then incubated on ice for 15 min. After aspiration, worms were incubated at room temperature (RT) for 3 min in 200 µL of 40% isopropanol. Once the supernatant was removed, 150 µL of a freshly prepared 3 µg/mL Nile Red solution in 40% isopropanol was added. After 30 min at 20 °C with constant agitation, the supernatant was removed to stop the reaction with the dye. Subsequently, worms were washed with PBST and mounted on slides with 2% agarose. Images were then taken immediately using a Nikon Eclipse 80i fluorescence microscope (Nikon Instruments Inc., Tokyo, Japan) coupled with a CCD camera with a FITC filter (Ex 465–495; DM 505; BA 515–555) at 4× magnification (40× total magnification) under the same conditions and the same integration time. The emitted fluorescence was quantified using the ImageJ version 1.48v analysis program [40].

4.10. Statistics

Statistical analysis was performed using StataSE v12 (StataCorp LP, College Station, TX, USA) and GraphPad Prism v8.0.2 (GraphPad Software, San Diego, CA, USA). The significance level (α) was set at 0.05. Differences were considered as non-significant (ns) when $p > 0.05$, significant (*) when $p < 0.05$, very significant (**) when $p < 0.01$, and highly significant (***) when $p < 0.001$.

The normality of the residuals of all the quantitative variables analyzed was assessed first. If the normality conditions of the residuals were met, strains were compared using a one-way ANOVA test (if homogeneity of variances was assumed) or Welch's test (if homogeneity of variances was not assumed), followed by multiple comparisons. Under these conditions, mean and standard deviation were used as descriptive statistics. If the normality conditions of the residuals were not met, the Kruskal–Wallis test (if distributions were similar) or the median test (if distributions were different) was conducted, followed by multiple comparisons. In this case, median and interquartile ranges were used as descriptive statistics.

For the qualitative variables, Pearson's chi-square test or Fisher's exact test was used to determine whether the strain affects the proportion of worms in each developmental stage, following Cochran's rule. Finally, the day on which individuals of each strain stopped laying eggs was evaluated using the survival curves generated with the Kaplan–Meier method. The survival curves of the strains were compared with the log-rank test.

5. Conclusions

Overall, the findings collectively support the notion that mutations in *CALR* could have significant effects on MPNs as a consequence of a loss of function of the protein. The further exploration of these effects for the advancement of novel therapies in these patients holds considerable promise and interest.

Supplementary Materials: The following supporting information can be downloaded at: https://www.mdpi.com/article/10.3390/ijms252111606/s1.

Author Contributions: Conceptualization, J.L.V.; methodology, J.L.V., A.G.-H., E.B. and J.C.; formal analysis, J.L.V., A.G.-H., E.B., B.E. and J.C.; investigation, A.G.-H., C.H., E.U.-C., and A.G.-S.; resources, J.L.V.; data curation, J.L.V. and A.G.-H.; writing—original draft preparation, A.G.-H.; writing—review and editing, J.L.V. and J.C.; supervision, J.L.V.; project administration, J.L.V.; funding acquisition, J.L.V. and J.C. All authors have read and agreed to the published version of the manuscript.

Funding: This research was funded by the PIUNA 2020 program of the University of Navarra (grant No. 15058203) and Ministerio de Ciencia e Innovación (Government of Spain, grant PID2021-127388NB-I00). Some strains were provided by the CGC, which is funded by the National Institutes of Health Office of Research Infrastructure Programs (P40 OD010440).

Institutional Review Board Statement: Not applicable.

Informed Consent Statement: Not applicable.

Data Availability Statement: All relevant data can be found within the article and its Supplementary Materials. The datasets generated during the current study are available from the corresponding author upon request.

Conflicts of Interest: The authors declare no conflicts of interest.

References

1. Cerón, J. *Caenorhabditis elegans* for research on cancer hallmarks. *Dis. Models Mech.* **2023**, *16*, dmm050079. [CrossRef] [PubMed]
2. Sendoel, A.; Kohler, I.; Fellmann, C.; Lowe, S.W.; Hengartner, M.O. HIF-1 antagonizes p53-mediated apoptosis through a secreted neuronal tyrosinase. *Nature* **2010**, *465*, 577–583. [CrossRef] [PubMed]
3. Possik, E.; Jalali, Z.; Nouët, Y.; Yan, M.; Gingras, M.C.; Schmeisser, K.; Panaite, L.; Dupuy, F.; Kharitidi, D.; Chotard, L.; et al. Folliculin regulates ampk-dependent autophagy and metabolic stress survival. *PLoS Genet.* **2014**, *10*, e1004273. [CrossRef]
4. Kyriakakis, E.; Markaki, M.; Tavernarakis, N. *Caenorhabditis elegans* as a model for cancer research. *Mol. Cell. Oncol.* **2015**, *2*, e975027. [CrossRef]
5. Kirienko, N.V.; Mani, K.; Fay, D.S. Cancer models in *Caenorhabditis elegans*. *Dev. Dyn.* **2010**, *239*, 1413–1448. [CrossRef]
6. McGary, K.L.; Park, T.J.; Woods, J.O.; Cha, H.J.; Wallingford, J.B.; Marcotte, E.M. Systematic discovery of nonobvious human disease models through orthologous phenotypes. *Proc. Natl. Acad. Sci. USA* **2010**, *107*, 6544–6549. [CrossRef]
7. Tefferi, A.; Vannucchi, A.M.; Barbui, T. Essential thrombocythemia: 2024 update on diagnosis, risk stratification, and management. *Am. J. Hematol.* **2024**, *99*, 697–718. [CrossRef]
8. Constantinescu, S.N.; Vainchenker, W.; Levy, G.; Papadopoulos, N. Functional consequences of mutations in myeloproliferative neoplasms. *Hemasphere* **2021**, *5*, e578. [CrossRef]
9. Pecquet, C.; Papadopoulos, N.; Balligand, T.; Chachoua, I.; Tisserand, A.; Vertenoeil, G.; Nédélec, A.; Vertommen, D.; Roy, A.; Marty, C.; et al. Secreted mutant calreticulins as rogue cytokines in myeloproliferative neoplasms. *Blood* **2023**, *141*, 917–929. [CrossRef]
10. Vadeikienė, R.; Jakštys, B.; Laukaitienė, D.; Šatkauskas, S.; Juozaitytė, E.; Ugenskienė, R. The Role of Mutated Calreticulin in the Pathogenesis of *BCR-ABL1*-Negative Myeloproliferative Neoplasms. *Int. J. Mol. Sci.* **2024**, *25*, 9873. [CrossRef]
11. Guijarro-Hernández, A.; Vizmanos, J.L. A broad overview of signaling in *Ph*-negative classic myeloproliferative neoplasms. *Cancers* **2021**, *13*, 984. [CrossRef] [PubMed]
12. Salati, S.; Genovese, E.; Carretta, C.; Zini, R.; Bartalucci, N.; Prudente, Z.; Pennucci, V.; Ruberti, S.; Rossi, C.; Rontauroli, S.; et al. Calreticulin Ins5 and Del52 mutations impair unfolded protein and oxidative stress responses in K562 cells expressing CALR mutants. *Sci. Rep.* **2019**, *9*, 10558. [CrossRef] [PubMed]
13. Guijarro-Hernández, A.; Eder-Azanza, L.; Hurtado, C.; Navarro-Herrera, D.; Ezcurra, B.; Novo, F.J.; Cabello, J.; Vizmanos, J.L. Transcriptomic analysis reveals JAK2/MPL-independent effects of calreticulin mutations in a *C. elegans* model. *Cells* **2023**, *12*, 186. [CrossRef] [PubMed]
14. Liu, P.; Zhao, L.; Loos, F.; Marty, C.; Xie, W.; Martins, I.; Lachkar, S.; Qu, B.; Waeckel-Énée, E.; Plo, I.; et al. Immunosuppression by Mutated Calreticulin Released from Malignant Cells. *Mol. Cell* **2020**, *77*, 748–760. [CrossRef]
15. Pronier, E.; Cifani, P.; Merlinsky, T.R.; Berman, K.B.; Somasundara, A.V.H.; Rampal, R.K.; LaCava, J.; Wei, K.E.; Pastore, F.; Maag, J.L.; et al. Targeting the CALR interactome in myeloproliferative neoplasms. *JCI Insight* **2018**, *3*, e122703. [CrossRef]
16. Arshad, N.; Cresswell, P. Tumor-associated calreticulin variants functionally compromise the peptide loading complex and impair its recruitment of MHC-I. *J. Biol. Chem.* **2018**, *293*, 9555–9569. [CrossRef]
17. Di Buduo, C.A.; Abbonante, V.; Marty, C.; Moccia, F.; Rumi, E.; Pietra, D.; Soprano, P.M.; Lim, D.; Cattaneo, D.; Iurlo, A.; et al. Defective interaction of mutant calreticulin and SOCE in megakaryocytes from patients with myeloproliferative neoplasms. *Blood* **2020**, *135*, 133–144. [CrossRef]
18. Eder-Azanza, L.; Navarro, D.; Aranaz, P.; Novo, F.J.; Cross, N.C.P.; Vizmanos, J.L. Bioinformatic analyses of CALR mutations in myeloproliferative neoplasms support a role in signaling. *Leukemia* **2014**, *28*, 2106–2109. [CrossRef]
19. Thiele, J.; Kvasnicka, H.M.; Orazi, A.; Gianelli, U.; Gangat, N.; Vannucchi, A.M.; Barbui, T.; Arber, D.A.; Tefferi, A. The international consensus classification of myeloid neoplasms and acute leukemias: Myeloproliferative neoplasms. *Am. J. Hematol.* **2023**, *98*, 166–179. [CrossRef]
20. Harrison, C.N.; Mead, A.J.; Panchal, A.; Fox, S.; Yap, C.; Gbandi, E.; Houlton, A.; Alimam, S.; Ewing, J.; Wood, M.; et al. Ruxolitinib *vs.* best available therapy for ET intolerant or resistant to hydroxycarbamide. *Blood* **2017**, *130*, 1889–1897. [CrossRef]
21. Park, B.J.; Lee, D.G.; Yu, J.R.; Jung, S.K.; Choi, K.; Lee, J.; Lee, J.; Kim, Y.S.; Lee, J.I.; Kwon, J.Y.; et al. Calreticulin, a calcium-binding molecular chaperone, is required for stress response and fertility in *Caenorhabditis elegans*. *Mol. Biol. Cell* **2001**, *12*, 2835–2845. [CrossRef] [PubMed]
22. Wang, W.A.; Liu, W.X.; Durnaoglu, S.; Lee, S.K.; Lian, J.; Lehner, R.; Ahnn, J.; Agellon, L.B.; Michalak, M. Loss of calreticulin uncovers a critical role for calcium in regulating cellular lipid homeostasis. *Sci. Rep.* **2017**, *7*, 5941. [CrossRef]

23. Sawa, M.; Suetsugu, S.; Sugimoto, A.; Miki, H.; Yamamoto, M.; Takenawa, T. Essential role of the *C. elegans* Arp2/3 complex in cell migration during ventral enclosure. *J. Cell Sci.* **2003**, *116*, 1505–1518. [CrossRef]
24. Szekely, T.; Wichmann, B.; Maros, M.E.; Csizmadia, A.; Bodor, C.; Timar, B.; Krenacs, T. Myelofibrosis progression grading based on type I and type III collagen and fibrillin 1 expression boosted by whole slide image analysis. *Histopathology* **2023**, *82*, 622–632. [CrossRef] [PubMed]
25. Delaval, B.; Lelièvre, H.; Birnbaum, D. Myeloproliferative disorders: The centrosome connection. *Leukemia* **2005**, *19*, 1739–1744. [CrossRef]
26. Prins, D.; Green, A.R. Mutant CALR functions: Gains and losses. *Blood* **2020**, *136*, 6–7. [CrossRef] [PubMed]
27. Van Duyn Graham, L.; Sweetwyne, M.T.; Pallero, M.A.; Murphy-Ullrich, J.E. Intracellular calreticulin regulates multiple steps in fibrillar collagen expression, trafficking, and processing into the extracellular matrix. *J. Biol. Chem.* **2010**, *285*, 7067–7078. [CrossRef]
28. Ibarra, J.; Elbanna, Y.A.; Kurylowicz, K.; Ciboddo, M.; Greenbaum, H.S.; Arellano, N.S.; Rodriguez, D.; Evers, M.; Bock-Hughes, A.; Liu, C.; et al. Type I but not type II calreticulin mutations activate the IRE1α/XBP1 pathway of the unfolded protein response to drive myeloproliferative neoplasms. *Blood Cancer Discov.* **2022**, *3*, 298–315. [CrossRef]
29. Yen, K.; Le, T.T.; Bansal, A.; Narasimhan, S.D.; Cheng, J.X.; Tissenbaum, H.A. A comparative study of fat storage quantitation in nematode *Caenorhabditis elegans* using label and label-free methods. *PLoS ONE* **2010**, *5*, e12810. [CrossRef]
30. Pernes, G.; Flynn, M.C.; Lancaster, G.I.; Murphy, A.J. Fat for fuel: Lipid metabolism in haematopoiesis. *Clin. Transl. Immunol.* **2019**, *8*, e1098. [CrossRef]
31. Mesaeli, N.; Nakamura, K.; Zvaritch, E.; Dickie, P.; Dziak, E.; Krause, K.H.; Opas, M.; MacLennan, D.H.; Michalak, M. Calreticulin is essential for cardiac development. *J. Cell Biol.* **1999**, *144*, 857–868. [CrossRef] [PubMed]
32. Guo, L.; Nakamura, K.; Lynch, J.; Opas, M.; Olson, E.N.; Agellon, L.B.; Michalak, M. Cardiac-specific expression of calcineurin reverses embryonic lethality in calreticulin-deficient mouse. *J. Biol. Chem.* **2002**, *277*, 50776–50779. [CrossRef] [PubMed]
33. Guijarro-Hernández, A.; Hurtado, C.; Martínez-Irujo, J.J.; Vizmanos, J.L. Monitoring *Caenorhabditis elegans* molting in a conventional luminometer. *MethodsX* **2023**, *10*, 102235. [CrossRef]
34. Mora-Lorca, J.A.; Sáenz-Narciso, B.; Gaffney, C.J.; Naranjo-Galindo, F.J.; Pedrajas, J.R.; Guerrero-Gómez, D.; Dobrzynska, A.; Askjaer, P.; Szewczyk, N.J.; Cabello, J.; et al. Glutathione reductase *gsr-1* is an essential gene required for *Caenorhabditis elegans* early embryonic development. *Free Radic. Biol. Med.* **2016**, *96*, 446–461. [CrossRef]
35. Escrich, V.; Ezcurra, B.; Gómez-Orte, E.; Romero-Aranda, C.; Miranda-Vizuete, A.; Cabello, J. 4D Microscopy: Unraveling *Caenorhabditis elegans* embryonic development using Nomarski microscopy. *J. Vis. Exp.* **2020**, *164*, e61736. [CrossRef]
36. Schnabel, R.; Hutter, H.; Moerman, D.; Schnabel, H. Assessing normal embryogenesis in *Caenorhabditis elegans* using a 4D microscope: Variability of development and regional specification. *Dev. Biol.* **1997**, *184*, 234–265. [CrossRef] [PubMed]
37. Woodruff, G.C.; Knauss, C.M.; Maugel, T.K.; Haag, E.S. Mating damages the cuticle of *C. elegans* hermaphrodites. *PLoS ONE* **2014**, *9*, e104456. [CrossRef]
38. Blaxter, M.L. Cuticle surface proteins of wild type and mutant *Caenorhabditis elegans*. *J. Biol. Chem.* **1993**, *268*, 6600–6609. [CrossRef]
39. Calvo, A.C.; Pey, A.L.; Ying, M.; Loer, C.M.; Martinez, A. Anabolic function of phenylalanine hydroxylase in *Caenorhabditis elegans*. *FASEB J.* **2008**, *22*, 3046–3058. [CrossRef]
40. Schneider, C.A.; Rasband, W.S.; Eliceiri, K.W. NIH Image to ImageJ: 25 years of image analysis. *Nat. Methods* **2012**, *9*, 671–675. [CrossRef]

International Journal of
Molecular Sciences

MDPI

Article

Immune Checkpoint Inhibitor Therapy and Associations with Clonal Hematopoiesis †

Abhay Singh [1,*], Nuria Mencia Trinchant [2], Rahul Mishra [3], Kirti Arora [4], Smit Mehta [1], Teodora Kuzmanovic [1], Maedeh Zokaei Nikoo [5], Inderpreet Singh [6], Amanda C. Przespolewski [7], Mahesh Swaminathan [7], Marc S. Ernstoff [7], Grace K. Dy [7], Lunbiao Yan [2], Eti Sinha [2], Shruti Sharma [6], Duane C. Hassane [2,8], Elizabeth A. Griffiths [7], Eunice Wang [7], Monica L. Guzman [2] and Swapna Thota [9]

1 Leukemia and Myeloid Disorders Program, Cleveland Clinic, Cleveland, OH 44106, USA
2 Division of Medicine, Weill Cornell Medical College, New York, NY 10065, USA
3 Department of Internal Medicine, Anne Arundel Medical Center, Annapolis, MD 21401, USA
4 Department of Medicine, Cleveland Clinic Akron General Hospital, Akron, OH 44307, USA
5 University Hospitals, Case Western Reserve University, Cleveland, OH 44106, USA
6 Upstate Community Hospital, SUNY Upstate Medical University, Syracuse, NY 13210, USA
7 Department of Medicine, Roswell Park Comprehensive Cancer Center, Buffalo, NY 14203, USA; grace.dy@roswellpark.org (G.K.D.)
8 Tempus Labs, Inc., Chicago, IL 60654, USA
9 Department of Medicine, The University of Tennessee Health Science Center, Memphis, TN 38103, USA
* Correspondence: singha21@ccf.org

† Presented at the Annual meeting of American Society of Hematology, Atlanta, GA, USA, 11–14 December 2021.

Abstract: Cancer cohorts are now known to be associated with increased rates of clonal hematopoiesis (CH). We sort to characterize the hematopoietic compartment of patients with melanoma and non-small cell lung cancer (NSCLC) given our recent population level analysis reporting evolving rates of secondary leukemias. The advent of immune checkpoint blockade (ICB) has dramatically changed our understanding of cancer biology and has altered the standards of care for patients. However, the impact of ICB on hematopoietic myeloid clonal expansion remains to be determined. We studied if exposure to ICB therapy affects hematopoietic clonal architecture and if their evolution contributed to altered hematopoiesis. Blood samples from patients with melanoma and NSCLC (n = 142) demonstrated a high prevalence of CH. Serial samples (or post ICB exposure samples; n = 25) were evaluated in melanoma and NSCLC patients. Error-corrected sequencing of a targeted panel of genes recurrently mutated in CH was performed on peripheral blood genomic DNA. In serial sample analysis, we observed that mutations in *DNMT3A* and *TET2* increased in size with longer ICB exposures in the melanoma cohort. We also noted that patients with larger size *DNMT3A* mutations with further post ICB clone size expansion had longer durations of ICB exposure. All serial samples in this cohort showed a statistically significant change in VAF from baseline. In the serial sample analysis of NSCLC patients, we observed similar epigenetic expansion, although not statistically significant. Our study generates a hypothesis for two important questions: (a) Can *DNMT3A* or *TET2* CH serve as predictors of a response to ICB therapy and serve as a novel biomarker of response to ICB therapy? (b) As ICB-exposed patients continue to live longer, the myeloid clonal expansion may portend an increased risk for subsequent myeloid malignancy development. Until now, the selective pressure of ICB/T-cell activating therapies on hematopoietic stem cells were less known and we report preliminary evidence of clonal expansion in epigenetic modifier genes (also referred to as inflammatory CH genes).

Keywords: immune checkpoint blockade; immune checkpoint inhibitor; clonal hematopoiesis of indeterminate potential; *DNMT3A*; TET2; non-small cell lung cancer; melanoma

1. Introduction

Selective expansion of clonal hematopoiesis (CH) mutations in DNA damage response pathway genes following chemotherapy, radiation therapy and radionuclide therapy exposure is well established among cancer survivors [1–4]. Analyzing exposures that lead to a selective growth advantage of CH is an active investigational focus [5,6]. Cancer survivors frequently harbor clonal hematopoiesis of indeterminate potential (CHIP or CH) mutations [7–10]. The number of cancer survivors living in the United States continues to increase each year as a result of the growth and aging of our population, as well as an increase in survival due to changes in early detection and treatment advances [11]. Immune checkpoint blockade (ICB) therapy has revolutionized outcomes among patients with various primary malignancies [12]. The selective pressures of T-cell activating therapies on the hematopoietic compartment are unclear. We previously reported a change in the landscape of secondary myeloid malignancies in a large US population database since the dawn of ICB therapy [13]. In the current study, we aimed to evaluate the impact of exposure to ICB therapy on hematopoietic clones (or CH) in patients with non-small cell lung cancer (NSCLC) and melanoma (MEL). In addition, some data suggest that CH mutations may have a role in preventing T-cell exhaustion and thereby, enhance antitumor activity [14,15]. Therefore, in a subset of patients, we studied the association between hematopoietic clones and duration of response to ICB, hypothesizing specific CH clones as potential novel biomarkers of response.

2. Results

We identified 167 samples from patients ($n = 142$) with a diagnosis of MEL ($n = 33$) and NSCLC ($n = 109$), treated with ICB at our institution. Forty-eight percent in MEL and 57% in NSCLC cohorts were females. Thirty percent of MEL and 85% of NSCLC cohorts had a history of smoking. The median ages of the MEL and the NSCLC cohorts were 63 and 68 years, respectively. Fifty-six percent and 55% of the MEL and the NSCLC cohorts, respectively, had metastatic disease (Table 1). Our cohort had minimal baseline chemotherapy and/or ICB exposure. Most baseline samples were collected prior to chemotherapy (CTX) or ICB exposure. Ten percent of the MEL cohort had CTX or targeted therapy exposure prior to initial sample collection and ICB treatment initiation. Forty-eight percent of the NSCLC cohort had prior CTX (Table 1).

Table 1. Characteristics of patients with non-small cell lung cancer (NSCLC) and Melanoma (MEL).

	NSCLC (n = 109)	MEL (n = 33 *)
Age (years)	67.6	62.5
Range	33–89	33–88
Gender		
Female (%)	62 (56.8%)	16 (48.5%)
Stage		
Metastatic (%)	60 (55%)	19 (57.5%)
Smoking		
Yes (%)	93 (85.3%)	10 (30.3%)
Vascular disease		
Yes (%)	21 (19.3%)	15 (45.5%)
Deep vein thrombosis/Pulmonary embolism		
Yes (%)	19 (17.4%)	2 (6%)
Exposures prior to baseline		
No exposure to chemo/targeted therapy	38 (34.9.9%)	29 (88%)
Radiotherapy exposure	51 (46.7%)	9 (27%)
Targeted and Chemotherapy exposure	4 (4%)	0 (0%)

Table 1. *Cont.*

	NSCLC (*n* = 109)	MEL (*n* = 33 *)
Treatment received		
Immune checkpoint blockade (ICB)	82 (75%)	29 (88%)
Number of ICB cycles (median)	13.6 (2–44)	22 (1–71)
Blood counts		
ANC (10^3/μL)	5.7 (1–20)	4.4 (1.9–7.6)
Platelets (10^3/μL)	306 (127–617)	238 (134–531)
Hemoglobin (gm/dL)	12.7 (8.2–16.8)	14 (8.4–16.6)
MCV (fL)	90.4 (3.5–107.8)	91.6 (82–102)
RDW (%)	14.5 (11.9–32.2)	13.5 (12–17.7)

* 1 patient with missing clinical data. ANC: Absolute neutrophil count; MCV: Mean corpuscular volume; RDW: Red cell distribution width.

2.1. CH in NSCLC and MEL

We identified CH at VAF > 1% in 22.6% (7 of 31 evaluable patients) and 37.6% (41/109) of the baseline MEL and NSCLC samples, respectively (Figure 1A,B). When using a VAF cut-off of >2%, CH incidence was 16.1% (5/31) in MEL and 24.7% (27/109) in patients with NSCLC. Ten percent and 19.5% of patients in the MEL and NSCLC samples, respectively, had mutations in more than one CH gene. In both groups, *DNMT3A* (*n* = 27), *TET2* (*n* = 7) and *ASXL1* (*n* = 6) were the most common genes found to be mutated. The mean VAF in the MEL cohort was 4.9% (1.01–19.1%) and 2.27% (1.01–26.4%) in the NSCLC cohort. We defined cohorts with CH at VAF > 2% compared to no CH cohorts in MEL and NSCLC patients. Patients with CH were older in age compared to those without CH, 70 vs. 62 years ($p = 0.12$) in the MEL cohort and 74 vs. 66 years ($p = 0.00012$) in the NSCLC cohort. CH patients had normal hematological parameters with the exception of increased red cell distribution width (RDW; a recently described progression predicting variable [16], RDW of 15.2 vs. 13.2 in MEL ($p = 0.0071$). Gender and other blood counts were assessed as a factor of CH, and no significant associations were noted.

2.2. Interaction of CH and ICB

Primary tumor responses in this cohort were defined as durable (receipt of ≥12 ICB cycles). All *DNMT3A* and *TET2* mutations expanded over time after ICB exposure (Figure 2a). In patients with MEL, CH with higher VAF was associated with longer duration of ICB therapy (as an example in Figure 2b; plot titled 'Immunotherapy_cycles'; PT-00298654 and PT-00306840 had VAFs 10% or more and received 25 or more ICB cycles). MEL patients with a *DNMT3A* mutation (*n* = 5) had a trend towards durable ICB responses (≥12 ICB cycles), i.e., received a higher median number of ICB cycles (21 cycles, range: 10–40) compared to non-*DNMT3A* CH mutant patients (7, range: 1–13; $p = 0.21$). Despite the significantly older age of the *DNMT3A* CH+ cohort (67.8 years; 52–88) versus the CH negative cohort (mean age 60.7; 33–77), both groups had an equivalent duration of ICB exposure (Supplemental Table S1). Additionally, as discussed above, patients with larger *DNMT3A* clones tended to receive a higher number of ICB cycles (Figure 2b). In the serial sample analysis, we observed that mutations in *DNMT3A* and *TET2* increased in size with longer ICB exposures in the MEL cohort (Figure 2a and Supplemental Figure S1, Supplemental Table S2). Three patients in the MEL cohort received >15 ICB cycles. Another patient (PT-00306840) with the most notable *DNMT3A* expansion received 40 ICB cycles (Figure 2a and Supplemental Figure S1). In the serial sample analysis for the NSCLC cohort, we observed that patients with ≥3 months of ICB exposure demonstrated a decrease in clone size in gene mutations such as *SRCAP*, *STK11* and *TPM1* (Supplemental Figure S2). Again, exceptions were *DNMT3A* and *TET2*, which showed stability or increase in size with longer ICB exposure. The characteristics of patients whose serial samples were available are shown in Supplemental Figure S2a (MEL) and Figure S2b (NSCLC).

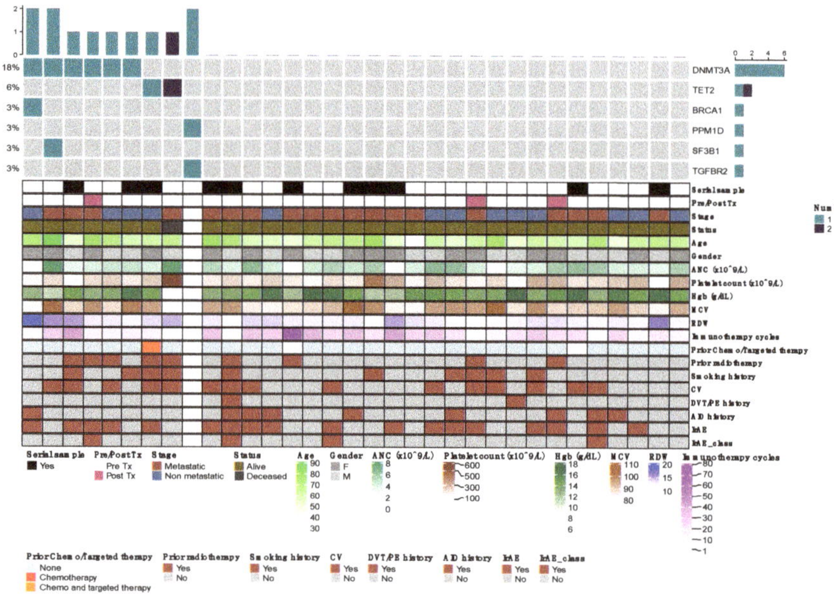

(A)

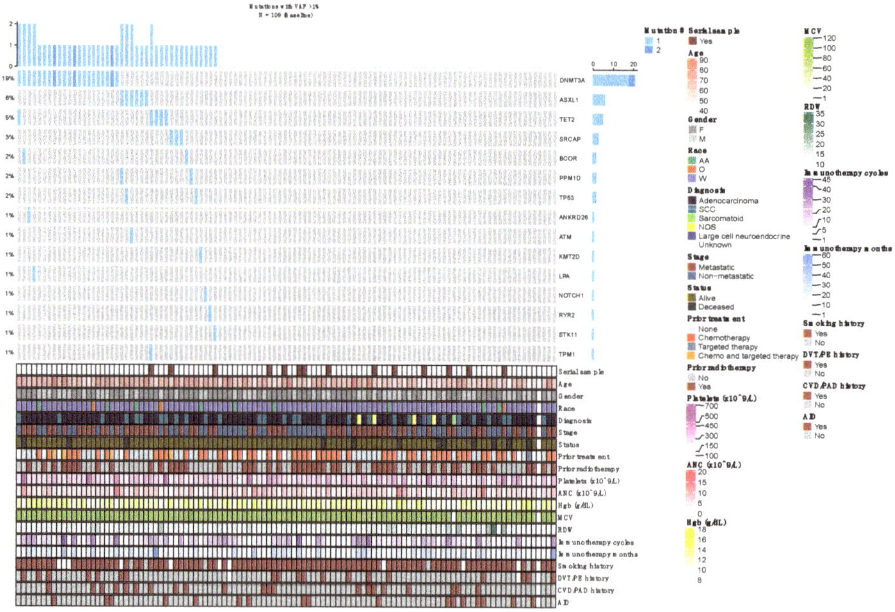

(B)

Figure 1. (**A**) Description of clinical, hematological, and genetic characteristics of patients with melanoma. (**B**) Description of clinical, hematological, and genetic characteristics of patients with non-small cell lung cancer. ANC (absolute neutrophil count); Hgb (hemoglobin); MCV (mean corpuscular volume, fL); RDW (red cell distribution width, %); CV (cardiovascular disease); DVT/PE (Deep vein thrombosis/Pulmonary embolism); AID (Autoimmune disease); IrAE (Immune-related adverse events). Race (AA: African American; O: other; W: White), SCC: Squamous cell cancer; NOS (Not otherwise specified); CVD/PAD (cardiovascular disease/Peripheral arterial disease).

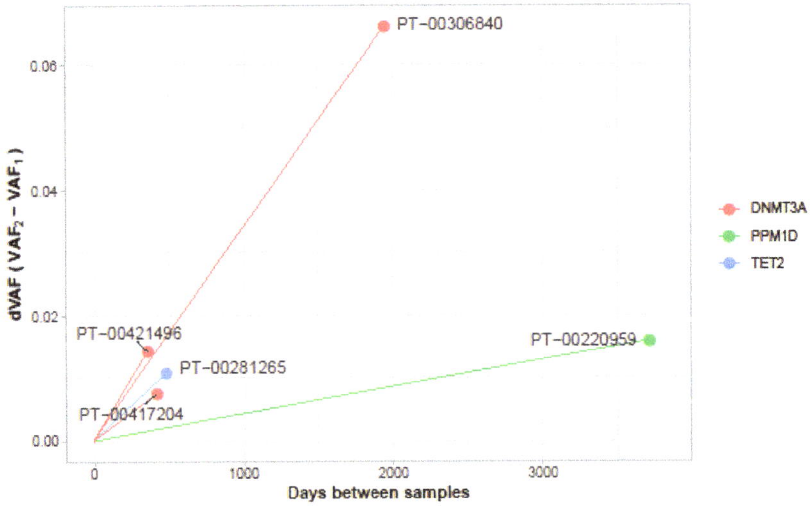

(a)

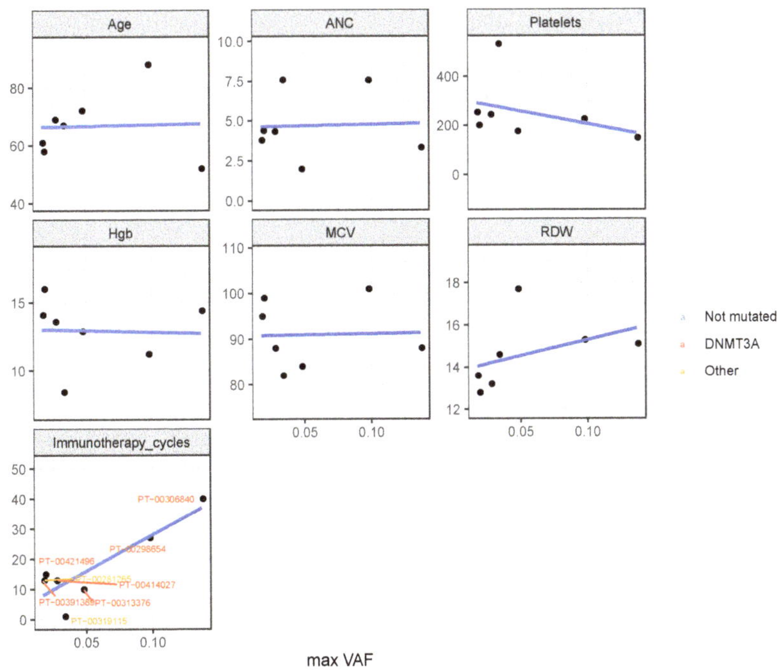

(b)

Figure 2. (**a**) Change in clonal architecture in serial blood samples after exposure to immune checkpoint inhibitor (ICB) in five patients with melanoma. Spider plot depicts difference in variant allele frequencies (VAF) (y-axis) in blood samples pre- and post-ICB therapy ICB (Immune checkpoint inhibitor) plotted against time between pre- and post-sample collection (x-axis); Pre-ICB sample collection at day 0. (**b**) Age, hematological and treatment characteristics in patients with melanoma and clonal hematopoiesis mutations, at baseline. ANC (absolute neutrophil count, $10^3/\mu L$); Hgb (hemoglobin, gm/dL); MCV (mean corpuscular volume, fL); RDW (red cell distribution width, %); VAF (Variant allele frequency).

3. Discussion

High CH prevalence was noted in solid malignancies and is associated with poor survival [8,17]. Receipt of CTX and RT has been associated with the emergence or propagation of DNA damage repair (DDR) pathway gene mutations [4,7,8]. Mutations in epigenetic modifiers, i.e., *DNMT3A* and *TET2* are not frequently affected by exposure to such therapy [7,18]. Large studies published thus far did include a subset that received ICB and targeted therapy. Associations of specific clonal dynamics for the patients on ICB have not been rigorously studied by serial sample analysis. In an attempt to answer this, a prior study investigated the impact of ICB on CH by analyzing blood samples from 91 patients with cutaneous melanoma and basal cell carcinoma before and after ICB treatment [17]. The results indicated that ICB treatment did not significantly affect the prevalence, size, or mutational landscape of CH and they concluded that ICB did not drive clonal evolution. This study, however, focused on clonal expansions in DDR pathway genes, such as *TP53* and *PPM1D* [17]. Our study performed sequential genomic sequencing and noted that VAFs either increased or decreased based on driver gene mutation while on ICB. We particularly noted expansions within genes involved in inflammatory pathways, i.e., *DNMT3A* and *TET2*. A plausible explanation for this discordance possibly stems from an insufficient time period to observe a meaningful clonal expansion in the prior study as well as the study question involving multiple CH mutations, as opposed to our serial cohort enriched with majorly inflammation-related mutations of *DNMT3A* and *TET2*.

DNMT3A clones originate at an early age and gradually expand at a steady rate [19]. The expected *DNMT3A* clonal expansion rate varies considerably with different exposures and mediators [19]. We demonstrate in our MEL cohort a significant *DNMT3A* clonal expansion among serial samples and a *TET2* clonal expansion (Supplemental Figure S1). An increase in VAF of CH-clones (predominantly *DNMT3A*) was associated with a longer duration of ICB therapy exposure. A certain limitation of our serial sample analysis is our inability to procure several serial samples on *DNMT3A/TET2* mutant patients in the NSCLC cohort. However, our study generates two essential and provocative hypotheses that warrant further investigation: (a) ICB and inflammatory-CH (iCH; *DNMT3A/TET2* related CH) share a bidirectional relationship where iCH may enhance the response to ICB and the response to ICB further drives iCH (as these mutant clones thrive under inflammation); (b) ICB-mediated iCH expansion may lead to a novel therapy-related myeloid neoplasm as patients on ICB therapies continue to live longer. To test the former, iCH as a potential novel biomarker of response, larger studies with numerous sequential samples are needed whereas, for the latter, several years of follow-up would be prudent. Overall, we noted that CH in epigenetic modifier genes (*DNMT3A*/*TET2*) was associated with a durable response to ICB therapy in ICB-exposed patients. The presence of *DNMT3A*/*TET2*-CH and their increasing clonal burden correlated with longer ICB exposure. The precise mechanisms behind these findings have not been clarified. One compelling hypothesis is that improved response to ICB and thus induction of inflammatory milieu provides selection pressure for fitter clones that thrive under inflammation.

It is important to note that, even in cases of ICB-sensitive disease, prolonged ICB therapy may not be feasible for some patients due to intolerable side effects, particularly those that are immune-mediated. A higher baseline iCH may not be able to predict ICB duration and response correctly in such cases. The inability to capture such cases is a limitation of our study. Another limitation is the lack of an external control group in our study. Ideally, a control group of patients with metastatic melanoma or NSCLC who had not received immune checkpoint inhibitors (ICBs) would have been included. However, this is challenging since ICBs are the current standard of care, especially for melanoma, and historical controls are hard to establish due to inconsistent sample availability in our biorepository or lack of comparable methods for assessing clonal hematopoiesis (CH), particularly when compared to chemotherapy. Given these limitations, we focused our conclusions on pre- and post-treatment changes in variant allele frequency (VAF), consistent with prior CH studies. Lastly, most baseline samples were collected prior to CTX or ICB exposure, however, ten percent of the MEL cohort had CTX or targeted therapy exposure prior to initial sample collection and ICB treatment initiation. Hence, part of the clone expansion observed maybe due to a previous insult in such patients, another limitation of this study.

Nonetheless, our findings and resultant hypothesis are well-supported by increasing evidence that CH modulates immune and inflammatory pathways in both clinical and in vivo settings [20]. Findings that support this observation include recent reports of *DNMT3A* CH in hematopoietic stem cell (HSC) grafts, which were shown to produce better outcomes in HSC transplant patients who did not receive post-transplant graft vs. host disease prevention with cyclophosphamide (PTCy) [15]. This observation suggests the role of T-cells and resultant inflammation as a permissive condition for the expansion of *DNMT3A* clones or vice versa. Whether heightened immune activation of T-cells in the setting of CH drives longer and better responses to ICB therapy, represents an important yet-to-be-answered question. Additionally, previously, *DNMT3A* CH evolving during effective ICB appeared to serve as a predictor of improved survival in NSCLC patients [21]. The precise mechanisms need clarification in future larger studies of sequential genomic analysis; however, our study generates a hypothesis that induction of pro-inflammatory milieu under ICB stress provides selection pressure for more fit HSC clones that thrive under inflammation or are less inflammation sensitive.

Preclinically, macrophages carrying the *DNMT3A* mutation enhance the inflammatory response in mouse models [22]. At the same time, pro-inflammatory states reciprocally were shown to enhance *DNMT3A* clonal expansion in pre-clinical and clinical models [22]. The loss of function *TET2* gene allows a switch of immunosuppressive tumor-associated macrophages to proinflammatory ones. It was also recently noted that deletion of *DNMT3A* in T-cells can prevent T-cell exhaustion and enhance anti-tumor activity [16]. In another study, a zebrafish model of CH suggested that the clonal fitness of mutant clones is driven by enhanced resistance to inflammatory signals from their *mutant* mature cell progeny. Using an approach called TWISTR (tissue editing with inducible stem cell tagging via recombination), authors identified a survival pathway within the mutant HSPCs involving inflammatory modulators. On a clinical level, in addition to the *DNMT3A*-PTCy discussion above, studies also suggest that deleting *DNMT3A* in CAR-T-cells prevents exhaustion and enhances antitumor activity [23]. The patients with prolonged cytopenia after CAR-T-cell therapy had bone marrow infiltration by interferon-gamma-producing CD8+ T-cells. In a remote way, this suggests that heightened T-cell activity, such as might occur with ICB treatment, could affect the bone marrow in a way that could favor and select certain CH clones [24]. These pre-clinical and clinical observations, including our study findings of *DNMT3A* expansion while on ICB therapy, provide ground for designing functional assays that link epigenetic modification from mutant *DNMT3A* to T-cell expansion; thereby setting grounds for evaluating iCH as a novel biomarker of ICB response.

4. Materials and Methods

4.1. Study Methods

We accessed and analyzed blood samples from the biorepository of Roswell Park Cancer Center (RPCCC) for patients with a diagnosis of NSCLC or MEL and treated with ICB. Patients were screened and identified through a clinical database as well as the biorepository for receipt of ICB therapy. Stored samples (n = 142); with a diagnosis of MEL (n = 33) and NSCLC (n = 109) treated with ICB at RPCCC were identified and analyzed. Additionally, serial prospective peripheral blood samples from subset of patients (NSCLC, n = 14, and MEL, n = 11) were obtained after informed consent. Clinical and laboratory variables were collected for the patients through retrospective chart review. Peripheral blood counts were determined using complete blood counts obtained at the time of sample collection (±30 days). Chemotherapy or radiotherapy exposure were based on receipt of any systemic therapy that patients had received at or after initial blood/DNA sampling. No patients in our analysis had another active hematologic malignancy or a precursor state such as monoclonal gammopathy of undetermined significance or monoclonal B-cell lymphocytosis at the time of peripheral blood sequencing. The study was approved by the Institutional Review Board (approval number BDR-113119).

4.2. Mutational Analysis

Genomic DNA from mononuclear cells or buffy coat was extracted. Illumina sequencing adapters containing unique dual sample indices (UDIs) were ligated onto fragments according to the Kapa Biosystems HyperPrep protocol. Targeted enrichment using a custom pool of biotinylated baits directed to 93 genes involved in clonal hematopoiesis, cancer, and cardiovascular disease (CVD) was performed according to the standard Twist Biosciences capture protocol. Sequencing was performed to 1800× mean overall depth of coverage using NovaSeq6000 (Illumina inc., San Diego, CA, USA) using 150 × 150 S4 chemistry. Clonal hematopoiesis (CH) detection followed the strategy in previous studies [25] for quality and filtration of artifacts. Gencore v0.13.0 [26] and fastp v0.20.1 [27] were used to trim adaptor sequences and remove duplicates. After alignment with BWA MEM v0.7.17 [28], VarDict-Java v1.7.0 [29], was used to call variants on reads. Bcftools v1.10.2 [30], SnpEff v4.3 [31], and Vcflib v1.0.1 [32], were used to filter out reads for mapping quality, depth, and strand bias. Variant-Effect-Predictor (VEP) v100.3 [33], was used to annotate variants. SNP were stringently filtered out when reported as >0.25% in population allele frequency databases. Variants with VAF $\geq$ 1% are being reported. The sensitivity of the test is estimated at >95% for mutations present at VAF > 1% (corresponding to 1/50 mutated cells).

4.3. Quantification and Statistical Analysis

Analysis was conducted in R environment (https://www.R-project.org; R: A language and environment for statistical computing. R Foundation for Statistical Computing, Vienna, Austria, accessed on 1 July 2021). Figures were produced using the package ggplot2 also in R v3.3.3 (Wickham, NZ, 2016). Statistical significance was defined as $p < 0.05$. Statistical tests were performed using R software. As per the procedure, we used a linear model for VAF changes. For each mutation in each individual with sequential sequencing data available, we modeled the growth rate of the mutation between the two time points according to the following formula: $a = \log (V/V0)/(T - T0)$ Where T and T0 indicate the age of the individual (in days) at the two measurement time points and V and V0 correspond to the VAF at T and T0, respectively. We also classified mutations as having increased, decreased, or remained constant during the follow-up period based on a binomial test comparing the two VAFs. Generalized estimating equations were used to test for an association between exposure to ICB and CH growth rate adjusting for age, gender, and smoking status accounting for correlation between the growth rate of mutations in the same person. A paired *t*-test was used to test for significance in the difference between growth rates of mutations within individuals who received ICB. List of genes in CH panel ($n = 93$) is in Supplemental Table S3.

5. Conclusions

To summarize, our study raises two important questions to be addressed: (a) Can *DNMT3A* or *TET2* CH serve as a predictor of response to ICB therapy? (b) As ICB-exposed patients continue to live longer, the myeloid clonal expansion may portend an increased risk for subsequent myeloid malignancy development. ICB-induced CH may predispose patients to a novel treatment-related hematopoietic neoplasm, which will need to be defined with longer follow-ups and larger studies. Additionally, our study, in alignment with prior studies, demonstrates *DNMT3A* and *TET2* to be the common genes to be mutated among cancer cohorts. Despite the small size of the cohort, owing to optimal latency time between serial samples, we noted *DNMT3A* clonal expansion while on ICB therapy. As a future direction, larger studies with sequential samples are needed to confirm this observation as well as functional assays to study the epigenetic advantage for T-cell expansion with mutant *DNMT3A* or *TET2*.

Supplementary Materials: The following supporting information can be downloaded at: https://www.mdpi.com/article/10.3390/ijms252011049/s1.

Author Contributions: Conceptualization, A.S. and S.T.; methodology, A.S., S.T. and N.M.T.; formal analysis, N.M.T.; investigation, A.S., S.T. and N.M.T.; resources, A.S., S.T., G.K.D., M.S.E., N.M.T., E.W. and M.L.G.; data curation, A.S., S.T., R.M., E.S. and L.Y.; writing—original draft preparation, A.S.; writing—review and editing, R.M., S.T., D.C.H., E.A.G., E.W., K.A., M.S., S.S., S.M., M.S.E., A.C.P., T.K., G.K.D., M.Z.N., I.S. and M.L.G.; visualization, N.M.T.; supervision, S.T., E.W., M.L.G., E.A.G., M.S.E. and D.C.H., project administration, S.T., E.W., D.C.H. and M.L.G.; funding acquisition, S.T. All authors have read and agreed to the published version of the manuscript.

Funding: This project was supported by KL2 BTC award from the University of Buffalo's CTSI (S.T.). Data Bank and BioRepository (DBBR) provided data and samples for this study. DBBR is funded by the National Cancer Institute (P30 CA016056) and is a Roswell Park Cancer Institute Cancer Center Support Grant shared resource.

Institutional Review Board Statement: The study was conducted in accordance with the Declaration of Helsinki, and approved by the Institutional Review Board of Roswell Park Comprehensive Cancer Center (BDR-113119, date of approval-15 April 2019).

Informed Consent Statement: Informed consent was obtained from all subjects involved in the study.

Data Availability Statement: The data presented in this study are available on request from the corresponding author. The data are not publicly available due to privacy or ethical restrictions.

Acknowledgments: We thank Roswell Park Cancer Institute Cancer Center research administration for continued support.

Conflicts of Interest: Dr. Duane C. Hassane was employed at Tempus Labs, Inc. The authors declare that this research was conducted in the absence of any commercial or financial relationships that could be construed as a potential conflict of interest. The funders had no role in the design of the study; in the collection, analyses, or interpretation of data; in the writing of the manuscript, or in the decision to publish the results.

References

1. Singh, A.; Mencia-Trinchant, N.; Griffiths, E.A.; Altahan, A.; Swaminathan, M.; Gupta, M.; Gravina, M.; Tajammal, R.; Faber, M.G.; Yan, L.; et al. Mutant *PPM1D*- and *TP53*-Driven Hematopoiesis Populates the Hematopoietic Compartment in Response to Peptide Receptor Radionuclide Therapy. *JCO Precis. Oncol.* **2022**, *6*, e2100309. [CrossRef] [PubMed]
2. Gibson, C.J.; Lindsley, R.C.; Tchekmedyian, V.; Mar, B.G.; Shi, J.; Jaiswal, S.; Bosworth, A.; Francisco, L.; He, J.; Bansal, A.; et al. Clonal Hematopoiesis Associated With Adverse Outcomes After Autologous Stem-Cell Transplantation for Lymphoma. *J. Clin. Oncol.* **2017**, *35*, 1598–1605. [CrossRef] [PubMed]
3. Mouhieddine, T.H.; Sperling, A.S.; Redd, R.; Park, J.; Leventhal, M.; Gibson, C.J.; Manier, S.; Nassar, A.H.; Capelletti, M.; Huynh, D.; et al. Clonal hematopoiesis is associated with adverse outcomes in multiple myeloma patients undergoing transplant. *Nat. Commun.* **2020**, *11*, 2996. [CrossRef] [PubMed]
4. Wong, T.N.; Miller, C.A.; Jotte, M.R.M.; Bagegni, N.; Baty, J.D.; Schmidt, A.P.; Cashen, A.F.; Duncavage, E.J.; Helton, N.M.; Fiala, M.; et al. Cellular stressors contribute to the expansion of hematopoietic clones of varying leukemic potential. *Nat. Commun.* **2018**, *9*, 455. [CrossRef] [PubMed]
5. Zhang, C.R.; Nix, D.; Gregory, M.; Ciorba, M.A.; Ostrander, E.L.; Newberry, R.D.; Spencer, D.H.; Challen, G.A. Inflammatory cytokines promote clonal hematopoiesis with specific mutations in ulcerative colitis patients. *Exp. Hematol.* **2019**, *80*, 36–41.e3. [CrossRef]
6. Higa, K.C.; Goodspeed, A.; Chavez, J.S.; De Dominici, M.; Danis, E.; Zaberezhnyy, V.; Rabe, J.L.; Tenen, D.G.; Pietras, E.M.; DeGregori, J. Chronic interleukin-1 exposure triggers selection for *Cebpa*-knockout multipotent hematopoietic progenitors. *J. Exp. Med.* **2021**, *218*, e20200560. [CrossRef]
7. Coombs, C.C.; Zehir, A.; Devlin, S.M.; Kishtagari, A.; Syed, A.; Jonsson, P.; Hyman, D.M.; Solit, D.B.; Robson, M.E.; Baselga, J.; et al. Therapy-Related Clonal Hematopoiesis in Patients with Non-hematologic Cancers Is Common and Associated with Adverse Clinical Outcomes. *Cell Stem Cell* **2017**, *21*, 374–382.e4. [CrossRef]
8. Olszewski, A.J.; Chorzalska, A.D.; Kim, A.S.; Quesenberry, P.J.; Lopresti, M.L.; Fenton, M.A.; Reagan, J.L.; Butera, J.N.; Sahin, I.; Hamel, C.; et al. Clonal haematopoiesis of indeterminate potential among cancer survivors exposed to myelotoxic chemotherapy. *Br. J. Haematol.* **2019**, *186*, e31–e35. [CrossRef]

9. Bewersdorf, J.P.; Ardasheva, A.; Podoltsev, N.A.; Singh, A.; Biancon, G.; Halene, S.; Zeidan, A.M. From clonal hematopoiesis to myeloid leukemia and what happens in between: Will improved understanding lead to new therapeutic and preventive opportunities? *Blood Rev.* **2019**, *37*, 100587. [CrossRef]
10. Singh, I.; Singh, A. Clonal Hematopoiesis of Indeterminate Potential: Current Understanding and Future Directions. *Curr. Oncol. Rep.* **2023**, *25*, 539–547. [CrossRef]
11. American Cancer Society. *Cancer Treatment & Survivorship Facts & Figures 2019–2021*; American Cancer Society: Atlanta, GA, USA, 2019.
12. Postow, M.A.; Callahan, M.K.; Wolchok, J.D. Immune Checkpoint Blockade in Cancer Therapy. *J. Clin. Oncol.* **2015**, *33*, 1974–1982. [CrossRef] [PubMed]
13. Singh, A.; Herr, M.M.; Griffiths, E.A.; Przespolewski, A.; Faber, M.G.; Mrad, C.; Wang, E.S.; Hahn, T.; Thota, S. Emerging trends of therapy related myeloid neoplasms following modern cancer therapeutics in the United States. *Sci. Rep.* **2021**, *11*, 23284. [CrossRef] [PubMed]
14. Prinzing, B.; Zebley, C.C.; Petersen, C.T.; Fan, Y.; Anido, A.A.; Yi, Z.; Nguyen, P.; Houke, H.; Bell, M.; Haydar, D.; et al. Deleting DNMT3A in CAR T cells prevents exhaustion and enhances antitumor activity. *Sci. Transl. Med.* **2021**, *13*, eabh0272. [CrossRef] [PubMed]
15. Gibson, C.J.; Kim, H.T.; Zhao, L.; Murdock, H.M.; Hambley, B.; Ogata, A.; Madero-Marroquin, R.; Wang, S.; Green, L.; Fleharty, M.; et al. Donor Clonal Hematopoiesis and Recipient Outcomes After Transplantation. *J. Clin. Oncol.* **2022**, *40*, 189–201. [CrossRef]
16. Weeks, L.D.; Niroula, A.; Neuberg, D.; Wong, W.; Lindsley, R.C.; Luskin, M.R.; Berliner, N.; Stone, R.M.; DeAngelo, D.J.; Soiffer, R.J.; et al. Prediction of Risk for Myeloid Malignancy in Clonal Hematopoiesis. *NEJM Evid.* **2023**, *2*, EVIDoa2200310. [CrossRef]
17. Miller, P.G.; Gibson, C.J.; Mehta, A.; Sperling, A.S.; Frederick, D.T.; Manos, M.P.; Miao, B.; Hacohen, N.; Hodi, F.S.; Boland, G.M.; et al. Fitness Landscape of Clonal Hematopoiesis Under Selective Pressure of Immune Checkpoint Blockade. *JCO Precis. Oncol.* **2020**, *4*, 1027–1033. [CrossRef]
18. Bolton, K.L.; Ptashkin, R.N.; Gao, T.; Braunstein, L.; Devlin, S.M.; Kelly, D.; Patel, M.; Berthon, A.; Syed, A.; Yabe, M.; et al. Cancer therapy shapes the fitness landscape of clonal hematopoiesis. *Nat. Genet.* **2020**, *52*, 1219–1226. [CrossRef]
19. Fabre, M.A.; de Almeida, J.G.; Fiorillo, E.; Mitchell, E.; Damaskou, A.; Rak, J.; Orrù, V.; Marongiu, M.; Chapman, M.S.; Vijayabaskar, M.S.; et al. The longitudinal dynamics and natural history of clonal haematopoiesis. *Nature* **2022**, *606*, 335–342. [CrossRef]
20. Pan, W.; Zhu, S.; Qu, K.; Meeth, K.; Cheng, J.; He, K.; Ma, H.; Liao, Y.; Wen, X.; Roden, C.; et al. The DNA Methylcytosine Dioxygenase Tet2 Sustains Immunosuppressive Function of Tumor-Infiltrating Myeloid Cells to Promote Melanoma Progression. *Immunity* **2017**, *47*, 284–297.e5. [CrossRef]
21. Ricciuti, B.; Alessi, J.V.M.; Li, Y.Y.; Lawrence, M.N.; Gupta, H.; Nishino, M.; Cherniack, A.D.; Sholl, L.M.; Awad, M.M. DNMT3A mutation to identify a subset of non-small cell lung cancers with increased sensitivity to PD-(L)1 blockade. *J. Clin. Oncol.* **2021**, *39* (Suppl. S15), 9113. [CrossRef]
22. Marnell, C.S.; Bick, A.; Natarajan, P. Clonal hematopoiesis of indeterminate potential (CHIP): Linking somatic mutations, hematopoiesis, chronic inflammation and cardiovascular disease. *J. Mol. Cell. Cardiol.* **2021**, *161*, 98–105. [CrossRef] [PubMed]
23. Singh, A.; Balasubramanian, S. The crossroads of cancer therapies and clonal hematopoiesis. *Semin. Hematol.* **2024**, *61*, 16–21. [CrossRef] [PubMed]
24. Strati, P.; Li, X.; Deng, Q.; Marques-Piubelli, M.L.; Henderson, J.; Watson, G.; Deaton, L.; Cain, T.; Yang, H.; Ravanmehr, V.; et al. Prolonged cytopenia following CD19 CAR T cell therapy is linked with bone marrow infiltration of clonally expanded IFNγ-expressing CD8 T cells. *Cell Rep. Med.* **2023**, *4*, 101158. [CrossRef] [PubMed]
25. Desai, P.; Mencia-Trinchant, N.; Savenkov, O.; Simon, M.S.; Cheang, G.; Lee, S.; Ritchie, E.K.; Guzman, M.L.; Ballman, K.V.; Roboz, G.J.; et al. Somatic mutations precede acute myeloid leukemia years before diagnosis. *Nat. Med.* **2018**, *24*, 1015–1023. [CrossRef] [PubMed]
26. Chen, S.; Zhou, Y.; Chen, Y.; Huang, T.; Liao, W.; Xu, Y.; Li, Z.; Gu, J. Gencore: An efficient tool to generate consensus reads for error suppressing and duplicate removing of NGS data. *BMC Bioinform.* **2019**, *20* (Suppl. S23), 606. [CrossRef]
27. Chen, S.; Zhou, Y.; Chen, Y.; Gu, J. fastp: An ultra-fast all-in-one FASTQ preprocessor. *Bioinformatics* **2018**, *34*, i884–i890. [CrossRef]
28. Li, H. Aligning sequence reads, clone sequences and assembly contigs with BWA-MEM. *arXiv* **2013**, arXiv:1303.3997.
29. Lai, Z.; Markovets, A.; Ahdesmaki, M.; Chapman, B.; Hofmann, O.; McEwen, R.; Johnson, J.; Dougherty, B.; Barrett, J.C.; Dry, J.R. VarDict: A novel and versatile variant caller for next-generation sequencing in cancer research. *Nucleic Acids Res.* **2016**, *44*, e108. [CrossRef]
30. Li, H. A statistical framework for SNP calling, mutation discovery, association mapping and population genetical parameter estimation from sequencing data. *Bioinformatics* **2011**, *27*, 2987–2993. [CrossRef]
31. Cingolani, P.; Platts, A.; Wang, L.L.; Coon, M.; Nguyen, T.; Wang, L.; Land, S.J.; Lu, X.; Ruden, D.M. A program for annotating and predicting the effects of single nucleotide polymorphisms, SnpEff: SNPs in the genome of Drosophila melanogaster strain w1118; iso-2; iso-3. *Fly* **2012**, *6*, 80–92. [CrossRef]

32. Garrison, E. *Vcflib, a Simple C++ Library for Parsing and Manipulating VCF Files*; MIT: Cambridge, MA, USA, 2016.
33. McLaren, W.; Gil, L.; Hunt, S.E.; Riat, H.S.; Ritchie, G.R.S.; Thormann, A.; Flicek, P.; Cunningham, F. The ensembl variant effect predictor. *Genome Biol.* **2016**, *17*, 122. [CrossRef]

International Journal of
Molecular Sciences

MDPI

Article

Biallelic Loss of 7q34 (*TRB*) and 9p21.3 (*CDKN2A/2B*) in Adult Ph-Negative Acute T-Lymphoblastic Leukemia

Natalya Risinskaya [1,*], Abdulpatakh Abdulpatakhov [1], Yulia Chabaeva [1], Olga Aleshina [1], Maria Gladysheva [1], Elena Nikulina [1], Ivan Bolshakov [1], Anna Yushkova [1], Olga Dubova [1,2], Anastasia Vasileva [1], Tatiana Obukhova [1], Hunan Julhakyan [1], Nikolay Kapranov [1], Irina Galtseva [1], Sergey Kulikov [1], Andrey Sudarikov [1] and Elena Parovichnikova [1]

1 National Medical Research Center for Hematology, 125167 Moscow, Russia; patakh1997@mail.ru (A.A.); uchabaeva@gmail.com (Y.C.); dr.gavrilina@mail.ru (O.A.); makislitsyna@gmail.com (M.G.); lenysh2007@rambler.ru (E.N.); julymbo04@gmail.com (I.B.); ann.unikova@bk.ru (A.Y.); doe30102001@gmail.com (O.D.); vasilnastia@yandex.ru (A.V.); obukhova_t@mail.ru (T.O.); oncohematologist@mail.ru (H.J.); immunophenotyping.lab@gmail.com (N.K.); irinagaltseva@gmail.com (I.G.); smkulikov@mail.ru (S.K.); dusha@blood.ru (A.S.)

2 Institute of Biodesign and Modeling of Complex Systems, I.M. Sechenov First Moscow State Medical University, 119991 Moscow, Russia

* Correspondence: risinska@gmail.com

Abstract: Tumor cells of acute lymphoblastic leukemia (ALL) may have various genetic abnormalities. Some of them lead to a complete loss of certain genes. Our aim was to reveal biallelic deletions of genes in Ph–negative T-ALL. Chromosomal microarray analysis (CMA) was performed for 47 patients with de novo Ph–negative T-ALL, who received treatment according to RALL-2016m clinical protocol at the National Medical Research Center for Hematology (Moscow, Russia) from 2017 to 2023. Out of forty-seven patients, only three had normal molecular karyotype. The other 44 patients had multiple gains, losses, and copy neutral losses of heterozygosity. Biallelic losses were found in 14 patients (30%). In ten patients (21%), a biallelic deletion of 9p21.3 involved a different number of genes, however *CDKN2A* gene loss was noted in all ten cases. For seven patients (15%), a biallelic deletion of 7q34 was found, including two genes—*PRSS1*, *PRSS2* located within the T-cell receptor beta (*TRB*) locus. A clonal rearrangement of the *TRB* gene was revealed in 6 out of 7 cases with 7q34 biallelic loss. Both biallelic deletions can be considered favorable prognostic factors, with an association with 9p21 being statistically significant ($p = 0.01$) and a trend for 7q34 ($p = 0.12$) being observed.

Keywords: biallelic loss; T-ALL; T-cell receptor beta (*TRB*); *CDKN2A*; chromosomal microarray (CMA); *TRB* clonality

1. Introduction

Acute T-cell lymphoblastic leukemia (T-ALL) is a type of aggressive hematological cancer that originates from early T-cell progenitor cells. In T-ALL, malignant hematopoietic cells with immature T-cell characteristics infiltrate the bone marrow. This type of leukemia accounts for approximately 20–25% of cases in adults [1–4]. The study of cytogenetic abnormalities in T-ALL cells is essential for classifying patients into specific risk groups. This information can help determine the overall treatment approach at the beginning of therapy. However, according to Parovichnikova et al. [5], karyotype abnormalities identified at the onset of T-ALL were not associated with improved or worse 5-year survival.

Over the past decade, researchers have conducted systematic screening of T-acute lymphoblastic leukemia (T-ALL) genomes using high-resolution microarray analysis and next-generation sequencing technologies. These studies have revealed that T-ALL is associated with the accumulation of genetic abnormalities that affect T-cell development. For example, deregulation of transcription factors and disruption of the CDKN2A/CDKN2B cell cycle regulators are found to play a significant role in the pathogenesis of T-ALL [2,4]. It has been found that the absence of biallelic deletion of *TCRG* (7p14), the surface expression of CD13, and heterozygous deletions of the short arm of chromosome 17, as well as mutations in the *IDH1/IDH2* and *DNMT3A* genes, are associated with a poor prognosis. In contrast, the expression of CD8 or CD62L, homozygous deletions of *CDKN2A/CDKN2B*, mutations of *NOTCH1* and/or *FBXW7*, and mutations or deletions of the tumor suppressor gene *BCL11B* have been associated with improved overall survival. It is important to note that the prognostic significance of homozygous *CDKN2A/CDKN2B* deletions is limited to cortical and mature T-cell acute lymphoblastic leukemia (T-ALL). Conversely, mutations in *ID1/ID2* and *DNMT3A* are specifically associated with poor outcomes in early, immature T-cell ALL in adults [4].

In this study, we focused on biallelic deletions detected by CMA and their occurrence in the population of T-ALL patients. We also analyzed the localization and association of these deletions with response to therapy. Earlier, the analysis of the 3-year relapse free survival (RFS) revealed a significant association with the absence of minimal residual disease (MRD) on day 70. These data allow us to consider day +70 as the most informative time point; the detection of MRD in the bone marrow at this time discriminates patients into a group with an unfavorable prognosis who might benefit from allogeneic HSCT, as the probability of RFS for these patients at this point is significantly lower (47% for B-ALL, 35% for T-ALL) compared to patients with negative MRD values (78% for B-ALL and 79% for T-ALL) ($p < 0.001$) [5]. Therefore, our goal was to identify biallelic deletions and assess the association between the most common ones and MRD status on day 70 after the start of treatment, as well as overall and event-free survival.

2. Results

The main characteristics of 47 patients included in the study are presented in Table 1.

Table 1. The main characteristics of the patients.

Parameters	T-ALL (n = 47)
Male:Female	34:13
Age, median	33 (19–53) years
Leukocytes, 10^9/L	44.59 (0.95–833.94)
LDH	1 207 (154–20,064)
Blast cells in peripheral blood, %	75 (0–97)
Blast cells in the bone marrow, %	86 (5.2–100)
Immunophenotype, EGIL, WHO	T-I 6 (12.7%)
	T-II 16 (34%)
	T-III 21 (44.6%)
	T-IV 1 (2.1%)
	MPAL(T-myelo) 3 (6.4%)
Standard cytogenetics	47
+mitosis	44 (93.6%)
−mitosis	3 (6.4%)
Karyotype	44
Normal	20 (20.0%)
Abnormal:	24 (80.0%)
CNS leukemia	10 (21.3%)
Extramedullary disease	34 (72.3%)
MRD-status (+70 day)	46
MRD+	13
MRD−	33
CR:	
After 2nd induction (+70 day)	16
Refractory disease	14
Early Death	1

T-ALL, T-cell lymphoblastic leukemia/lymphoma; LDH, lactate dehydrogenase; EGIL, European Group on Immunological Classification of Leukemia; WHO, World Health Organization; MPAL, mixed phenotype acute leukemia; CNS, central nervous system; CR, complete remission.

In the first stage, we compared the results obtained by the CMA with the results of CCA and FISH performed for patients on RALL-2016 treatment protocol (Supplementary Figure S1) at the onset of the disease. Usually, when analyzing the tumor genome by CMA, aberrations larger than 5 MB and additional microdeletions involving the *CDKN2A/B*, *BTG1*, *EBF1*, *ETV6*, *ERG*, *IKZF1*, *PAX5*, and *RB1* genes are taken into account. Aberrations smaller than 5 MB in size should be considered only if they are associated with known leukemia-associated genes or other neoplasia-associated genes, including cell cycle regulators, oncogenes and tumor suppressor genes [6]. However, since our focus was on biallelic deletions, a combination of two events that could be germinal in origin, we used thresholds for detecting deletions and duplications greater than 50,000 base pairs (bp) and greater than 3 million bp for cnLOH, as proposed for the study of hereditary aberrations [7]. A complete data on the dimensions and localization of the detected aberrations is presented in Table S1. Of the forty-seven patients, only three had a normal molecular karyotype. The other 44 patients had multiple deletions, duplications, and copy neutral loss of heterozygosity. Biallelic deletions were found in 14 patients (30%) (Table 2). Data on the T-ALL immunophenotype and MRD status on day 70 are also provided in Supplementary Table S1.

2.1. *Biallelic Deletions in the Study Cohort*

Ten patients (21%) had a biallelic deletion of 9p21.3 involving a different number of genes, but in all cases it included the loss of the *CDKN2A* gene. The combination of events leading to the complete loss of fragment 9p21.3 is shown in Table 2. In six cases, overlapping deletions led to complete allele loss, in one case, duplication of a deletion was due to copy neutral LOH, and in three cases, biallelic deletion was the result of two aberrations whose boundaries coincided. We also found monoallelic deletions of 9p21.3 in patients 7, 11, 19, 21, 39, and 40 (Supplementary Table S1). In patients #7 and #21, the deletions occurred within the cnLOH region. It is possible that the two aberrations occurred in reverse order, resulting in a monoallelic deletion rather than a biallelic variant.

Seven patients (15%) had a biallelic 7q34 loss (Table 2). Only in one case this was a result from overlapping deletions of different lengths (patient #14). In other cases, the boundaries of deletions on homologous chromosomes matched. Additionally, we found a monoallelic deletion in seven other patients (patients 1, 5, 21, 24, 28, 31, and 32). The location and size of this deletion was approximately 126,000 base pairs, similar to the biallelic deletions in other patients. This deletion includes only two genes—*PRSS1*, *PRSS2*, a part of the trypsinogen cluster located at the T-cell receptor beta (*TRB*) locus. In one patient (#27), the biallelic loss identified by CMA was combined with the t(6;7)(q23;q34) translocation, revealed by CCA. In the remaining patients with bi- and monoallelic deletions, no additional 7q34 aberrations were found (See Supplementary Material Table S1).

Four patients had both biallelic deletions of 7q34 and 9p21.3 (Figure 1).

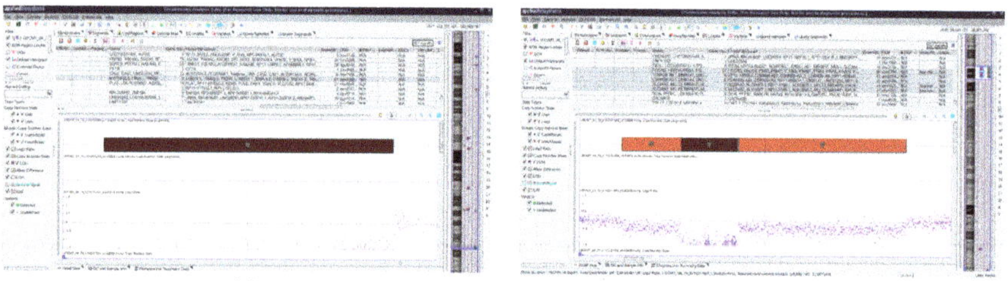

(a) (b)

Figure 1. Molecular karyotype of patient # 27 with biallelic deletions of 9p21.3 (**a**) and 7q34 (**b**). Chromosomes 7 and 9 are highlighted in blue frames, and the deepred indicate the loci of the biallelic deletions. A standard cytogenetic study also revealed a translocation t(6;7)(q23;q34) in this patient, as shown in the Supplementary Table S1.

Table 2. Biallelic losses in a cohort of patients with T-ALL. The aberrations flanking the biallelic deletion are also shown. Deletions are marked in yellow, cnLOH are marked in purple. * Patient with translocation t(6;7)(q23;q34).

Patient#	Age	Gender	Immunophenotype	% of Blast Cells in Bone Marrow	9p21.3 (Start-End Position of Genomic Coordinates)	7q34 (Start-End Position of Genomic Coordinates)	12p13.2 (Start-End Position of Genomic Coordinates)	13q14.2 (Start-End Position of Genomic Coordinates)
12	47	m	T-III	80.1	9p21.3(21972814_22025494)x0	7q34(142610489_142796623)x0		
14	40	m	T-II	84.9		7q34(142538468_142787265)x0, 7q34q36.1(142792254_151451166)x1		
15	23	m	T-III	96.5		7q34(142438198_142787265)x0		
23	41	m	T-II	81.2	9p24.3p13.3(204082_33290534)x2 hmz, 9p21.3(21682143_22103814)x0	7q34(142659319_142785320)x0		
26	20	m	T-III	94.9	9p21.3(21471728_22313094)x0	7q34(142637680_142796623)x0		13q14.2(48411504_48496038)x0
27	40	m	T-III	87.5	9p22.1p21.3(19703574_20908514)x1, 9p21.3(20914896_22056500)x0, 9p21.3(22061616_25458801)x1	7q34(142309952_142795256)x0 *		
28	42	f	T-III	61.5	9p21.3(21052665_21865843)x1, 9p21.3(21866502_21996864)x0, 9p21.3(21998037_25552602)x1			
30	54	f	T-II	86			12p13.2(11592806_11983676)x0	
36	40	m	T-II	38	9p24.3p21.3(204083_21635941)x1 [0.76], 9p21.3(20272224_22647015)x0 [0.5], 9p21.3p13.1(22681778_38780194)x1 [0.76]			
38	21	f	T-III	59.3	9p24.3p21.3(204082_21905380)x1, 9p21.3(21909980_22233512)x0, 9p21.3p11.2(22238596_40880243)x1			
43	33	f	T-III	89.3	9p24.3p21.3(203862_20710799)x1, 9p21.3(20719868_22088261)x0, 9p21.3p11.2(22283154_41008724)x1			
44	30	f	T-III	71		7q34(142353951_142785767)x0		
45	29	m	T-II	94.8	9p22.3p21.3(14432343_22130515)x1, 9p21.3p21.2(22137086_25938431)x0, 9p21.2q13(25944009_67986968)x1			
46	23	m	T-III	66	9p21.3(21720109_22502487)x0			

Patient No. 26 had three biallelic deletions: additionally, deletion of 13q14.2, which included the *RB1*, *LPAR6*, and *RCBTB2* genes, was revealed. Patient # 30 had a deletion of 12p13.2 that resulted in the complete loss of the *ETV6* gene. No other biallelic deletions were found in any of the patients.

2.2. Association between 7q34 Loss and Clonal TRB Rearrangement

T-ALL is characterized by T-cell clonality associated with TRG gene (7p14) rearrangement, as well as TRB gene (7q34) rearrangement in some cases. It is likely that the clonal rearrangement appears as a deletion on CMA. Therefore, we tested TRB clonality for 47 patients using the same DNA samples taken on CMA. Examples of clonal variants associated with biallelic 7q34 loss are shown in Figure 2.

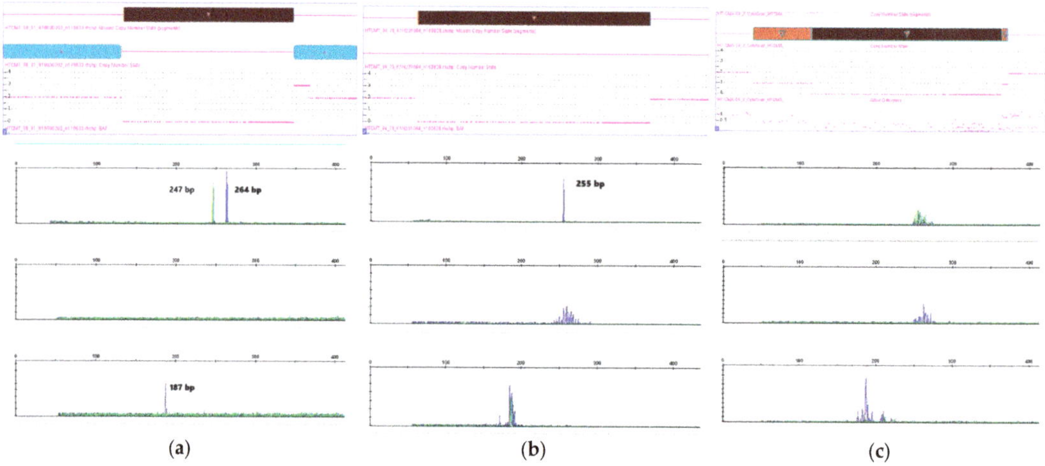

Figure 2. Detail views of biallelic loss 7q34 and TRB clonality assay with monoclonal peaks for patients 15 (**a**) and 27 (**b**) and polyclonal Gaussian curves for patient 44 (**c**).

In the group of patients with 7q34 biallelic loss, the majority of patients had TRB clonality, except for one patient. The same result was obtained in the group with monoallelic deletion. Groups without 7q34 genetic abnormalities (33 patients) include patients with polyclonal result (23 patients) and TRB-clonality (10 patients) (69.7% vs. 30.3%). The data are presented as a histogram in Figure 3a.

We hypothesized that patients with a normal 7q34 locus and *TRB* clonality might have smaller deletions than the threshold of 50 kb we chose for deletions. We analyzed CMA data for all samples in our cohort, with a minimum threshold of 1 kb or less for deletions. We found additional seven biallelic and four monoallelic deletions of 7q34 of 5 kb or more in eleven patients. However, these findings did not confirm a direct association between *TRB* clonality and deletions of 7q34. As a result, 10 of the 25 patients (40%) with confirmed biallelic or monoallelic deletion of 7q34 had no *TRB* clonality, while 6 of the 22 patients (27.3%) with a normal 7q34 locus did have this clonality. The data are presented in Figure 3b and Supplementary Table S2.

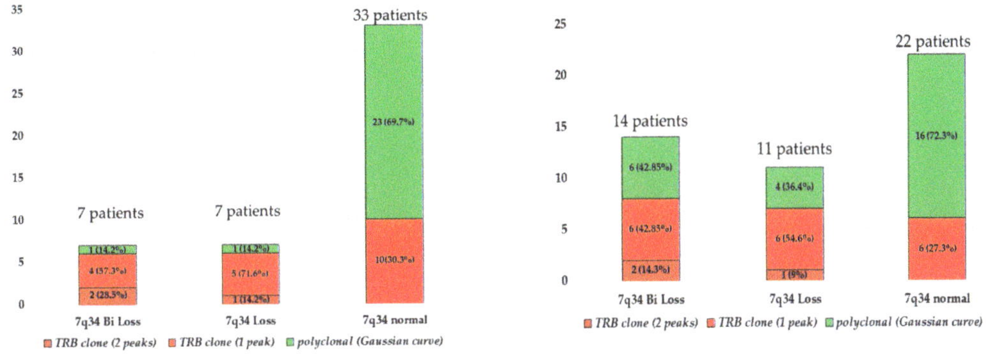

(a) (b)

Figure 3. Histogram of the distribution of *TRB* clonality in groups of patients with biallelic loss of 7q34, monoallelic loss of 7q34, and intact 7q34 locus. (**a**)—CMA results with a cutoff of 50 kb for losses, (**b**)—a cutoff of 1 kb for losses. Dark red color indicates biallelic *TRB* clonality, red indicates *TRB* clonality with one monoclonal PCR peak, green indicates polyclonal samples. On the *X*-axis, the groups are arranged in the following order: with biallelic 7q34 loss, monoallelic 7q34 loss, no 7q34 lesions.

2.3. Association between 7q34 and 9p21.3 Losses and MRD Status at Day 70

We used MRD status on day 70 as a surrogate endpoint. This choice was based on the fact that some patients received treatment according to the RALL-2016 protocol, which does not include additional targeted therapy, and some patients were treated under a modified version of the RALL-2016 protocol that includes targeted therapy for patients with MRD. Up to day 70, all patients were treated according to a unified protocol, there were no cases of early mortality before day 70. We analyzed the association between biallelic and monoallelic loss and MRD status on day 70. One patient was transplanted before the 70th day and her MRD status was not determined on the 70th day, so she was excluded from the analysis. The frequency analysis of the association of MRD status on day 70 and the presence of deletion 7q34 ($p = 0.1262$) and 9p21.3 ($p = 0.0119$) is illustrated by Figure 4.

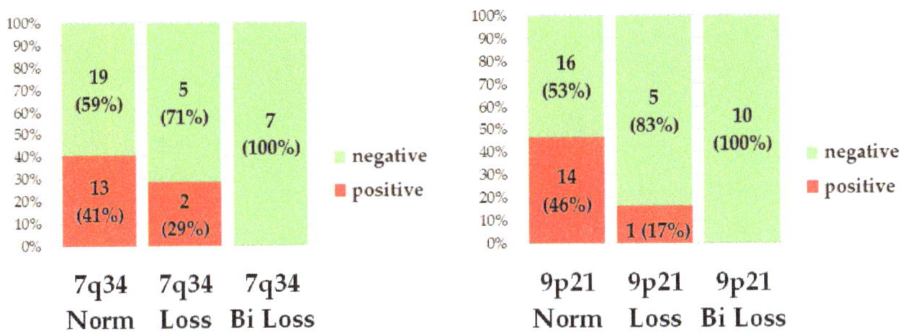

(a) (b)

Figure 4. Diagrams of the distribution of the MRD status depending on the presence of loss 7q34 (**a**) or 9p23.1 (**b**). The number of patients and percentage are indicated on the bars. Green indicates MRD-negative patients, red indicates MRD-positive patients. Along the X axis the bars are arranged in the following order—without loss, with monoallelic loss, with biallelic loss.

Following MRD detection on the 70th day, patients 3, 5, 6, 16, 20, 21, and 29 were transferred to other treatment protocols due to complications and for medical reasons according to the decision of the expert commission. Therefore, it is difficult to estimate the overall survival rate (Figure 5) accurately. We did not find any significant differences in patients' outcomes depending on the presence of deletions. This may be due to the fact that a number of patients received targeted therapy or allogeneic HSCT in the case of MRD positivity.

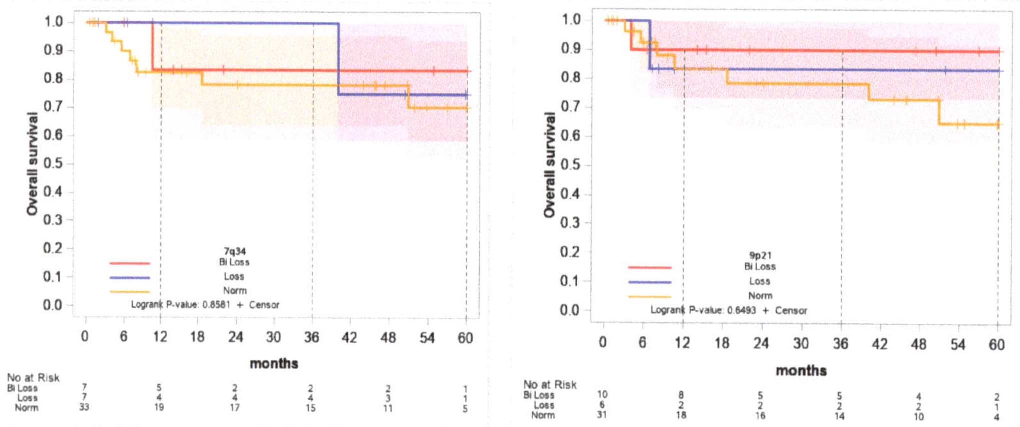

(a) (b)

Figure 5. Overall survival curves of patients depending on the presence of 7q34 (**a**) and 9p21.3 (**b**) deletions. Patients with biallelic loss (red curve), monoallelic loss (blue curve) and patients without deletions (yellow curve) were analyzed. The *X*-axis indicates the time after the start of therapy (months).

3. Discussion

Cytoband 9p21.3 is expected to play a significant role in the formation of biallelic deletions. Cyclin-dependent kinase inhibitor 2A/B (*CDKN2A/B*) genes are frequently altered in acute lymphoblastic leukemia (ALL) patients. Data on the prognostic value of the *CDKN2A/B* deletion are contradictory. Zhang et al. showed by meta-analysis that *CDKN2A/B* deletions were independent poor prognostic markers for both adult and pediatric ALL patients [8]. According to Wang et al. the most common type of *CDKN2A* deletion was homozygous loss and adult T-ALL patients with *CDKN2A* loss had a poor prognosis. These patients might benefit from intensive chemotherapy or allogeneic hematopoietic stem-cell transplantation [9]. Remke et al. noted when compared within child patients with 9q21.3 balanced leukemias, neither heterozygous nor homozygous deletions of the *CDKN2A* gene locus were associated with a differential treatment response [10]. According to VanVlierberghe homozygous loss of *CDKN2A/CDKN2B* is associated with a favorable outcome [4]. We have also shown that biallelic 9p21.3 loss can be considered as a statistically significant (p = 0.0119) favorable prognostic factor.

We have noted a surprisingly high incidence of 7q34 biallelic deletions and their repeated localization in our cohort. The patients in this study were selected randomly, with the main criteria being initiation of therapy according to the RALL-2016m protocol and availability of archived bone marrow DNA at the onset of disease. Nevertheless, 15% of patients showed complete loss of genetic material in a small segment of chromosome 7 (Figure 6). Additionally, seven more patients (15%) had a monoallelic deletion in the same *TRB* locus.

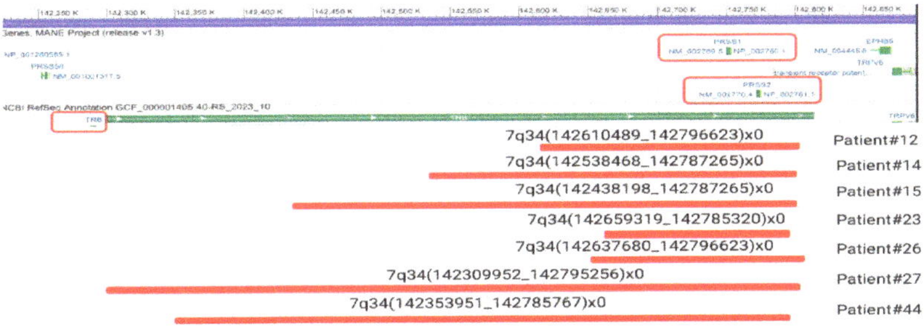
7q34(142610489_142796623)x0
Patient#12
7q34(142538468_142787265)x0
Patient#14
7q34(142438198_142787265)x0
Patient#15
7q34(142659319_142785320)x0
Patient#23
7q34(142637680_142796623)x0
Patient#26
7q34(142309952_142795256)x0
Patient#27
7q34(142353951_142785767)x0
Patient#44

Figure 6. The location of biallelic deletions of 7q34 in the studied cohort of patients, relative to the *TRB* locus, is shown in red lines. This figure was adapted from https://www.ncbi.nlm.nih.gov/gene/6957 (accessed on 19 August 2024).

The beta locus of T-cell receptor located at 7q34 includes segments V, J, D and C. During the development of T cells, the beta chain is synthesized as a result of recombination at the DNA level, connecting segment D to segment J; then segment V is attached to the DJ gene. The beta locus also includes eight trypsinogen genes, three of which encode functional proteins and five of them are pseudogenes [11]. It is likely that the result of recombination looks like a deletion when analyzing gene copy number alterations using CMA. In the majority of patients with deletions, we revealed *TRB* clonality in our study. However, we also encountered patients with deletions but no *TRB* clonality, as well as patients with clonality but without deletions. It is not clear whether the biallelic loss is caused by a rearrangement of *TRB* on one chromosome and deletion on another, or by a biallelic rearrangement leading to the production of amplicons with the same length during PCR for T-cell clonality analysis. 7q34 loss may be a favorable molecular prognostic marker associated with T-I and T-II variants of T-ALL according to our data (Supplementary Table S1). We previously conducted a similar study on a cohort of patients with B-ALL and have found a similar frequency of biallelic deletions at 9p23.1 (5 out of 36 patients, 14%). The 7q34 locus was virtually unaffected in B-ALL, with only one out of thirty-six patients (less than 3%) showing any changes [12]. We have now investigated the *TRB* clonality in this patient as well and identified a biallelic clonal rearrangement of *TRB*. We have not found any similar studies in the literature on biallelic deletions at this locus. However, the participation of the *TRB* locus in translocations in T-ALL was noted [13–18]. Raimondi notes that even early cytogenetic studies of the T-ALL genome showed non-random breakpoints in the following three clusters of T cell receptor genes *TRA*, *TRD* (14q11.2) or *TRB* (7q34). *TCR* breakpoints are present in about 30–35% of ALL [14].

During translocations, the elements of the *TRB* promoter and enhancer are combined with a relatively small number of genes encoding transcription factors, which can lead to malignancy of T cells. Chromosomal aberrations that affect *TRB* loci were among the first reported in T-ALL. Subsequently, these and other rare translocations facilitated the identification of genes that affected during T-ALL, many of which are also transcriptionally activated without any detectable chromosomal rearrangements in these loci. Several recurrent translocations like t(1;7)(p32;q34)/*TRB::TAL1*, t(7;9)(q34;q32)/*TRB::TAL2*, t(7;12)(q34;p12) *TRB::LMO3*, inversions inv(7)(p15q34) and translocations t(7;7)(p15;q34) *TRB::HOXA10*, as well as t(6;7)(q23;q34) [*TRB::MYB*] with overexpression of MYB have been reported in T-ALL [2,15]. *TRB::TLX1*, *TRB::NOTCH1*, *TRB::NKX2* are also described [16]. Molecular study of t(7;19)(q34;p13) in a pediatric patient with acute T-cell lymphoblastic leukemia led to the identification of a translocation between the *TRB* and *LYL1* loci [17]. Variants of T-ALL with inv(7) (p15q34;*TRB::TLX1*) in combination with del*CDKN2AB*/9p21 and cases of translocation of *TRB::TLX1* in combination with del*CDKN2AB*/9p21 and del *TP53*/17p13 are also described [18]. In general, the abundance of chimeric genes involving *TRB* indicates genetic instability of this locus in T-ALL. Similarly, our data support the assumption that the existence of DNA breakpoint hotspots also result in mono- and biallelic deletions covering *TRB* locus.

4. Materials and Methods

The study included 47 patients with Ph-negative T-ALL who received therapy at the National Medical Research Center for Hematology according to the RALL-2016m protocol from 2017 to 2023 and had available tumor DNA material at the onset of the disease. The RALL-2016m protocol is a modification of the previous RALL-2009/2016 protocols, based on the principle of low intensity and non-interruptive treatment. MRD assessment is carried out on days +70 of therapy in accordance with the protocol.

All patients included in the protocol underwent immunophenotyping, cytogenetic and molecular tests of bone marrow samples at the onset of the disease. Bone marrow cells obtained from patients during the initial examination were analyzed using G-differential chromosome staining and FISH. The FISH method was performed to excluded BCR-ABL1-positive ALL (BCR/ABL (DF) Gene Fusion Probe Detection Kit (Wuhan HealthCare Biotechnology Co., Ltd., Wuhan, China)). After a standard cytogenetic test, additional FISH tests were used to identify rearrangements of *KMT2A*/11q23 (*MLL*) (XL *MLL* plus Break Apart Probe (Metasystems, Altlussheim, Germany)), *TCRAD*/14q11 (*TCRA/D* Break Apart Probe (Metasystems, Altlussheim, Germany)), *TP53*/17p13 (*P53/CEP17* chromosome and gene anomaly detection probe Deletion Probe (Wuhan HealthCare Biotechnology Co., Ltd., Wuhan, China)), *IGH*/14q32 (IGH Break Apart Probe (Metasystems, Altlussheim, Germany)), *BCL11B*/14q32 (BCL11B Break Apart FISH Probe (Empire Genomics, New York, NY, USA)), *PDGFRA* (*PDGFRA* Gene Break Apart Probe Detection Kit, (Wuhan HealthCare Biotechnology Co., Ltd., Wuhan, China)), *PDGFRB* (*PDGFRB* Gene Break Apart Probe Detection Kit, (Wuhan HealthCare Biotechnology Co., Ltd., Wuhan, China)) genes. The karyotype and results of FISH analysis were described in accordance with the criteria of the International Cytogenomic Nomenclature ISCN, 2020 [19].

In patients who met T-ALL criteria, we performed an additional analysis to determine the immunophenotype associated with leukemia for further assessment of MRD using flow cytometry. MRD was assessed using the "different from normal" method and identification immunophenotypically immature T-cells in bone marrow [20]. Tests before 2020 were performed with BD FACSCanto II flow cytometer with 2-tube 6-color panel, which includes antibodies against CD99, CD7, CD3 (cytoplasmic and surface), CD5, CD45, CD8. Studies after 2021 were performed with BC CytoFLEX flow cytometer with single-tube 10-color panel, which includes antibodies against CD99, CD7, CD34, CD56, CD3 (cytoplasmic and surface), CD4, CD5, CD45, CD8. MRD was assessed at the end of induction (day 70) using 6- or 10-color flow cytometry of the bone marrow specimens.

CMA was carried out with Thermo Fisher Scientific (Santa Clara, CA 95151, USA) equipment using the CytoScan™ HT-CMA 96F array SNP-oligonucleotide microarray (Thermo Fisher Scientific, Waltham, MA, USA) in accordance with the manufacturer's protocol. The analysis was performed at the "Genomed" laboratory of Molecular Pathology (Moscow, Russia). Material for analysis—DNA isolated from bone marrow cells in patients with ALL before therapy, in an amount of not less than 100 ng and not more than 200 ng with an A260/A280 ratio of not less than 1.8 and reference male DNA of a similar concentration (Thermo Fisher Scientific, Waltham, MA, USA). The scanning results were processed with the Multi Sample Viewer Software (v.1.1.0.11) and Chromosome Analysis Suite (ChAS 4.3.0.71) (Thermo Fisher Scientific, Waltham, MA, USA). Cutoff of $\geq$3 Mb for LOH and $\geq$50 kb for losses and gains was used according to Gonzales et al. [7].

PCR analysis of TRB clonality was performed according to the BIOMED-2 Concerted Action BMH4-CT98-3936 protocol [21]. Primers for multiplex PCR were synthesized by Syntol LLC (Moscow, Russia). For PCR we used the same DNA samples as for CMA.

The achievement of MRD-negative status on day 70 (end of induction) was used as surrogate endpoint to study the prognostic significance of aberrations. Categorical variables were analyzed by frequencies. We use Fisher Exact Test to test hypotheses about differences in distributions of categorical features in comparison groups. The survival analysis with Kaplan-Maier estimates and log-rank test were used for the comparison of overall survival (OS) in different groups of patients. All calculations were made using SAS 9.4.

5. Conclusions

According to the literature, translocations involving 7q34 are common in T-ALL. In this study, we present data on the abundance of biallelic deletions at 7q34 for the first time in T-ALL patients. The frequency of these deletions is similar to that of 9p21 deletions, which have been reported in numerous studies. We have demonstrated that the boundaries of 7q34 deletions are highly conserved and affect almost the complete beta chain of the T-cell receptor. Most of them look like the result of clonal rearrangement of TRB (6 out of 7 cases of biallelic loss in 7q34). However, it is not clear whether biallelic loss is caused by a rearrangement of the TRB on one chromosome and a deletion on another chromosome, or by a biallelic rearrangement that leads to the production of amplicons with the same length during PCR analysis for T-cell clonality. We also analyzed the association between these deletions and minimal residual disease (MRD) in T-ALL. Both biallelic deletions can be considered favorable prognostic factors, with an association with 9p21 being statistically significant and a trend for 7q34 ($p = 0.12$).

Supplementary Materials: The following supporting information can be downloaded at: https://www.mdpi.com/article/10.3390/ijms251910482/s1.

Author Contributions: Conceptualization, N.R. and O.A.; methodology, N.R., T.O., I.G. and S.K.; formal analysis, Y.C. and S.K.; investigation, N.R., A.A., O.D., A.Y., N.K., I.B., E.N. and M.G.; resources, A.A., A.V. and H.J.; data curation, O.A.; writing—original draft preparation, N.R. and Y.C.; writing—review and editing, A.S.; supervision, O.A.; project administration, E.P.; funding acquisition, N.R. All authors have read and agreed to the published version of the manuscript.

Funding: This research was funded by Russian Science Foundation (RSF) project No. 23-25-00490 https://www.rscf.ru/en/project/23-25-00490/ (accessed on 14 August 2024).

Institutional Review Board Statement: This study was conducted in accordance with the Declaration of Helsinki and approved by the Ethics Committee of the National Research Center for Hematology (protocol #175/25 October 2023).

Informed Consent Statement: Informed consent was obtained from all subjects involved in the study.

Data Availability Statement: Data are contained within the article and Supplementary Materials.

Conflicts of Interest: The authors declare no conflicts of interest.

References

1. Gianni, F.; Belver, L.; Ferrando, A. The Genetics and Mechanisms of T-Cell Acute Lymphoblastic Leukemia. *Cold Spring Harb. Perspect. Med.* **2020**, *10*, a035246. [CrossRef] [PubMed]
2. De Bie, J.; Quessada, J.; Tueur, G.; Lefebvre, C.; Luquet, I.; Toujani, S.; Cuccuini, W.; Lafage-Pochitaloff, M.; Michaux, L. Cytogenetics in the management of T-cell acute lymphoblastic leukemia (T-ALL): Guidelines from the Groupe Francophone de Cytogénétique Hématologique (GFCH). *Curr. Res. Transl. Med.* **2023**, *71*, 103431. [CrossRef] [PubMed]
3. Girardi, T.; Vicente, C.; Cools, J.; De Keersmaecker, K. The genetics and molecular biology of T-ALL. *Blood* **2017**, *129*, 1113–1123. [CrossRef] [PubMed]
4. Van Vlierberghe, P.; Ambesi-Impiombato, A.; De Keersmaecker, K.; Hadler, M.; Paietta, E.; Tallman, M.S.; Rowe, J.M.; Forne, C.; Rue, M.; Ferrando, A.A. Prognostic relevance of integrated genetic profiling in adult T-cell acute lymphoblastic leukemia. *Blood* **2013**, *122*, 74–82. [CrossRef] [PubMed]
5. Parovichnikova, E.N.; Aleshina, O.A.; Troitskaya, V.V.; Chabaeva, Y.A.; Sokolov, A.N.; Isinova, G.A.; Kotova, E.S.; Akhmerzaeva, Z.H.; Klyasova, G.A.; Galtseva, I.V.; et al. Comparison of the treatment results in adult patients with acute Ph-negative lymphoblastic leukemia on protocols of the Russian multicenter studies ALL-2009 and ALL-2016. *Russ. J. Hematol. Transfusiol.* **2022**, *67*, 460–477. (In Russian) [CrossRef]
6. Schoumans, J.; Suela, J.; Hastings, R.; Muehlematter, D.; Rack, K.; van den Berg, E.; Berna Beverloo, H.; Stevens-Kroef, M. Guidelines for genomic array analysis in acquired haematological neoplastic disorders. *Genes Chromosomes Cancer* **2016**, *55*, 480–491. [CrossRef] [PubMed]

7. Gonzales, P.R.; Andersen, E.F.; Brown, T.R.; Horner, V.L.; Horwitz, J.; Rehder, C.W.; Rudy, N.L.; Robin, N.H.; Thorland, E.C.; On behalf of the Acmg Laboratory Quality Assurance Committee. Interpretation and reporting of large regions of homozygosity and suspected consanguinity/uniparental disomy, 2021 revision: A technical standard of the American College of Medical Genetics and Genomics (ACMG). *Genet. Med. Off. J. Am. Coll. Med. Genet.* **2022**, *24*, 255–261. [CrossRef] [PubMed]
8. Zhang, W.; Kuang, P.; Liu, T. Prognostic significance of CDKN2A/B deletions in acute lymphoblastic leukaemia: A meta-analysis. *Ann. Med.* **2019**, *51*, 28–40. [CrossRef] [PubMed]
9. Wang, H.P.; Zhou, Y.L.; Huang, X.; Zhang, Y.; Qian, J.J.; Li, J.H.; Li, X.Y.; Li, C.Y.; Lou, Y.J.; Mai, W.Y.; et al. CDKN2A deletions are associated with poor outcomes in 101 adults with T-cell acute lymphoblastic leukemia. *Am. J. Hematol.* **2021**, *96*, 312–319. [CrossRef] [PubMed]
10. Remke, M.; Pfister, S.; Kox, C.; Toedt, G.; Becker, N.; Benner, A.; Werft, W.; Breit, S.; Liu, S.; Engel, F.; et al. High-resolution genomic profiling of childhood T-ALL reveals frequent copy-number alterations affecting the TGF-beta and PI3K-AKT pathways and deletions at 6q15-16.1 as a genomic marker for unfavorable early treatment response. *Blood* **2009**, *114*, 1053–1062. [CrossRef] [PubMed]
11. TRB T Cell Receptor Beta Locus [Homo Sapiens (Human)] Gene ID: 6957. Available online: https://www.ncbi.nlm.nih.gov/gene/6957 (accessed on 17 August 2024).
12. Risinskaya, N.; Gladysheva, M.; Abdulpatakhov, A.; Chabaeva, Y.; Surimova, V.; Aleshina, O.; Yushkova, A.; Dubova, O.; Kapranov, N.; Galtseva, I.; et al. DNA Copy Number Alterations and Copy Neutral Loss of Heterozygosity in Adult Ph-Negative Acute B-Lymphoblastic Leukemia: Focus on the Genes Involved. *Int. J. Mol. Sci.* **2023**, *24*, 17602. [CrossRef] [PubMed]
13. Raimondi, S. Acute T-type lymphoblastic leukemia (T-ALL). *Atlas Genet. Cytogenet. Oncol. Hematol.* **2007**, *11*, 328–339. Available online: http://atlasgeneticsoncology.org/haematological/1374/t-lineage-acute-lymphoblastic-leukemia-(t-all) (accessed on 20 August 2024).
14. Yamamoto, K.; Nakamachi, Y.; Yakushijin, K.; Miyata, Y.; Okamura, A.; Kawano, S.; Matsuoka, H.; Minami, H. A novel TRB@/NOTCH1 fusion gene in T-cell lymphoblastic lymphoma with t(7;9)(q34;q34). *Eur. J. Haematol.* **2013**, *90*, 68–75. [CrossRef] [PubMed]
15. Bardelli, V.; Arniani, S.; Pierini, V.; Di Giacomo, D.; Pierini, T.; Gorello, P.; Mecucci, C.; La Starza, R. T-Cell Acute Lymphoblastic Leukemia: Biomarkers and Their Clinical Usefulness. *Genes* **2021**, *12*, 1118. [CrossRef]
16. Homminga, I.; Vuerhard, M.J.; Langerak, A.W.; Buijs-Gladdines, J.; Pieters, R.; Meijerink, J.P. Characterization of a pediatric T-cell acute lymphoblastic leukemia patient with simultaneous LYL1 and LMO2 rearrangements. *Haematologica* **2012**, *97*, 258–261. [CrossRef] [PubMed]
17. Müller, J.; Walter, W.; Haferlach, C.; Müller, H.; Fuhrmann, I.; Müller, M.L.; Ruge, H.; Meggendorfer, M.; Kern, W.; Haferlach, T.; et al. How T-lymphoblastic leukemia can be classified based on genetics using standard diagnostic techniques enhanced by whole genome sequencing. *Leukemia* **2023**, *37*, 217–221. [CrossRef] [PubMed]
18. Pasquini, A.; Ciolli, G.; Mannelli, F.; Scappini, B.; Gianfaldoni, G.; Pilerci, S.; Fasano, L.; Quinti, E.; Paradiso, V.; Crupi, F.; et al. ALL-256 Nelarabine, Etoposide, and Cyclophosphamide for Adult T Cell Acute Lymphoblastic Leukemia/Lymphoma Relapsing After Pediatric-Inspired Frontline Approaches: Report of 3 Cases From a Real-Life Setting. *Acute Lymphoblastic Leuk.* **2023**, *23* (Suppl. S1), S242–S243. [CrossRef]
19. McGowan-Jordan, J.; Ros, J. *ISCN 2020: An International System for Human Cytogenomic Nomenclature*, 1st ed.; S. Karger AG: Basel, Switzerland, 2020.
20. Porwit-MacDonald, A.; Björklund, E.; Lánczky, A.; Tsao, L.; Fioretos, T.; Bahram, F.; Book, M.; Wang, Y.-H.; Kim, W.Y.; Hasselblom, S.; et al. Genomic features of T-cell acute lymphoblastic leukemia patients harboring NUP214-ABL1 or ETV6-JAK2 fusions. *Blood Cancer J.* **2022**, *12*, 7.
21. van Dongen, J.J.; Langerak, A.W.; Brüggemann, M.; Evans, P.A.; Hummel, M.; Lavender, F.L.; Delabesse, E.; Davi, F.; Schuuring, E.; García-Sanz, R.; et al. Design and standardization of PCR primers and protocols for detection of clonal immunoglobulin and T-cell receptor gene recombinations in suspect lymphoproliferations: Report of the BIOMED-2 Concerted Action BMH4-CT98-3936. *Leukemia* **2003**, *17*, 2257–2317. [CrossRef] [PubMed]

International Journal of
Molecular Sciences

MDPI

Article

Mycovirus-Containing *Aspergillus flavus* Alters Transcription Factors in Normal and Acute Lymphoblastic Leukemia Cells

Cameron K. Tebbi [1,*], Jiyu Yan [1], Eva Sahakian [2], Melanie Mediavilla-Varela [2], Javier Pinilla-Ibarz [2], Saumil Patel [3], George E. Rottinghaus [4], Rachel Y. Liu [1] and Clare Dennison [5]

1 Children's Cancer Research Group Laboratory, Tampa, FL 33613, USA; jiyuyanshine@gmail.com (J.Y.); rachelliu1957@gmail.com (R.Y.L.)
2 Moffitt Cancer Center, Tampa, FL 33612, USA; eva.sahakian@moffitt.org (E.S.); melanie.mediavilla-varela@moffitt.org (M.M.-V.); javier.pinilla@moffitt.org (J.P.-I.)
3 Tampa General Hospital, Tampa, FL 33606, USA; spatel@tgh.org
4 Electron Microscopy Department, University of Missouri, Columbia, MO 65211, USA; rottinghausg@missouri.edu
5 Diagnostic Laboratories, College of Veterinary Medicine, University of South Florida, Tampa, FL 33620, USA; clareldennison@gmail.com
* Correspondence: ctebbi@childrenscancerresearchgrouplaboratory.org

Abstract: Transcription factors control genes to maintain normal hemopoiesis, and dysregulation of some factors can lead to acute lymphoblastic leukemia (ALL). Mycoviruses are known to alter the genetics of their fungal host. The present study evaluates the effects of the products of a mycovirus-containing *Aspergillus flavus* (MCAF), isolated from the home of a patient with ALL, on certain transcription factors of normal and ALL cell lines. Our published studies have shown that ALL patients have antibodies to MCAF, and that exposure of the mononuclear leukocytes of patients in complete remission to its products, unlike controls, results in the re-development of genetic and cell surface phenotypes characteristic of ALL. For the present study, normal, pre-B, and B-cell leukemia cell lines were exposed to the culture of MCAF. Pre- and post-exposure levels of PAX5, Ikaros, and NF-κB were assessed. Exposure to MCAF resulted in apoptosis, cell cycle changes, and complete downregulation of all transcription factors in normal cell lines. In acute leukemia cell lines, cellular apoptosis and alterations in the cell cycle were also noted; however, while there was downregulation of all tested transcription factors, residual levels were retained. The noted alterations in the transcription factors caused by MCAF are novel findings. The possible role of MCAF in leukemogenesis needs to be further investigated. Mycovirus-containing *Aspergillus flavus* was initially isolated from a leukemia patient's home. Our prior published studies have illuminated intriguing associations of this organism with leukemia. Unlike controls, patients diagnosed with acute lymphoblastic leukemia (ALL) harbor antibodies to this organism. Furthermore, the exposure of mononuclear cells from patients with ALL in complete remission to the products of this organism reproduced genetic and cell phenotypes characteristic of ALL. These findings underscore the potential role of environmental factors in leukemogenesis and hint at novel avenues for therapeutic intervention and preventive strategies.

Keywords: leukemia; acute lymphoblastic leukemia; cause of leukemia; etiology of leukemia; mycovirus; fungi; virus; *Aspergillus flavus*; genetics; transcription factors; environment; PAX5; IKAROS; NF-κB

1. Introduction

Leukemia ranks as the fifteenth most diagnosed human cancer and the eleventh cause of death due to a malignant disorder and affects both sexes and all age groups [1,2]. Acute lymphoblastic leukemia (ALL), with an incidence of 1.7 per 100,000 population per year, is seen at any age but is most commonly diagnosed in children, constituting 25–30% of all pediatric malignant disorders [1]. ALL originates from the transformation of B-cell progenitors. Many pre-B and B-cell acute leukemias have specific genetic changes and altered regulators of normal B-cell development. The exact mechanism by which these factors drive the leukemic transformation is unclear. Alteration in the normal differentiation process may be critical in the development of this disease [3–6].

Transcription factors have a vital role in normal lymphoid cell development. The actions of these factors include the integration of external signals to gene expression, programs that reconstruct cellular physiology at a basic level, and an array of post-transcriptional modifications (PTMs). The formation of lineage-restricted progenitors is a part of the function of several transcription factors that activate B-cell genes, including the restriction of alternative cell fates. Some factors reported to be consequential in promoting B cell differentiation include *PAX5*, *Ebf1*, and *Ikaros*.

PAX5 transcription factor, also known as B-cell specific activator protein (BSAP), is a master regulator of the normal development, differentiation, maturation, and maintenance of B-cells. Deletion or inactivating mutations of PAX5 results in chromosomal rearrangements, translocations, and cell arrest. The mutation of PAX5 is one of the consistent genetic alterations found in B-cell acute lymphoblastic leukemia (B-ALL). This transcription factor, and others, form a network that promotes B cell differentiation [4,7–10]. Experimentally and clinically, transcription factors have been found to play an essential role in ALL, where several of these factors are often downregulated [7,11]. Based on animal studies, the alterations and graded reduction of lineage are some of the factors that can induce leukemia [12,13]. In pre-B cell ALL, genes encoding some transcription factors are usually altered or deleted, indicating their role in this disease. It has been postulated that haploinsufficiency for *PAX5* or *Ebf1* synergizes with *STAT5* activation and can initiate the process of ALL development [14,15]. Furthermore, several common genetic variants associated with increased risk for ALL have been recognized [16–18]. In children with ALL, it is estimated that at least 4% are likely to have functional germline mutations [19,20]. In familial ALL, predisposing germline mutations in the hematopoietic regulator genes *PAX5, SH2B3, ETV6*, and *Ikzf1* have been reported [21–27]. Alteration in the *Ikaros* transcription factors also occurs in T-cell acute lymphoblastic leukemia [28]. It is proposed that the etiology of ALL involves a combination of genetic predisposition followed by a provoking event such as an infection [1,29–34]. We have previously shown that using the ELISA technique, patients with ALL in complete remission and long-term survivors have antibodies to the supernatant of the culture of a certain mycovirus-containing *Aspergillus flavus* (SMCAF) [35]. Multiple sets of controls, including normal individuals, patients with a variety of solid tumors, and those with sickle cell disease, lack such antibodies [35]. Interestingly, the organism used was isolated from the home of a patient with ALL. The isolated organism does not produce any aflatoxin, possibly due to its infestation with a mycovirus. Mycoviruses are shown to suppress the production of aflatoxin in their fungal host, which is attributed to the virus/virus and virus/host interactions [36–39]. Our previous studies have also revealed that exposure of the mononuclear cells from ALL patients in complete remission to the SMCAF results in the re-development of the cell surface phenotypes and genetic markers characteristic of ALL, while the controls remain unchanged [40].

Fungal agents in general, and the Aspergillus species in particular, are ubiquitous microorganisms, spread worldwide, and can be present indoors or outdoors. It has been estimated that between 30 to 80% of fungal species are infected with mycoviruses [41]. These are found to have the potential to cause significant changes in the genetics of their fungal host. Some mycoviruses have been shown to induce the transcriptional rewiring of their residing fungi [42]. The level expression of specific host genes differs in mycovirus-free and infected fungi. Alterations in transcription factors in mycovirus-infected fungi have been reported [43,44]. Experimentally, the transcriptome sequencing (RNA-seq) of mycovirus-infected *Malassezia sympodialis* has also been shown to result in an upregulation of several ribosomal components as compared to the virus-cured control, indicating that the mycovirus can modify the transcriptional and translational aspects of the host [42,45–47].

Only limited data regarding the effects of mycoviruses-infected fungi on human health are available.

The present study was designed to evaluate if the supernatant of a mycovirus-containing *Aspergillus flavus* (SMCAF) has any effects on the cellular transcription factors of pre-B and B-cell ALL compared to other leukemias and 'normal' control cell lines. The investigations also examine the impact of the SMCAF on the survival rate and cell cycle of established pre-B and B-cell ALL cell lines, compared to the 'normal' B-lymphocyte, T-cell leukemia, and chronic myelogenous leukemia cell lines.

2. Results

2.1. Chemical Analysis

Repeated evaluation of the supernatant of the culture of mycovirus-containing *Aspergillus flavus* revealed that this organism does not produce any aflatoxin.

2.2. Electron Microscopy

Transmission electron microscopy examination of the culture of *Aspergillus flavus* demonstrated the existence of the virus-like particles within the body of the organism and the culture supernatant (Figure 1). The sizes of the particles observed ranged between 30–50 nm and were in single or aggregate form, with or without patent dense cores. Particles ranging from 20–25 nm and 60–80 nm containing dense cores were seen in the hyphae.

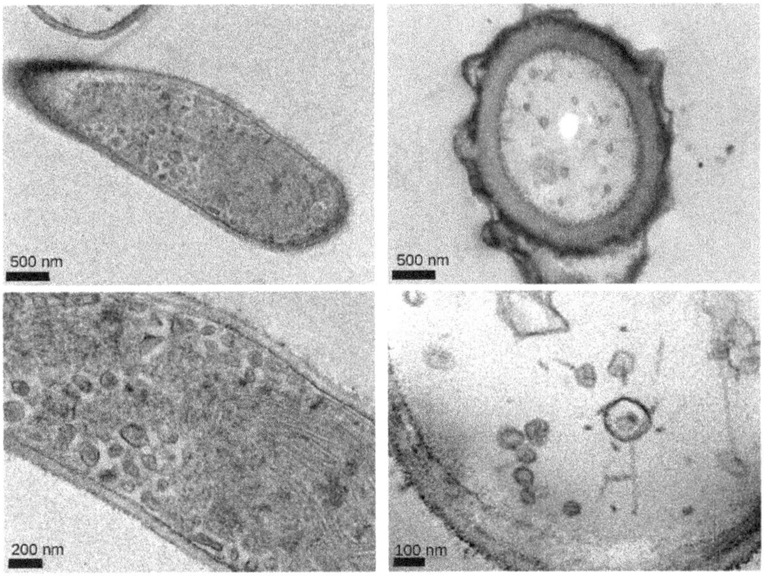

Figure 1. Viral particles measuring 20–80 nm in diameter found in the transmission electron microscopy evaluation of the culture of *Aspergills flavus* isolated from home of a patient with acute lymphoblastic leukemia. The sample was collected from the suspension culture of *Aspergillus flavus* and was glutaraldehyde-fixed. Transmission electron microscopy is a micrograph of a formvar-coated copper grid preparation that is contrast-enhanced with aqueous uranyl acetate. Scale bars are indicated at the bottom of each panel.

2.3. Transcription Factors

Normal cell line: In the RPMI 1788 cell line, which was used as a 'normal' B-cell control cell line, the addition of SMCAF resulted in a dose-dependent downregulation of all transcription factors tested, i.e., *PAX5*, *Ikaros* 55 kD and 75 kD and *NF-κB p65*. No detectable levels remained with the 0.4 mg/mL ($p < 0.01$) (Figures 2–5).

Pre-B and B-cell lines: A dose-dependent downregulation of *PAX5* in NALM6 clone G5 (CRL-3273) and GM20390 cell lines was noted (Figure 2). The pattern in the downregulation of *PAX5* was similar for the NALM6 and GM20390, pre-B and B-cell leukemia cell lines (Figure 2). However, unlike RPMI-1788, where doses of greater than 0.2 mg/mL of SMCAF resulted in the complete abolition of this transcription factor, in GM20390 and NALM6 cell lines, with the dose of 0.2 mg/mL, a statistically insignificant downregulation of PAX5 was noted ($p = 0.23$ and $p = 0.65$, respectively) (Figure 2). Even with doses of 0.4 mg/mL, while a statistically significant downregulation occurred ($p = 0.006$ and $p < 0.0001$, respectively), a residual PAX5 transcription factor could still be detected (Figure 2).

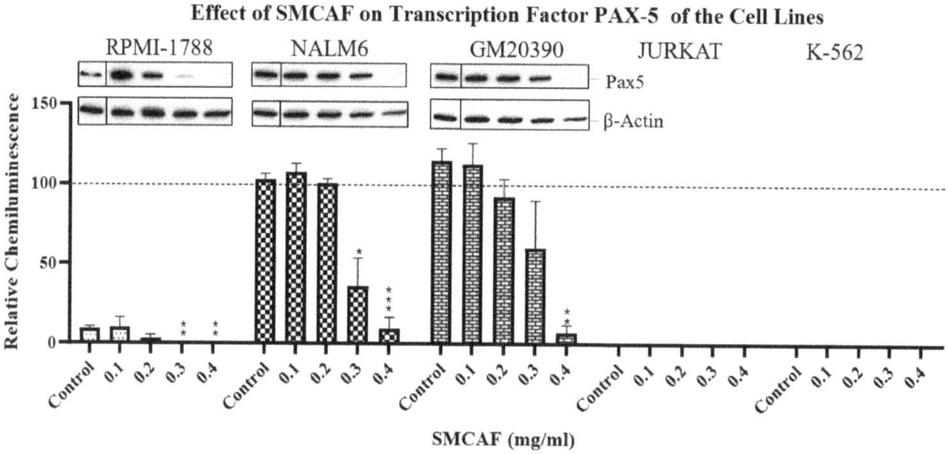

Figure 2. The effects of mycovirus-containing *Aspergillus flavus* on the 'normal' control cell line (RPMI-1788), pre-B (NALM6) and B-cell (GM20390) cell lines. Basal levels of the *PAX5* transcription factor, which are lower in the 'normal' cell line, completely receded at the highest dose of SMCAF. PAX5 basal levels are higher in pre-B ALL and B-cell ALL lines and are significantly downregulated by SMCAF, but not completely lost. Jurkat and K-562 cells did not express PAX5 under any conditions tested. Error bars represent the mean (SEM) standard error for three replicates. The dotted line represents the normalized value of 100 for a NALM6 control sample from each blot. Asterisks denote statistical significance relative to its own control (* $p < 0.05$; ** $p < 0.01$, *** $p < 0.001$). For each cell line, Western blot images include the control bands in a separate box from the treated bands; these images are from the same blot and exposure but reflect the cropping out of additional lines that were not used in this evaluation.

An evaluation of the effects of SMCAF on the *Ikaros* 55 kD transcription factor in NALM6 and GM20390 revealed that the downregulation was gradual and incomplete (Figure 3). This contrasts with RPMI-1788, a 'normal' cell line, where statistically significant downregulation of *Ikaros* 55 kD and 75 kD was noted by adding 0.1 mg/mL ($p = 0.034$ and $p = 0.009$, respectively). In the NALM6 cell line, with the doses of 0.1 to 0.3 mg/mL of SMCAF, downregulation of *Ikaros* 55 kD was not statistically significant ($p = 0.9165$, 0.8946 and 0.2725, respectively); however, with a dose of 0.4 mg /mL, the changes became substantial, but incomplete ($p = 0.0411$). In the GM20390 cell line, with doses of 0.1–0.4 mg/mL of the SMCAF, a gradual but incomplete downregulation of *Ikaros* 55 kD was noted ($p = 0.0436$, $p = 0.0148$, $p = 0.0103$, and $p = 0.0091$, respectively) (Figure 3). A similar finding was observed on the effects of SMCAF on *Ikaros* 75 kD on pre-B and B-cell lines, albeit with a more gradual downregulation of this transcription factor. In NALM6 and GM20390, statistically significant downregulation of *Ikaros* 75 kD was found with the addition of 0.3 and 0.4 mg/mL of SMCAF ($p = 0.5787$ and 0.0447 for NALM6; $p = 0.0184$ and 0.0238 for GM20390, respectively) (Figure 4).

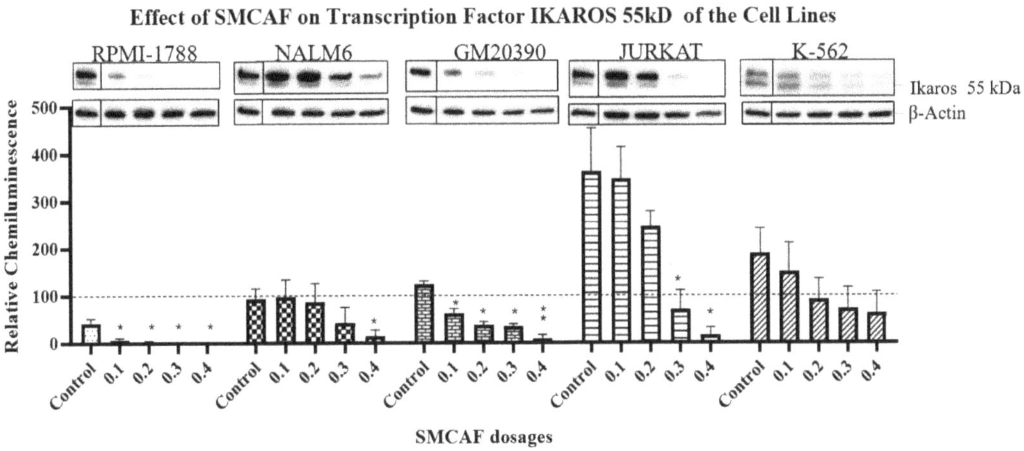

Figure 3. The effects of mycovirus-containing *Aspergillus flavus* on the 'normal' control B-cells (RPMI-1788), pre-B ALL (NALM6), B-cell ALL (GM20390), T-cell leukemia (Jurkat) and CML (K-562) cell lines. In the *Ikaros* 55 kDa transcription factor is downregulated in a dose-dependent manner and is completely eradicated at the highest dose of SMCAF. *Ikaros* 55 kDa basal levels are highest in Jurkat cells and downregulated in a dose-dependent manner in pre-B ALL, B-cell ALL, T-cells, and CML cells. Error bars represent standard error of the mean (SEM) for three replicates. The dotted line represents the normalized value of 100 for a NALM6 control sample from each blot. Asterisks denote statistical significance relative to its own control (* $p < 0.05$; ** $p < 0.01$). For each cell line, Western blot images include the control bands in a separate box from the treated bands; these images are from the same blot and exposure but reflect the cropping out of additional lines that were not used in this evaluation.

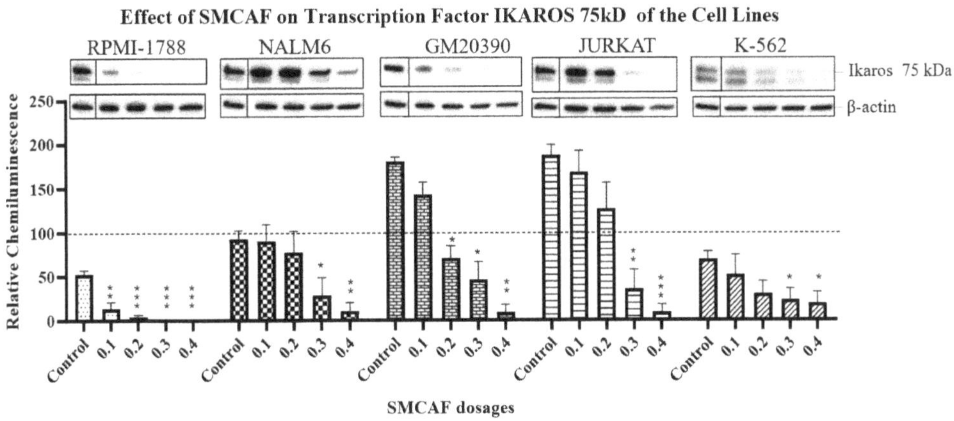

Figure 4. The effects of mycovirus-containing *Aspergillus flavus* on 'normal' control (RPMI-1788), pre-B (NALM6), B-cell (GM20390), T-cell leukemia (Jurkat) and CML (K-562) cell lines. Basal levels of the *Ikaros* 75 kDa transcription factor are highest in the T-cell line. *Ikaros* 75 kDa is downregulated in a dose-dependent manner in all five cell lines. Error bars represent the standard error of the mean (SEM) for three replicates. The dotted line represents the normalized value of 100 for a NALM6 control sample from each blot. Asterisks denote statistical significance relative to its own control (* $p < 0.05$; ** $p < 0.01$, *** $p < 0.001$). For each cell line, Western blot images include the control bands in a separate box from the treated bands; these images are from the same blot and exposure but reflect the cropping out of additional lines that were not used in this evaluation.

Exposure of RPMI-1788 to SMCAF resulted in the downregulation of transcription factor *NF-κB p65* to the extent that no levels were detectable with SMCAF doses greater than 0.2 mg/mL ($p = 0.0204$). The effects were less significant in the pre-B cell NALM6 cell line, where only with SMCAF doses of 0.3 and 0.4 mg/mL did levels of this transcription factor significantly decline ($p = 0.0014$ and $p < 0.0001$, respectively). No significant changes of *NF-κB* found in GM20390 cells with any doses of SMCAF ranging from 0.1 to 0.4 mg/mL were noted ($p = 0.5193$, $p = 0.9831$, $p = 0.5187$ and $p = 0.0625$, respectively) (Figure 5).

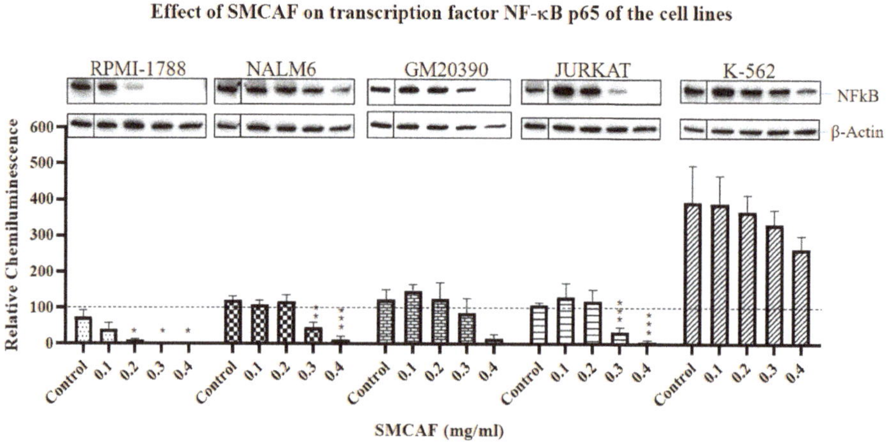

Figure 5. The effects of mycovirus-containing *Aspergillus flavus* on 'normal' control (RPMI-1788), pre-B (NALM6), B-cell (GM20390), T-cell leukemia (Jurkat) and CML (K-562) cell lines. While the downregulation of *NF-κB p65* transcription factor in the 'normal' cell line is complete with no residual remaining, this is significantly less and incomplete in the pre-B, B-cell, and T-cell cell lines. No statistically significant reduction in the *NF-κB p65* transcription factor was noted in the CML cell line. The *NF-κB p65* transcription factor is significantly downregulated by SMCAF in a dose-dependent manner in normal B-cells, pre-B ALL, B-cell ALL, and T-cell leukemia cell lines. The CML cells line showed a reduction in *NF-κB p65* that was not statistically significant. Error bars represent the mean (SEM) standard error for three replicates. The dotted line represents the normalized value of 100 for a NALM6 control sample from each blot. Asterisks denote statistical significance relative to its own control (* $p < 0.05$; ** $p < 0.01$, *** $p < 0.001$). For each cell line, Western blot images include the control bands in a separate box from the treated bands; these images are from the same blot and exposure but reflect the cropping out of additional lines that were not used in this evaluation.

T and CML Cell lines: The control cell lines Jurkat and K562 do not have the expression of the *PAX5* transcription factor. In the Jurkat cell line, upon exposure to the SMCAF, transcription factor *Ikaros* 55 kD downregulated; however, with doses of 0.1 to 0.2 mg/mL, this was not significant ($p = 0.9016$ and 0.3031, respectively). A considerable downregulation was noted with doses of 0.3 and 0.4 mg/mL ($p = 0.0453$ and $p = 0.0214$, respectively) (Figure 3). The transcription factor *Ikaros* 55 kD in K-562 cells showed no statistically significant changes with any doses of the SMCAF (Figure 3). In the Jurkat line, the addition of SMCAF resulted in a very gradual downregulation of the transcription factor *Ikaros* 75 kD, and only with doses of 0.3 and 0.4 mg/mL did the downregulation become significant ($p = 0.0037$ and $p = 0.0003$, respectively) (Figure 4). Similarly, the *Ikaros* 75 kD level in the K562 cell line was gradual, and it was only significantly downregulated with SMCAF doses of 0.3 and 0.4 mg/mL ($p = 0.0425$ and $p = 0.0313$) (Figure 4). The downregulation of *NF-κB p65* in the Jurkat cell line was only significant with SMCAF doses of 0.3 and 0.4 mg/mL ($p = 0.0051$ and $p = 0.0003$, respectively). In the K-562 cell line, with all SMCAF doses used, the *NF-κB p65* level was not significantly altered ($p > 0.29$) (Figure 5).

Culture media used as a control for SMCAF had no significant effects on the levels of any transcription factors in any of the cell lines tested (Figures 2–5).

2.4. Apoptosis and Cell Cycle

Upon exposure to SMCAF, analyses revealed notable changes in the leukemic cell lines. The results of the apoptosis studies, conducted with annexin V/PI staining, showed that there was a significant increase in the early apoptosis in the GM20390, NALM6, and K562 cell lines after 72 h of treatment with the SMCAF (Figure 6A,B,D). In addition, a significant increase in late apoptosis was observed in the cell line GM16726 after the treatment (Figure 6C). Cell cycle analysis was performed after 72 h of supernatant in the culture of the mycovirus-containing *Aspergillus flavus* treatment. An increase in the G1 phase was observed in the GM20390 cell line (33.9% to 41.6%) (Figure 6E). In addition, an increase in the S phase was noted in the NALM6 (47.9% to 55.7%) cell line (Figure 6F). No changes were observed in the control cell lines. Corroboration of apoptotic cell death was observed while analyzing the cell cycle, in the increase in cells in G0 after treatment with the supernatant of the culture of mycovirus-containing *Aspergillus flavus* in NALM6 Jurkat cells. (Representative data from 2 independent experiments). Of course, the apoptosis and cell cycle studies were preliminary studies and not subject to statistical evaluations.

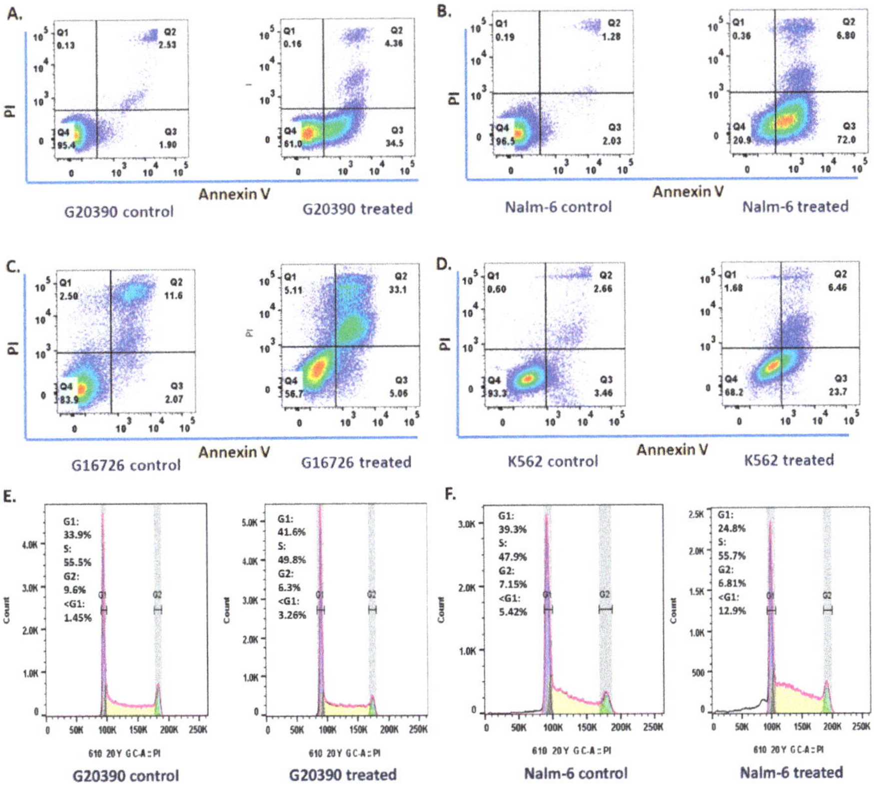

Figure 6. To demonstrate the effects of SMCAF on cell cycle and apoptosis, a single study was performed using GM16726, an acute lymphoblastic leukemia cell line with lymphomatous features: (**A–D**) annexin/PI analysis; and (**E**,**F**) cell cycle analysis of leukemic cells after 72 h of treatment with SMCAF. GM16726 is an acute lymphoblastic leukemia cell line with lymphomatous features isolated from a 27-year-old Black patient in the leukemic phase of B-cell lymphoma. The information provided is based on a single investigation.

3. Discussion

The novel finding that products of a mycovirus-containing *Aspergillus flavus* can alter transcription factors in normal and leukemia cell lines is significant. The normal development, differentiation, and maintenance of the hematopoietic system require the activity of several signaling pathways, epigenetics, and transcription factors. These factors recognize and bind to specific DNA sequences and can control chromatin and transcription, resulting in a system that guides various genomic expressions. Transcription factors are essential in regulating cellular growth and developing hemopoietic cells. The chromosomal translocations and aberrant expression of transcription factors can potentially be associated with leukemogenesis. Transcription factors are shown to have a role in the cancer cell cycle, progression, metastasis, and resistance to treatment [48]. For example, the PAX5 gene, located at chromosome 9q13, is a member of the paired box (PAX) transcription factors that regulate early development and differentiation of B-cell lineage in the hemopoietic system. This transcription factor activates B cell-specific genes and represses those specific for other hematopoietic lineages. PAX5 regulates its target genes via recruiting chromatin-modifying proteins in the committed B cells. The PAX5 gene encodes the B-cell lineage-specific protein (BSAP), expressed during the early stages of B-cell development. Alteration in PAX5 has been implicated in developing human B-cell malignancies, including precursor B-cell acute lymphoblastic leukemia.

Our findings, for the first time, indicate that exposure to mycovirus-containing *Aspergillus flavus* can alter the transcription factors. In the described experiments, the exposure altered most transcription factors and resulted in cellular apoptosis and cell cycle alteration. These novel findings may indicate that mycovirus-containing fungi may have the potential to modulate the rate of gene transcription, altering cellular division, proliferation, differentiation, metabolism, function, and apoptosis. These findings may have therapeutic and etiological significance. In our experiments, changes in the transcription factors were not uniform, and the effects significantly differed between the 'normal' and leukemia cell lines. Significant differences in acute versus chronic leukemias were noted within the leukemia cell lines. In the *RPMI-1788*, which was used as a 'normal' control, exposure to lower doses of SMCAF resulted in the downregulation of all transcription factors tested to the point of non-detection (Figures 2–5). In contrast, even with the highest dose utilized, some transcription factors were detectable in all leukemia cell lines. Interestingly, the effects of the supernatant of the mycovirus-containing *Aspergillus flavus* on the transcription factors, such as *NF-κB p65*, were significantly different in acute and chronic leukemia cell lines. In the chronic myelogenous leukemia cell line, K-562, used as a control, transcription factors were still detectable even with the highest doses of SMCAF. In this cell line, *NF-κB p65*, downregulation with all the doses used was not statistically significant.

Specifically, in the pre-B and B-cell lines, the downregulation of *PAX5* was only seen with much higher doses of SMCAF compared to *RPMI-1788*, a 'normal' control cell line. In the pre-B and B-cell leukemia cell lines, with doses of 0.1–0.2 mg/mL, statistically significant downregulation of *PAX5* was not noted; even with the highest dose of SMCAF, this transcription factor was still detectable. Located on chromosome 9 p13, *PAX5* is known to act as a transcriptional activator or repressor of the genes involved in the B-lineage development. PAX5 functions as a master regulator and a factor for IgH locus rearrangement. In addition, it inhibits the differentiation toward other lineages. The CD19 expression, which occurs in the later stages of B-cell development, is controlled by this transcription factor. Alterations and loss of the *PAX5* are suggested to contribute to leukemogenesis [14]. Loss-of-function mutations in *PAX5* transcription factor occur in B-progenitor acute lymphoblastic leukemia [49–51]. In childhood B-cell progenitor ALL, genome-wide analysis using oligo SNP arrays, *PAX5* was found to be the main target of somatic mutations, which was altered in 38.9% of the cases [8]. In one adult study of ALL, PAX5 was found to be mutated in 34% of the patients [49]. The mutation reduces levels of *PAX5* protein or the generation of hypomorphic alleles [8]. This is due to a partial, rather than complete, loss of function of this transcription factor. In some studies, a *PAX5* fusion product, P5-C20orf112, induces downregulation of pre-B cell receptor genes and causes differential proliferation patterns in B-cell lymphoblastic cell lines [52–54]. *PAX5* is found to be involved in several leukemia-associated rearrangements, resulting in the fusion genes encoding chimeric proteins that antagonize *PAX5* transcriptional activity. It is shown that individuals with loss-of-function variants and those with somatic deletion of the wild type of *PAX5* allele can develop ALL [55]. Therefore, the downregulation of this transcription factor upon exposure to SMCAF is a significant finding.

In a reported study of a murine model, transgenic RNAi was used to reversibly suppress endogenous *PAX5*, which cooperates with an activated signal transducer and activator of transcription 5 (STAT5) to induce B-ALL [14]. In this model, the restoration of endogenous *PAX5*, even temporarily, reversed the process, allowing for the surface expression of mature B cell markers and release of the pre-B stage differentiation block. This and similar studies have established a contributory relationship between the PAX5 and the development of pre-B ALL [14,52,56]. In this regard, the data presented in this manuscript, which for the first time show that exposure to SMCAF results in the downregulation of this transcription factor, is of importance.

In our studies, *Ikaros* transcription factors were tested in all our experimental cell lines, as these are essential regulators of lymphopoiesis and are known to be involved in ALL [57]. Upon exposure to the products of MCAF, the downregulation of *Ikaros* 55 kD/*Ikaros* 75 kD was seen to occur in all cell lines tested. In RPMI-1788, a 'normal' cell line, with the addition of 0.1 mg/mL or a higher amount of SMCAF, the downregulation of *Ikaros* 55 kD and 75 kD were statistically significant. Higher doses resulted in the total elimination of these factors (Figures 3 and 4). Downregulations in the leukemia cell lines were less intense and were, even with the largest dose of 0.4 mg/mL, incomplete. In GM20390 and NALM6 clone G5 (CRL-3273), the downregulation of *Ikaros* 55 kD occurred after exposure to doses greater than 0.1 and 0.4 mg/mL of SMCAF, respectively (Figure 3). Likewise, statistically significant downregulation of *Ikaros* 75 kD was found with 0.2 and 0.3 mg/mL of SMCAF, respectively (Figure 4). In these cell lines, *Ikaros* 55 kD, and more noticeably, *Ikaros* 75 kD, were still detectable even with 0.4 mg/mL, which was the highest dose used. The effect of SMCAF on the Jurkat, and K-562 cell lines was less intense than those of the pre-B and B-cell lines and did not result in the total elimination of the *Ikaros* 55 kD and 75 kD transcription factors, with a significant residual detectable with the highest dose utilized.

Our finding demonstrates for the first time that the product of mycovirus-containing *Aspergillus flavus* can alter and downregulate *Ikaros* 55 kDa and 75 kDa. *Ikaros*, a zinc finger transcription factor, is a significant hematopoiesis regulator and is frequently deleted or mutated in B-cell precursor acute lymphoblastic leukemia [58–60]. Somatic mutations or an alteration of *Ikzf1* is seen in 15–20% of childhood B-cell ALL; its deletion is seen in over 75% of BCR-ABL positive disease [8,57,60–65]. *Ikzf1* mutations occur in up to approximately 50% of adults with ALL [66,67]. The mechanisms involved in *Ikaros* regulation of the gene expression and cellular proliferation in T-ALL are unknown. It has been shown that the reintroduction of *Ikaros* into *Ikaros*-null T-ALL cells result in the termination of cellular proliferation and the induction of T-cell differentiation [68].

As transcription factors, *Ikaros* are critical regulators of lymphocyte ontogeny and differentiation [69–74]. During hematopoiesis, Ikaros functions as a transcriptional activator or repressor for B and T cell differentiation by recruitment of chromatin remodeling complexes [69]. The IKZF1 gene encodes the Ikaros protein, a hemopoiesis regulator. It is essential in developing all lymphoid lineages and functions as a tumor suppressor [70].

In our studies, upon exposure to SMCAF, downregulation of *NF-κB* was noted, on a dose-dependent basis, in all cell lines, except K562 (Figure 4). This downregulation was most notable in RPMI-1788, where smaller doses of SMCAF resulted in the total elimination of *NF-κB*. In the Pre-B and B-cell cell lines, while the levels of this transcription factor steadily declined with doses of 0.3 mg/mL and 0.4 mg/mL of SMCAF (p = 0.062 and p = 0.001, respectively), it was not completely eliminated with the highest doses utilized.

Of interest is that, in the K562, a CML cell line, there was no statistically significant decline in the levels of *NF-κB p65*, even with the highest dose of SMCAF, i.e., 0.4 mg/mL used (Figure 4). Constitutive activation of *NF-κB* complexes has been reported in most (39/42) ALL patients without subtype restriction [9].

NF-κB and its associated regulatory factors are involved in cell proliferation and in the control of apoptosis in leukemias [75–79]. Given the role of the *NF-κB* pathway in leukemia, it is essential to investigate the inhibition of its activity by agents capable of blocking its pathway. NF-κB inhibitory molecules may be used, singularly, or in combination with chemotherapeutic agents, to treat hematological malignancies [80–83]. The finding of the downregulation of *NF-κB*, *PAX5*, and *Ikaros* 55 and 75 kD under the influence of SMCAF in certain acute leukemia cell lines is of significance. The fact that SMCAF can change various transcription factors in these cell lines is novel and is of value. This, along with our prior published findings revealing that patients with B-cell ALL, in complete remission and long-term survivors, unlike controls, uniformly have antibodies to SMCAF, and that the exposure of their mononuclear leukocytes to these products results in the re-development of characteristic genetics and cell surface phenotypes of this disease, is of interest and requires further investigation [35,40]. In light of the hypotheses indicating that the development of ALL is due to a combination of the genetic predisposition followed by a provoking event such as an infection [1,13,29–34], the role of a mycovirus-containing *Aspergillus flavus* in leukemogenesis needs to be further investigated.

Microorganisms have been implicated in the etiology of malignant disorders, mainly due to their various effects resulting in genetic or epigenetic changes [84–87]. It has been estimated that infectious microorganisms cause 18% of all malignant disorders [88]. This is more pronounced in developing countries, where 26% of cancers are attributed to infections compared to 8% in developed nations [89–93]. Some viruses are known to have the ability to alter the genetics of their host as a part of their cytopathogenesis. The incorporation of the viral genome into the host chromosome can be incidental or occur as part of the life cycle of these organisms. Viral genome integration can potentially lead to significant cellular consequences, including gene disruption, insertional mutagenesis, oncogenesis, and apoptosis [94–96]. As noted previously, mycoviruses can alter their fungal host's phenotype, including the host's pigmentation, morphology, sexual and asexual sporulation, production of aflatoxin, and growth. Some dsRNA mycovirus-containing fungal agents have been shown to alter the expression of genes involved in the ribosomal synthesis and programmed cell death of the fungal host. Whether these organisms can exert any changes in humans or animals infected with mycovirus-containing fungi has not been explored and requires investigation.

In the past, the carcinogenic effects of fungi have been generally attributed to their mycotoxin production, and in the case of *Aspergillus* species, to the aflatoxin [36,93,97]. *Aspergillus* infected with a mycovirus, as is the case in that investigated in the above studies, does not produce any aflatoxin. This is attributed to the mycovirus infection, the removal of which results in the reproduction of aflatoxin. Indeed, this phenomenon is used to take advantage of controlling aflatoxin in grain crops. Therefore, the effects of up- and downregulation of the transcription factors in our experiments cannot be attributed to aflatoxin. Rare reports of mycovirus-containing fungi affecting humans as a pathogen and their effects on the infected individuals are available. An example is the Malassezia species, which produces various skin diseases including dandruff, seborrheic dermatitis, and atopic dermatitis. In one study, this organism contained MrV40 mycovirus, which belongs to the Totiviridae family [98].

Prior attempts to alter transcription factor activities for therapeutic purposes have been made in several types of cancer by direct mechanisms such as amplification or deletion of genes, point mutations, chromosome translocations, and alteration of expression, or indirectly via non-coding DNA mutations, which can alter binding of the transcription factor. Attempts to change the mode or levels of transcription factors for therapeutic purposes also have been made. This has included blockage of transcription factor–cofactor protein–protein interactions, the prevention of transcription factor–DNA binding, and modulating the levels of transcription factors. The latter has been attempted by altering levels of ubiquitylation and ensuing proteasome degradation or by inhibiting regulators of transcription factor expression [99]. Other efforts to change the transcription factors have included targeting small-molecule-based heterobifunctional proteolysis targeting chimera (PROTACs), which modulates protein target levels by taking over the ubiquitin–proteasome system to bring about degradation of the target [100–102]. Several new approaches aimed at transcription factors have recently emerged. These include, as follows: PROTAC-mediated protein degradation; modulation of auto-inhibition; the use of cysteine reactive inhibitors targeting intrinsically disordered regions of transcription factors; and combinations of transcription factor inhibitors with kinase inhibitors to block the development of resistance.

In the light of prior findings showing that patients with ALL have antibodies to the SMCAF and that exposure to this product can cause the re-development of cell surface phenotypes in those in remission, but not in controls, the alteration of the transcription factors noted in this report is of significance. Further investigation of the possible relationship between mycovirus-containing filamentous fungi and leukemogenesis is warranted.

4. Materials and Methods

4.1. Mycovirus-Containing *Aspergills flavus*

This organism was isolated from the home of a patient with ALL and cultured in an underlayer of 1% solid agar with an overlayer of 3.5% Czapek-Dox broth (Difco; Becton Dickinson, Sparks, MD, USA) in a glass bottle, incubated at 28 °C and sub-cultured at approximately four-week intervals. To ensure the persistence of the mycovirus in the *Aspergillus flavus*, the cultures were periodically checked by transmission electron microscopy. For the described studies, a portion of the supernatant of mycovirus-containing *Aspergillus flavus* was collected after approximately four weeks of culture, filtered through a 0.45 µm filter (Thermo Scientific, Swedesboro, NJ, USA. Catalogue #169-0045), and concentrated via a centrifugal filter device with 3K of nominal molecular weight limit (NMWL) (Amicon Ultra-15 centrifugation device, EMD Millipore, EMD Millipore Corporation, Taunton, MA, USA) at 4000× *g* for 55 min. The concentrated SMCAF was quantitated by a BCA protein assay kit (Thermo Fisher Scientific, Pittsburgh, PA, USA) and had an approximate total protein concentration of 3–4 mg/mL.

Cell lines were initially obtained from the Coriell Institute for Medical Research (Camden, NJ, USA). The pre-B and B-cell ALL cell lines were GM20390 and NALM6 clone G5 (CRL-3273). For comparison, RPMI-1788, which is a 'normal' cell line, BCL2 Jurkat, an acute T-cell lymphoblastic leukemia cell line, and K562-S (CRL-3343), a chronic myelogenous leukemia (CML) cell line, were used. All cell lines were cultured in RPMI-1640 (Thermo Fisher Scientific, Waltham, MA, USA) with 10% fetal calf serum (Thermo Fisher Scientific, Waltham, MA, USA) and penicillin/streptomycin antibiotics and incubated at 37 °C with 5% CO_2. Cells were harvested, counted, adjusted, and seeded at 2.4×10^4/mL for culture. For the described studies, each cell line was cultured for three days with concentrated SMCAF using 0.1, 0.2, 0.3, and 0.4 mg SMCAF protein per milliliter. In a limited study, the effects of doses ranging from 0.01 to 0.05 of SMCAF were initially tested using the same condition to evaluate the impact of smaller doses. The culture media was used as the control. Upon harvest, cell count and viability were tested for each culture performed. For measurement of the cell viability rate, pre- and 72 h post-treatment of each cell line cultured with SMCAF were stained with methylene blue and counted using a hemocytometer. The percentage of survival was recorded.

4.2. Electron Microscopy

To evaluate the *Aspergillus flavus* for the presence of mycoviruses, the culture's fungal growth and supernatant were analyzed for viral contents by electron microscopy. The culture-grown organism was fixed in glutaraldehyde and osmium tetroxide. Before transmission electron microscopy observation, this was placed into resin blocks suitable for ultramicrotomy sectioning at 70 nm, collected on copper grids, and contrast-enhanced with uranyl acetate.

4.3. Cell Cycle Studies

For the cell cycle and apoptotic studies, GM16726, which is an acute lymphoblastic leukemia cell line with lymphomatous features, was used. Cell cycle analysis studies were performed to characterize the effect of the SMCAF on the cells. Cells were washed and resuspended in 200 µL of PBS, followed by the dropwise addition of 2 mL of ice-cold 70% ethanol during vortex mixing. The cell suspension was incubated at −20 degrees centigrade for two hours. The cells then were washed with PBS and resuspended in 400 µL of a staining solution containing 0.6 mM of propidium iodide (PI) (Invitrogen P3566, Invitrogen, Carlsbad, CA, USA), 0.2 mg/mL of RNAse (ThermoFisher, R1253, ThermoFisher Scientific, Pittsburgh, PA, USA) and 0.1% v/v of Triton X100 (ThermoFisher, BP151-100, ThermoFisher Scientific, Pittsburgh, PA, USA). Cells were incubated at 37 degrees centigrade for 30 min before measurement of fluorescence using an LSR II flow cytometer (BD Bioscience, Franklin Lakes, NJ, USA). Data were analyzed using FlowJo 10.7 software (Tree Star Watson model, Tree Star, Inc., San Carlos, CA, USA).

4.4. Annexin V/PI Analysis

To examine the apoptotic cell death, cells were seeded at 2×10^5/well in a T75 flask in RPMI 1640 media with 10% fetal calf serum and 1% Penicillin/Streptomycin and incubated at 37 °C with 5% CO_2. The cells were treated with SMCAF with protein concentrations, as outlined above. Cultures were collected after 72 h of incubation. Cells were resuspended in 100 µL of Annexin V binding buffer (component no. 51-66121E, BD Biosciences, San Diego, CA, USA) with 5 µL of Annexin V-FITC (component no. 556419, BD Biosciences, San Diego, CA, USA) and incubated for 15 min at room temperature. At this point, 200 µL of Annexin V staining buffer was added, and fluorescence was measured using an LSR II flow cytometer (BD Biosciences, San Diego, CA, USA) and data were analyzed using FlowJo software (Tree Star, Inc., San Carlos, CA, USA). Annexin V positive, PI negative cells were identified as early apoptotic while Annexin V positive, PI positive cells were identified as late apoptotic.

4.5. Analysis for Detection of Aflatoxin

For the detection of aflatoxin in the supernatant of the culture of the mycovirus-containing *Aspergillus flavus*, a method commonly used for the quantitation of this toxin in cereal grains and complex feedstuffs was used. Samples were extracted with acetonitrile-water (7:3). The extracts were passed through EASI-EXTRACT aflatoxin immunoaffinity cleanup columns. The HPLC analyzed samples with Kobra cell post-column derivatization with fluorescence detection at 365 nm excitation and 440 nm emission. The detection limit was set at ten ppb total aflatoxins. It should be noted that periodically, the SMCAF was tested to ensure that it did not contain any aflatoxin.

4.6. Western Blot

The levels of transcription factors *PAX5*, *Ikaros* 55 kD and 75 kD, and *NF-κB p65* were measured, with and without exposure to SMCAF, using an immunoblotting technique. For Western blot, each cell line was harvested and centrifuged at 2000 RPM at 20 °C for five minutes and the pellets were washed twice with 4 mL of ice-cold Tris-buffered saline (TBS) (ThermoFisher Scientific, Pittsburgh, PA, USA). Cells were treated with a specified amount of SMCAF, as described above, or culture media, which was used as a control. Radio-immune precipitation assay (RIPA) lysis buffer (ThermoFisher Scientific, Pittsburgh, PA, USA) was used at a final 3×10^7 cells/mL concentration. The RIPA consisted of 50 mM Tris–HCl (pH 7.4), 1.0% NP–leupeptin, and pepstatin (ThermoFisher Scientific, Pittsburgh, PA, USA). Each cell lysate was mixed on a shaker for 15 min at 4 °C, sonicated twice for 10 s at 50 kHz, shaken for 15 min on ice, and then centrifuged at $12{,}000\times g$ at 4 °C for 20 min.

The total protein was measured using a bicinchoninic acid (BCA) assay, aliquoted in 10 μg/μL in the loading buffer, and then denatured at boiling water for five minutes before being subjected to the Western blot analysis. The precast mini tris–glycine gel 4–20% (Bio-Rad, Hercules, CA, USA) was utilized to perform protein electrophoresis. A 0.22 μm nitrocellulose membrane and Efficient Western Transfer Buffer (Bioscience, St Louis, MO, USA) were used for protein transfer. 5% dry milk in 1x TBST wash buffer (tris-buffered saline with 0.05% Tween 20) was utilized for the membrane blocking. To detect transcription factors, *Ikaros*, *NF-κB p65*, and *PAX5*, appropriate primary monoclonal antibodies, and the secondary antibody HRP-linked anti-rabbit IgG were used (Cell Signaling Technology, Danvers, MA, USA). The enhanced chemiluminescence system (Viagene Biotech, Tampa, FL, USA) detected specific antibody binding and was read on the FlourChem E system (ProteinSimple, San Jose, CA, USA). The Western blot images were analyzed using FIJI/Imaging V1.52P-Win 64 software. Each study was repeated four times, and statistical analyses were performed based on these repeats. The chemiluminescent signal intensity for each transcription factor was measured and divided by the signal intensity for actin in the same blot lane to arrive at a transcription factor/actin ratio. These values were normalized to a NALM6 control sample on each blot to yield relative chemiluminescence values. These values were graphed using GraphPad Prism 8 software with representative blot images included in the figures.

4.7. Statistical Analysis

The GraphPad Prism two-tail unpaired t-test between control and SMCAF treatment groups was used for statistical analysis of the data. The statistical significance was set at p-value < 0.05.

Author Contributions: C.K.T. conceived, designed, and drafted the protocol, provided the culture of mycovirus-containing *Aspergillus flavus*, and prepared the manuscript. J.Y. performed transcription experiments, performed statistical analyses of the data, and prepared the figures and tables relating to the studies. E.S. contributed to the planning of the cell cycle studies, analyzed, and interpreted the data, and assisted with the preparation of the figures and revisions of the manuscript. M.M.-V. performed experiments regarding cell cycle studies, prepared the related graphs, and analyzed and interpreted the data. J.P.-I. contributed to the interpretation of data and review of the manuscript. S.P. contributed to the interpretation of the data and review of the manuscript. G.E.R. performed chemical analysis to rule out the existence of aflatoxin. R.Y.L. helped with the performance of the Western blot studies. C.D. performed the electron microscopy studies. All authors have read and agreed to the published version of the manuscript.

Funding: This work was supported by the Children's Cancer Research Group, 1Voice Foundation, Susan, and Gerald Horton Foundation.

Institutional Review Board Statement: Not applicable.

Informed Consent Statement: Not applicable.

Data Availability Statement: The data that support the findings of this study are available from the corresponding author upon request.

Acknowledgments: We acknowledge the technical assistance of Amanda Garces, at the Morsani College of Medicine University of South Florida. Lauren Busciglio's assistance in preparing the manuscript is appreciated.

Conflicts of Interest: The authors declare no conflict of interest.

References

1. Tebbi, C.K. Etiology of Acute Leukemia: A Review. *Cancers* **2021**, *13*, 2256. [CrossRef] [PubMed]
2. Bray, F.; Ferlay, J.; Soerjomataram, I.; Siegel, R.L.; Torre, L.A.; Jemal, A. Global cancer statistics 2018: GLOBOCAN estimates of incidence and mortality worldwide for 36 cancers in 185 countries. *CA A Cancer J. Clin.* **2018**, *68*, 394–424. [CrossRef] [PubMed]
3. Gocho, Y.; Yang, J.J. Genetic defects in hematopoietic transcription factors and predisposition to acute lymphoblastic leuke-mia. *Blood* **2019**, *134*, 793–797. [CrossRef] [PubMed]

4. Nutt, S.L.; Kee, B.L. The Transcriptional Regulation of B Cell Lineage Commitment. *Immunity* **2007**, *26*, 715–725; Erratum in *Immunity* **2017**, *27*, 361. [CrossRef] [PubMed]
5. Greaves, M. Leukaemia Firsts' in cancer research and treatment. *Nat. Rev. Cancer* **2016**, *16*, 163–172. [CrossRef]
6. Wagener, R.; Elitzur, S.; Brozou, T.; Borkhardt, A. Functional damaging germline variants in ETV6, IKZF1, PAX5 and RUNX1 predisposing to B-cell precursor acute lymphoblastic leukemia. *Eur. J. Med. Genet.* **2023**, *66*, 104725. [CrossRef]
7. Somasundaram, R.; Prasad, M.A.J.; Ungerbäck, J.; Sigvardsson, M. Transcription factor networks in B-cell differentiation link development to acute lymphoid leukemia. *Blood* **2015**, *126*, 144–152. [CrossRef]
8. Mullighan, C.G.; Goorha, S.; Radtke, I.; Miller, C.B.; Coustan-Smith, E.; Dalton, J.D.; Girtman, K.; Mathew, S.; Ma, J.; Pounds, S.B.; et al. Genome-wide analysis of genetic alterations in acute lymphoblastic leukaemia. *Nature* **2007**, *446*, 758–764. [CrossRef]
9. Kordes, U.; Krappmann, D.; Heissmeyer, V.; Ludwig, W.D.; Scheidereit, C. Transcription factor NF-κB is constitutively activated in acute lymphoblastic leukemia cells. *Leukemia* **2000**, *14*, 399–402. [CrossRef]
10. Schinnerl, D.; Fortschegger, K.; Kauer, M.; Marchante, J.R.M.; Kofler, R.; Boer, M.L.D.; Strehl, S. The role of the Janus-faced transcription factor PAX5-JAK2 in acute lymphoblastic leukemia. *Blood* **2015**, *125*, 1282–1291. [CrossRef]
11. Lee, T.I.; Young, R.A. Transcriptional Regulation and Its Misregulation in Disease. *Cell* **2013**, *152*, 1237–1251. [CrossRef] [PubMed]
12. Takahashi, K.; Yamanaka, S. A decade of transcription factor-mediated reprogramming to pluripotency. *Nat. Rev. Mol. Cell Biol.* **2016**, *17*, 183–193. [CrossRef] [PubMed]
13. Rosenbauer, F.; Wagner, K.; Kutok, J.L.; Iwasaki, H.; Le Beau, M.M.; Okuno, Y.; Akashi, K.; Fiering, S.; Tenen, D.G. Acute myeloid leukemia induced by graded reduction of a lineage-specific transcription factor, PU. *Nat. Genet.* **2004**, *36*, 624–630. [CrossRef] [PubMed]
14. Heltemes-Harris, L.M.; Willette, M.J.; Ramsey, L.B.; Qiu, Y.H.; Neeley, E.S.; Zhang, N.; Thomas, D.A.; Koeuth, T.; Baechler, E.C.; Kornblau, S.M.; et al. *Ebf1* or *Pax5* haploinsufficiency synergizes with STAT5 activation to initiate acute lymphoblastic leukemia. *J. Exp. Med.* **2011**, *208*, 1135–1149. [CrossRef] [PubMed]
15. de Smith, A.J.; Lavoie, G.; Walsh, K.M.; Aujla, S.; Evans, E.; Hansen, H.M.; Smirnov, I.; Kang, A.Y.; Zenker, M.; Ceremsak, J.J.; et al. Predisposing germline mutations in high hyperdiploid acute lymphoblastic leukemia in children. *Genes Chromosomes Cancer* **2019**, *58*, 723–730. [CrossRef]
16. Papaemmanuil, E.; Hosking, F.J.; Vijayakrishnan, J.; Price, A.; Olver, B.; Sheridan, E.; E Kinsey, S.; Lightfoot, T.; Roman, E.; Irving, J.A.; et al. Loci on 7p12.2, 10q21.2 and 14q11.2 are associated with risk of childhood acute lymphoblastic leukemia. *Nat. Genet.* **2009**, *41*, 1006–1010. [CrossRef]
17. Sherborne, A.L.; Hosking, F.J.; Prasad, R.B.; Kumar, R.; Koehler, R.; Vijayakrishnan, J.; Papaemmanuil, E.; Bartram, C.R.; Stanulla, M.; Schrappe, M.; et al. Variation in CDKN2A at 9p21.3 influences childhood acute lymphoblastic leukemia risk. *Nat. Genet.* **2010**, *42*, 492–494. [CrossRef]
18. Migliorini, G.; Fiege, B.; Hosking, F.J.; Ma, Y.; Kumar, R.; Sherborne, A.L.; da Silva Filho, M.I.; Vijayakrishnan, J.; Koehler, R.; Thomsen, H.; et al. Variation at 10p12.2 and 10p14 influences risk of childhood B-cell acute lymphoblastic leukemia and phe-notype. *Blood* **2013**, *122*, 3298–3307. [CrossRef]
19. Zhang, J.; Walsh, M.F.; Wu, G.; Edmonson, M.N.; Gruber, T.A.; Easton, J.; Hedges, D.; Ma, X.; Zhou, X.; Yergeau, D.A.; et al. Germline Mutations in Predisposition Genes in Pediatric Cancer. *N. Engl. J. Med.* **2015**, *373*, 2336–2346. [CrossRef]
20. Gröbner, S.N.; Worst, B.C.; Weischenfeldt, J.; Buchhalter, I.; Kleinheinz, K.; Rudneva, V.A.; Johann, P.D.; Balasubramanian, G.P.; Segura-Wang, M.; Brabetz, S.; et al. The landscape of genomic alterations across childhood cancers. *Nature* **2018**, *555*, 321–327. [CrossRef]
21. Perez-Garcia, A.; Ambesi-Impiombato, A.; Hadler, M.; Rigo, I.; LeDuc, C.A.; Kelly, K.; Jalas, C.; Paietta, E.; Racevskis, J.; Rowe, J.M.; et al. Genetic loss of SH2B3 in acute lymphoblastic leukemia. *Blood* **2013**, *122*, 2425–2432. [CrossRef]
22. Shah, S.; A Schrader, K.; Waanders, E.; E Timms, A.; Vijai, J.; Miething, C.; Wechsler, J.; Yang, J.; Hayes, J.; Klein, R.J.; et al. A recurrent germline PAX5 mutation confers susceptibility to pre-B cell acute lymphoblastic leukemia. *Nat. Genet.* **2013**, *45*, 1226–1231. [CrossRef] [PubMed]
23. Moriyama, T.; Metzger, M.L.; Wu, G.; Nishii, R.; Qian, M.; Devidas, M.; Yang, W.; Cheng, C.; Cao, X.; Quinn, E.; et al. Germline genetic variation in ETV6 and risk of childhood acute lymphoblastic leukemia: A systematic genetic study. *Lancet Oncol.* **2015**, *16*, 1659–1666. [CrossRef]
24. Noetzli, L.; Lo, R.W.; Lee-Sherick, A.B.; Callaghan, M.; Noris, P.; Savoia, A.; Rajpurkar, M.; Jones, K.; Gowan, K.; Balduini, C.L.; et al. Germline mutations in ETV6 are associated with thrombocytopenia, red cell macrocytosis and predisposition to lymphoblastic leukemia. *Nat. Genet.* **2015**, *47*, 535–538. [CrossRef]
25. Zhang, M.Y.; E Churpek, J.; Keel, S.B.; Walsh, T.; Lee, M.K.; Loeb, K.R.; Gulsuner, S.; Pritchard, C.C.; Sanchez Bonilla, M.; Delrow, J.J.; et al. Germline ETV6 mutations in familial thrombocytopenia and hematologic malignancy. *Nat. Genet.* **2015**, *47*, 180–185. [CrossRef] [PubMed]
26. Topka, S.; Vijai, J.; Walsh, M.F.; Jacobs, L.; Maria, A.; Villano, D.; Gaddam, P.; Wu, G.; McGee, R.B.; Quinn, E.; et al. Germline ETV6 Mutations Confer Susceptibility to Acute Lymphoblastic Leukemia and Thrombocytopenia. *PLoS Genet.* **2015**, *11*, e1005262. [CrossRef] [PubMed]
27. Yoshida, N.; Sakaguchi, H.; Muramatsu, H.; Okuno, Y.; Song, C.; Dovat, S.; Shimada, A.; Ozeki, M.; Ohnishi, H.; Teramoto, T.; et al. Germline IKAROS mutation associated with primary immunodeficiency that progressed to T-cell acute lymphoblastic leukemia. *Leukemia* **2017**, *31*, 1221–1223. [CrossRef]

28. Kastner, P.; Chan, S. Role of Ikaros in T-cell acute lymphoblastic leukemia. *World J. Biol. Chem.* **2011**, *2*, 108–114. [CrossRef]
29. Wiemels, J. Perspectives on the causes of childhood leukemia. *Chem. Interact.* **2012**, *196*, 59–67. [CrossRef]
30. Greaves, M.F. Speculations on the cause of childhood acute lymphoblastic leukemia. *Leukemia* **1988**, *2*, 120–125.
31. Greaves, M. A causal mechanism for childhood acute lymphoblastic leukemia. *Nat. Rev. Cancer* **2018**, *18*, 471–484, Correction in *Nat. Rev. Cancer* **2018**, *18*, 526. [CrossRef] [PubMed]
32. Greaves, M.; Cazzaniga, V.; Ford, A. Can we prevent childhood Leukaemia? *Leukemia* **2021**, *35*, 1258–1264. [CrossRef] [PubMed]
33. Zhao, X.; Qian, M.; Goodings, C.; Zhang, Y.; Yang, W.; Wang, P.; Xu, B.; Tian, C.; Pui, C.-H.; Hunger, S.P.; et al. Molecular Mechanisms of *ARID5B*-Mediated Genetic Susceptibility to Acute Lymphoblastic Leukemia. *JNCI J. Natl. Cancer Inst.* **2022**, *114*, 1287–1295. [CrossRef] [PubMed]
34. Martín-Lorenzo, A.; Hauer, J.; Vicente-Dueñas, C.; Auer, F.; González-Herrero, I.; García-Ramírez, I.; Ginzel, S.; Thiele, R.; Constantinescu, S.N.; Bartenhagen, C.; et al. Infection Exposure Is a Causal Factor in B-cell Precursor Acute Lymphoblastic Leukemia as a Result of *Pax5*-Inherited Susceptibility. *Cancer Discov.* **2015**, *5*, 1328–1343. [CrossRef] [PubMed]
35. Tebbi, C.K.; Badiga, A.; Sahakian, E.; Arora, A.I.; Nair, S.; Powers, J.J.B.; Achille, A.N.B.; Jaglal, M.V.; Patel, S.; Migone, F. Plasma of Acute Lymphoblastic Leukemia Patients React to the Culture of a Mycovirus Containing *Aspergillus flavus*. *J. Pediatr. Hematol.* **2020**, *42*, 350–358. [CrossRef]
36. Tebbi, C.K. Mycoviruses in Fungi: Carcinogenesis of Fungal Agents May Not Always Be Mycotoxin Related. *J. Fungi* **2023**, *9*, 368. [CrossRef]
37. Kotta-Loizou, I.; Coutts, R.H.A. Mycoviruses in Aspergilli: A Comprehensive Review. *Front. Microbiol.* **2017**, *8*, 1699. [CrossRef]
38. Schmidt, F.R. The RNA interference-virus interplay: Tools of nature for gene modulation, morphogenesis, evolution, and a possible mean for aflatoxin control. *Appl. Microbiol. Biotechnol.* **2009**, *83*, 611–615. [CrossRef]
39. Schmidt, F.R.; Lemke, P.A.; Esser, K. Viral influences on aflatoxin formation by Aspergillus flavus. *Appl. Microbiol. Biotechnol.* **1986**, *24*, 248–252. [CrossRef]
40. Tebbi, C.K.; Badiga, A.; Sahakian, E.; Powers, J.J.; Achille, A.N.; Patel, S.; Migone, F. Exposure to a mycovirus containing Aspergillus Flavus reproduces acute lymphoblastic leukemia cell surface and genetic markers in cells from patients in remission and not controls. *Cancer Treat. Res. Commun.* **2021**, *26*, 100279. [CrossRef]
41. Ghabrial, S.A.; Suzuki, N. Viruses of Plant Pathogenic Fungi. *Annu. Rev. Phytopathol.* **2009**, *47*, 353–384. [CrossRef] [PubMed]
42. Clancey, S.A.; Ruchti, F.; LeibundGut-Landmann, S.; Heitman, J.; Ianiri, G. A Novel Mycovirus Evokes Transcriptional Rewir-ing in the Fungus Malassezia and Stimulates Beta Interferon Production in Macrophages. *MBio* **2020**, *11*, e01534-20.
43. Sun, Q.; Choi, G.H.; Nuss, D.L. Hypovirus-responsive transcription factor gene pro1 of the chestnut blight fungus Cryphonectria parasitica is required for female fertility, asexual spore development, and stable maintenance of hypovirus in-fection. *Eukaryot Cell* **2009**, *8*, 262–270. [CrossRef] [PubMed]
44. Son, M.; Yu, J.; Kim, K.H. Five Questions about Mycoviruses. *PLoS Pathog.* **2015**, *11*, e1005172. [CrossRef] [PubMed]
45. Nuss, D.L. Hypovirulence: Mycoviruses at the fungal–plant interface. *Nat. Rev. Microbiol.* **2005**, *3*, 632–642. [CrossRef]
46. Jiang, D.; Fu, Y.; Guoqing, L.; Ghabrial, S.A. Viruses of the plant pathogenic fungus Sclerotinia sclerotiorum. *Adv. Virus Res.* **2013**, *86*, 215–248.
47. Pearson, M.N.; Beever, R.E.; Boine, B.; Arthur, K. Mycoviruses of filamentous fungi and their relevance to plant pathology. *Mol. Plant Pathol.* **2009**, *10*, 115–128. [CrossRef]
48. Filtz, T.M.; Vogel, W.K.; Leid, M. Regulation of transcription factor activity by interconnected post-translational modifications. *Trends Pharmacol. Sci.* **2014**, *35*, 76–85. [CrossRef]
49. Familiades, J.; Bousquet, M.; Lafage-Pochitaloff, M.; Béné, M.-C.; Beldjord, K.; De Vos, J.; Dastugue, N.; Coyaud, E.; Struski, S.; Quelen, C.; et al. PAX5 mutations occur frequently in adult B-cell progenitor acute lymphoblastic leukemia and PAX5 haploinsufficiency is associated with BCR-ABL1 and TCF3-PBX1 fusion genes: A GRAALL study. *Leukemia* **2009**, *23*, 1989–1998. [CrossRef]
50. Cobaleda, C.; Jochum, W.; Busslinger, M. Conversion of mature B cells into T cells by dedifferentiation to uncommitted progenitors. *Nature* **2007**, *449*, 473–477. [CrossRef]
51. Cobaleda, C.; Schebesta, A.; Delogu, A.; Busslinger, M. Pax5: The guardian of B cell identity and function. *Nat. Immunol.* **2007**, *8*, 463–470. [CrossRef] [PubMed]
52. Liu, G.J.; Cimmino, L.; Jude, J.G.; Hu, Y.; Witkowski, M.T.; McKenzie, M.D.; Kartal-Kaess, M.; Best, S.A.; Tuohey, L.; Liao, Y.; et al. Pax5 loss imposes a reversible differentiation block in B-progenitor acute lymphoblastic leukemia. *Genes Dev.* **2014**, *28*, 1337–1350. [CrossRef] [PubMed]
53. Nakitandwe, J.; Chen, S.-C.; Lenny, N.T.; Miller, C.B.; Su, X.; Mullighan, C.G.; Downing, J.R. Acute Lymphoblastic Leukemia-Associated PAX5 Mutations Induce Aberrant B Cell Development. *Blood* **2010**, *116*, 10. [CrossRef]
54. Nowak, D.; Kawamata, N.; Niebuhr, B.; Nowak, V.; Mossner, M.; Nahar, R.R.; Thoennissen, N.H.; Iwanski, G.B.; Stocking, C.; Dugas, M.; et al. The Pax5 Fusion Product Pax5-C20orf112 Causes Downregulation of Pre-B Cell Receptor Genes and Induces Differential Proliferation Patterns in B-Lymphoblastic Cell Lines. *Blood* **2009**, *114*, 1284. [CrossRef]
55. Jia, Z.; Gu, Z. PAX5 alterations in B-cell acute lymphoblastic leukemia. *Front. Oncol.* **2022**, *12*, 1023606. [CrossRef]
56. Mullighan, C.G.; Downing, J.R. Genome-wide profiling of genetic alterations in acute lymphoblastic leukemia: Recent insights and future directions. *Leukemia* **2009**, *23*, 1209–1218. [CrossRef]

57. Mullighan, C.G.; Miller, C.B.; Radtke, I.; Phillips, L.A.; Dalton, J.; Ma, J.; White, D.; Hughes, T.P.; Le Beau, M.M.; Pui, C.H. BCR–ABL1 lymphoblastic leukaemia is charac-terized by the deletion of Ikaros. *Nature* **2008**, *453*, 110–114. [CrossRef]
58. Yoshida, T.; Georgopoulos, K. Ikaros fingers on lymphocyte differentiation. *Int. J. Hematol.* **2014**, *100*, 220–229. [CrossRef]
59. John, L.B.; Ward, A.C. The Ikaros gene family: Transcriptional regulators of hematopoiesis and immunity. *Mol. Immunol.* **2011**, *48*, 1272–1278. [CrossRef]
60. Marke, R.; van Leeuwen, F.N.; Scheijen, B. The many faces of IKZF1 in B-cell precursor acute lymphoblastic leukemia. *Haematologica* **2018**, *103*, 565–574. [CrossRef]
61. Kuiper, R.P.; Schoenmakers, E.F.P.M.; Van Reijmersdal, S.V.; Hehir-Kwa, J.Y.; van Kessel, A.G.; Van Leeuwen, F.N.; Hoogerbrugge, P.M. High-resolution genomic profiling of childhood ALL reveals novel recurrent genetic lesions affecting path-ways involved in lymphocyte differentiation and cell cycle progression. *Leukemia* **2007**, *21*, 1258–1266. [CrossRef] [PubMed]
62. Iacobucci, I.; Storlazzi, C.T.; Cilloni, D.; Lonetti, A.; Ottaviani, E.; Soverini, S.; Astolfi, A.; Chiaretti, S.; Vitale, A.; Messa, F.; et al. Identification and molecular characterization of recurrent genomic de-letions on 7p12 in the IKZF1 gene in a large cohort of BCR-ABL1-positive acute lymphoblastic leukemia patients: On behalf of Gruppo Italiano Malattie Ematologiche dell'Adulto Acute Leukemia Working Party (GIMEMA AL WP). *Blood* **2009**, *114*, 2159–2167. [PubMed]
63. Kastner, P.; Dupuis, A.; Gaub, M.-P.; Herbrecht, R.; Lutz, P.; Chan, S. Function of Ikaros as a tumor suppressor in B cell acute lymphoblastic leukemia. *Am. J. Blood Res.* **2013**, *3*, 1–13. [PubMed]
64. Vairy, S.; Tran, T.H. IKZF1 alterations in acute lymphoblastic leukemia: The good, the bad and the ugly. *Blood Rev.* **2020**, *44*, 100677. [CrossRef]
65. Stanulla, M.; Cave, H.; Moorman, A.V. IKZF1 deletions in pediatric acute lymphoblastic leukemia: Still a poor prognostic marker? *Blood* **2020**, *135*, 252–260. [CrossRef]
66. Mi, J.Q.; Wang, X.; Yao, Y.; Lu, H.J.; Jiang, X.X.; Zhou, J.F.; Wang, J.H.; Jiao, B.; Shen, S.H.; Tang, J.Y.; et al. Newly diagnosed acute lymphoblastic leukemia in China (II): Prognosis related to genetic abnormalities in a se-ries of 1091 cases. *Leukemia* **2012**, *26*, 1507–1516. [CrossRef]
67. Dupuis, A.; Gaub, M.P.; Legrain, M.; Drenou, B.; Mauvieux, L.; Lutz, P.; Herbrecht, R.; Chan, S.; Kastner, P. Biclonal and biallelic deletions occur in 20% of B-ALL cases with IKZF1 mutations. *Leukemia* **2012**, *27*, 503–507. [CrossRef]
68. Ding, Y.; Zhang, B.; Payne, J.L.; Song, C.; Ge, Z.; Gowda, C.; Iyer, S.; Dhanyamraju, P.K.; Dorsam, G.; Reeves, M.E.; et al. Ikaros tumor suppressor function includes induction of active enhancers and super-enhancers along with pio-neering activity. *Leukemia* **2019**, *33*, 2720–2731. [CrossRef]
69. Davis, K.L. Ikaros: Master of hematopoiesis, agent of leukemia. *Ther. Adv. Hematol.* **2011**, *2*, 359–368. [CrossRef]
70. Georgopoulos, K.; Moore, D.D.; Derfler, B. Ikaros, an early lymphoid-specific transcription factor and a putative mediator for T cell commitment. *Science* **1992**, *258*, 808–812. [CrossRef]
71. Kim, J.; Sif, S.; Jones, B.; Jackson, A.; Koipally, J.; Heller, E.; Winandy, S.; Viel, A.; Sawyer, A.; Ikeda, T.; et al. Ikaros DNA-Binding Proteins Direct Formation of Chromatin Remodeling Complexes in Lymphocytes. *Immunity* **1999**, *10*, 345–355. [CrossRef] [PubMed]
72. Koipally, J.; Renold, A.; Kim, J.; Georgopoulos, K. Repression by Ikaros and Aiolos is mediated through histone deacetylase complexes. *EMBO J.* **1999**, *18*, 3090–3100. [CrossRef] [PubMed]
73. Boutboul, D.; Kuehn, H.S.; Van de Wyngaert, Z.; Niemela, J.E.; Callebaut, I.; Stoddard, J.; Lenoir, C.; Barlogis, V.; Farnarier, C.; Vely, F.; et al. Dominant-negative IKZF1 mutations cause a T, B, and myeloid cell combined immunodeficiency. *J. Clin. Investig.* **2018**, *128*, 3071–3087. [CrossRef] [PubMed]
74. Churchman, M.L.; Qian, M.; Kronnie, G.T.; Zhang, R.; Yang, W.; Zhang, H.; Lana, T.; Tedrick, P.; Baskin, R.; Verbist, K.; et al. Germline Genetic IKZF1 Variation and Predisposition to Childhood Acute Lymphoblastic Leukemia. *Cancer Cell* **2018**, *33*, 937–948.e8. [CrossRef]
75. Espinosa, L.; Cathelin, S.; D'Altri, T.; Trimarchi, T.; Statnikov, A.; Guiu, J.; Rodilla, V.; Inglés-Esteve, J.; Nomdedeu, J.; Bellosillo, B.; et al. The Notch/Hes1 pathway sustains NF-kappaB activation through CYLD repression in T cell leukemia. *Cancer Cell* **2010**, *18*, 268–281. [CrossRef]
76. Bellavia, D.; Campese, A.F.; Alesse, E.; Vacca, A.; Felli, M.P.; Balestri, A.; Stoppacciaro, A.; Tiveron, C.; Tatangelo, L.; Giovarelli, M.; et al. Constitutive activation of NF-kappaB and T-cell leukemia/lymphoma in Notch3 transgenic mice. *EMBO J.* **2000**, *19*, 3337–3348. [CrossRef]
77. Beg, A.A.; Baltimore, D. An essential role for NF-kappaB in preventing TNF-alpha-induced cell death. *Science* **1996**, *274*, 782–784. [CrossRef]
78. Aggarwal, B.B. Nuclear factor-κB: The enemy within. *Cancer Cell* **2004**, *6*, 203–208. [CrossRef]
79. Jeremias, I.; Kupatt, C.; Baumann, B.; Herr, I.; Wirth, T.; Debatin, K.M. Inhibition of nuclear factor kappaB activation attenuates apoptosis resistance in lymphoid cells. *Blood* **1998**, *91*, 4624–4631. [CrossRef]
80. Greten, F.R.; Karin, M. The IKK/NF-kappaB activation pathway-a target for prevention and treatment of cancer. *Cancer Lett.* **2004**, *206*, 193–199. [CrossRef]
81. Turco, M.C.; Romano, M.F.; Petrella, A.; Bisogni, R.; Tassone, P.; Venuta, S. NF-kappaB/Rel-mediated regulation of apoptosis in hematologic malignancies and normal hematopoietic progenitors. *Leukemia* **2004**, *18*, 11–17. [CrossRef] [PubMed]
82. Braun, T.; Carvalho, G.; Fabre, C.; Grosjean, J.; Fenaux, P.; Kroemer, G. Targeting NF-kappaB in hematologic malignancies. *Cell Death Differ.* **2006**, *13*, 748–758. [CrossRef] [PubMed]

83. Munzert, G.; Kirchner, D.; Ottmann, O.; Bergmann, L.; Schmid, R.M. Constitutive NF-kappab/Rel activation in philadelphia chromosome positive (Ph+) acute lymphoblastic leukemia (ALL). *Leuk. Lymphoma* **2004**, *45*, 1181–1184. [CrossRef] [PubMed]
84. Luria, S. Viruses, Cancer Cells, and the Genetic Concept of Virus Infection. *Cancer Res.* **1960**, *20*, 677–688. [PubMed]
85. Melana, S.M.; Nepomnaschy, I.; Sakalian, M.; Abbott, A.; Hasa, J.; Holland, J.F.; Pogo, B.G. Characterization of Viral Particles Isolated from Primary Cultures of Human Breast Cancer Cells. *Cancer Res.* **2007**, *67*, 8960–8965. [CrossRef]
86. Pogo, B.G.; Holland, J.F. Possibilities of a viral etiology for human breast cancer. *Biol. Trace Element Res.* **1997**, *56*, 131–142. [CrossRef]
87. Li, H.P.; Leu, Y.W.; Chang, Y.S. Epigenetic changes in virus-associated human cancers. *Cell Res.* **2005**, *15*, 262–271. [CrossRef]
88. Burnett-Hartman, A.N.; Newcomb, P.A.; Potter, J.D. Infectious agents, and colorectal cancer: A review of Helicobacter pylori, Streptococcus bovis, JC virus, and human papillomavirus. *Cancer Epidemiol. Biomark. Prev.* **2008**, *17*, 2970–2979. [CrossRef]
89. Parsa, N. Environmental Factors Inducing Human Cancers. *Iran. J. Public Health* **2012**, *41*, 1–9.
90. Parsa, N.Z.; Mukherjee, A.B.; Chaganti, R.S.K.; Gaidano, G.; Hauptschein, R.S.; Dalla-Favera, R.; Lenoir, G. Cytogenetic and molecular analysis of 6q deletions in Burkitt's lymphoma cell lines. *Genes Chromosomes Cancer* **1994**, *9*, 13–18. [CrossRef]
91. Mager, D.L. Bacteria and cancer: Cause, coincidence, or cure? A review. *J. Transl. Med.* **2006**, *4*, 14. [CrossRef] [PubMed]
92. Egi, Y.; Ito, M.; Tanaka, S.; Imagawa, S.; Takata, S.; Yoshihara, M.; Haruma, K.; Chayama, K. Role of Helicobacter pylori Infection and Chronic Inflammation in Gastric Cancer in the Cardia. *Ultrasound Med. Biol.* **2007**, *37*, 365–369. [CrossRef] [PubMed]
93. Tebbi, C. Carcinogenesis and Leukemogenesis of Microorganisms. *J. 21st Century Pathol.* **2022**, *2*, 109.
94. Lyles, D.S. Cytopathogenesis and Inhibition of Host Gene Expression by RNA Viruses. *Microbiol. Mol. Biol. Rev.* **2000**, *64*, 709–724. [CrossRef] [PubMed]
95. Desfarges, S.; Ciuffi, A. Viral integration and consequences on host gene expression. In *Viruses: Essential Agents of Life*; Springer: Dordrecht, The Netherlands, 2012; pp. 147–175. [CrossRef]
96. Her, L.-S.; Lund, E.; Dahlberg, J.E. Inhibition of Ran guanosine triphosphatase-dependent nuclear transport by the matrix protein of vesicular stomatitis virus. *Science* **1997**, *276*, 1845–1848. [CrossRef]
97. Ahmed Adam, M.A.; Tabana, Y.M.; Musa, K.B.; Sandai, D.A. Effects of different mycotoxins on humans, cell genome and their involvement in cancer. *Oncol. Rep.* **2017**, *37*, 1321–1336. [CrossRef]
98. Park, M.; Cho, Y.-J.; Kim, D.; Yang, C.-S.; Lee, S.M.; Dawson, T.L.; Nakamizo, S.; Kabashima, K.; Lee, Y.W.; Jung, W.H. A Novel Virus Alters Gene Expression and Vacuolar Morphology in *Malassezia* Cells and Induces a TLR3-Mediated Inflammatory Immune Response. *MBio* **2020**, *11*, e01521-20. [CrossRef]
99. Bushweller, J.H. Targeting transcription factors in cancer—From undruggable to reality. *Nat. Rev. Cancer* **2019**, *19*, 611–624. [CrossRef]
100. Lebraud, H.; Wright, D.J.; Johnson CNHeightman, T.D. Protein Degradation by In-Cell Self-Assembly of Proteolysis Tar-geting Chimeras. *ACS Cent. Sci.* **2016**, *2*, 927–934. [CrossRef]
101. Zeng, S.; Huang, W.; Zheng, X.; Cheng, L.; Zhang, Z.; Wang, J.; Shen, Z. Proteolysis targeting chimera (PROTAC) in drug discovery paradigm: Recent progress and future challenges. *Eur. J. Med. Chem.* **2021**, *210*, 112981. [CrossRef]
102. Burslem, G.M.; Crews, C.M. Proteolysis-Targeting Chimeras as Therapeutics and Tools for Biological Discovery. *Cell* **2020**, *181*, 102–114. [CrossRef] [PubMed]

International Journal of
Molecular Sciences

MDPI

Article

The Role of Mutated Calreticulin in the Pathogenesis of *BCR-ABL1*-Negative Myeloproliferative Neoplasms

Roberta Vadeikienė [1,*,†], Baltramiejus Jakštys [2,†], Danguolė Laukaitienė [1], Saulius Šatkauskas [2], Elona Juozaitytė [3] and Rasa Ugenskienė [1,4]

1 Oncology Research Laboratory, Institute of Oncology, Lithuanian University of Health Sciences, LT-50161 Kaunas, Lithuania
2 Research on Delivery of Medicine and Genes Cluster, Faculty of Natural Sciences, Vytautas Magnus University, LT-44001 Kaunas, Lithuania; saulius.satkauskas@vdu.lt (S.Š.)
3 Institute of Oncology, Lithuanian University of Health Sciences, LT-50161 Kaunas, Lithuania
4 Department of Genetics and Molecular Medicine, Lithuanian University of Health Sciences, LT-50161 Kaunas, Lithuania
* Correspondence: roberta.vadeikiene@lsmuni.lt
† These authors contributed equally to this work.

Abstract: Myeloproliferative neoplasms (MPNs) are characterized by increased proliferation of myeloid lineages in the bone marrow. Calreticulin (*CALR*) 52 bp deletion and *CALR* 5 bp insertion have been identified in essential thrombocythemia (ET) and primary myelofibrosis (PMF). There is not much data on the crosstalk between mutated *CALR* and MPN-related signaling pathways, such as JAK/STAT, PI3K/Akt/mTOR, and Hedgehog. Calreticulin, a multifunctional protein, takes part in many cellular processes. Nevertheless, there is little data on how mutated *CALR* affects the oxidative stress response and oxidative stress-induced DNA damage, apoptosis, and cell cycle progression. We aimed to investigate the role of the *CALR* 52 bp deletion and 5 bp insertion in the pathogenesis of MPN, including signaling pathway activation and functional analysis in *CALR*-mutated cells. Our data indicate that the JAK/STAT and PI3K/Akt/mTOR pathways are activated in *CALR*-mutated cells, and this activation does not necessarily depend on the CALR and MPL interaction. Moreover, it was found that *CALR* mutations impair calreticulin function, leading to reduced responses to oxidative stress and DNA damage. It was revealed that the accumulation of G2/M-*CALR*-mutated cells indicates that oxidative stress-induced DNA damage is difficult to repair. Taken together, this study contributes to a deeper understanding of the specific molecular mechanisms underlying *CALR*-mutated MPNs.

Keywords: calreticulin; myeloproliferative neoplasms; JAK/STAT; PI3K/Akt/mTOR; Hedgehog; oxidative stress; DNA damage; apoptosis; cell cycle

1. Introduction

Myeloproliferative neoplasms (MPNs) are a heterogeneous group of hematologic malignancies resulting from mutant hematopoietic stem/progenitor cells. According to the World Health Organization (WHO), classical Philadelphia chromosome-negative (*BCR-ABL1*-negative) MPNs are classified into primary myelofibrosis (PMF), essential thrombocythemia (ET), and polycythemia vera (PV). PMF is characterized by excessive bone marrow scarring and fibrosis, ET by excessive platelet production, and PV by excessive red cell production [1,2]. Clinically, *BCR-ABL1*-negative MPNs share the features of bone marrow hypercellularity and an increased risk of thrombosis or hemorrhage; incurable MPNs can lead to acute leukemia [3,4]. In addition to being classified as a myeloproliferative neoplasm, chronic myeloid leukemia (CML) is distinguished by being *BCR-ABL1* positive [1,2].

Each MPN has unique clinical features with a unifying theme of somatic acquisition of a mutation in either *JAK2* (Janus kinase 2), *MPL* (thrombopoietin receptor), or *CALR* (calreticulin) in hematopoietic stem cells. Carriers of the mentioned genetic mutations have a higher risk of developing PMF, PV, and ET; however, the exact cause of these diseases remains unknown. Environmental and behavioral risk factors, e.g., exposure to ionizing radiation, carcinogenic and immunotoxic agents, as well as a history of smoking, have also been associated with an increased risk of *BCR-ABL1* negative MPNs [5,6]. While analyzing the genetic basis of MPNs, it was determined that more than 90% of PV patients carry the *JAK2* p.V617F mutation; however, around 2% of PV patients do not have *JAK2* p.V617F, but insertions and deletions in exon 12 [7–9]. About 90% of ET cases represent a molecular clonal marker: *JAK2* p.V617F (50–60%), *MPL* p.W515L/K (3–15%) mutations, and *CALR* 52 bp deletion or 5 bp insertion (20–25%) [10–12]. Patients with PMF harbor one of three somatic mutations: *JAK2* p.V617F (up to 60%), *MPL* p.W515L/K (up to 15%), and *CALR* 52 bp deletion or 5 bp insertion (up to 20%) [13]. Recently, mutations in epigenetic regulators and RNA splicing genes, e.g., *TET2*, *SRSF2*, *IDH2*, and *ASXL1*, have also been found in patients with MPNs. However, the mentioned mutations do not have any diagnostic impact in most cases because of their low frequency and specificity [14]. In the last decade, advances in understanding the molecular mechanisms underlying excessive myeloproliferation have been achieved, and novel targeted therapies for MPNs have been developed, e.g., ruxolitinib, a specific JAK1/2 inhibitor, is the first agent approved to treat high-risk patients with PV and PMF [15]. However, ruxolitinib has limited use in that most patients with MPN progress or become intolerant within 2–3 years [16]. Considering the heterogeneous genomic landscape, additional mutations in MPN could represent diagnostic and prognostic value, leading to the risk of progression and informing decisions on therapeutic management. Therefore, there is still a need for novel MPN therapeutic options rationally designed based on recent molecular mechanistic insights.

The first findings of somatic mutations in the calreticulin gene that drive myeloproliferation were reported in 2013. *CALR* mutations are found in a significant proportion of patients with PMF and ET and, as mentioned before, are the second most common gene alterations that drive myeloproliferation [17]. Changes in *CALR* are mutually exclusive with mutations in *JAK2* and *MPL* genes [10,18]. Although the coexistence of the two driver mutations has been reported, these are rare events, and their clinical-prognostic implications are under investigation [19]. More than 50 *CALR* mutations have been identified, and all known variants cause a +1 bp frameshift in the reading frame of exon 9 and generate a novel terminal amino acid sequence common to all mutant calreticulin proteins [20]. A 52 bp deletion (type 1: c.1092_1143del) and a 5 bp insertion (type 2: c.1154_1155insTTGTC) are accepted as the most frequent forms of mutated *CALR* found in PMF and ET patients. It has been determined that the aforementioned phenotypic driver mutations in MPNs have an impact on genes that are directly involved in cytokine signaling (e.g., *JAK2*, *MPL*, *BCR-ABL1*) [21–23]. *CALR* instead encodes an endoplasmic reticulum (ER) chaperone that functions in calcium ion homeostasis, cell adhesion, antigen presentation, danger signaling, and cell death, and assists glycoproteins in obtaining their mature structure [24,25]. A systematic investigation of *CALR* mutations revealed that the loss of the C-terminal KDEL motif leads to reduced endoplasmic reticulum retention of mutated calreticulin and impairs the aforementioned multiple native calreticulin functions [26]. From a clinical viewpoint, it was observed that the presence of *CALR* mutations is related to a clinically distinctive and good prognosis of ET and PMF, compared to *JAK2*-mutated ones. However, it is important to note that a worse MPN course, i.e., increased risk of transformation of ET to secondary myelofibrosis, splenomegaly, aspirin-induced hemorrhage, and worsened survival, was also observed in patients harboring a *CALR* 52 bp deletion and 5 bp insertion [10,17,18,27–32]. In addition, it was observed that *CALR* gene mutations appear early in ET and PMF; hence, this could be used as a transformation marker [33]. Active investigations on how mutated *CALR* induces cell transformation are being carried out, yet there are no conclusive data about mutated *CALR's* contribution to MPN pathogenesis. Therefore, the need arises for a deeper understanding of the molecular mechanisms underlying the characteristics of *CALR*-mutated MPNs. The identification of aberrant mechanisms of mutated calreticulin and its role in MPN etiopathogenesis would serve to develop novel molecular targeted therapy approaches for MPNs in the future.

The analysis of the molecular mechanism of mutated calreticulin is complicated because a commercial cell line carrying a *CALR* 52 bp deletion or 5 bp insertion has not yet been established. To our knowledge, the only commercial cell line to harbor *CALR* mutation is MARIMO. However, this cell line is characterized by a 61 bp deletion in exon 9 [34–37]. The function of *CALR* 61 bp deletion in the MARIMO cell line remains unclear, and the authors question the use of these cells as a model for the malign function of *CALR* mutants. The way out of the problem of lacking a commercial cell line is to initiate common *CALR* mutations in relatively easy-to-transfect cells, such as HEK293, 32D, or Ba/F3 cells [10,38,39]. Recently, several studies have been conducted with human suspension cell lines that were also transfected, and an analysis related to *CALR*'s mutation role in MPNs was performed [40–42]. Nevertheless, the use of suspension cell lines is complicated because these cells are difficult to transfect using conventional transfection methods, such as liposomal or calcium phosphate methods [43]. It is difficult to find an appropriate cellular model reflecting the genetic basis and molecular profiling of MPNs, so a few research groups have analyzed calreticulin's role in these diseases using circulating $CD34^+$ cells or cells cultured from blood or bone marrow samples of patients with MPN [38,44–47]. It can be added that the amount of research related to patient cell samples is limited because not all research institutions have access to patient blood and bone marrow samples. Furthermore, the preparation and cultivation of cells derived from patients is complicated, cost-effective, and has technical limitations compared to commercial cell lines. Considering that originally, mutationally, and adhesively different cellular models have been used in previous studies, mutated *CALR*-related research data remains conflicting.

The Janus kinase/signal transducer and activator of the transcription (JAK/STAT) pathway is one of the central junctions of interaction in cell functions, e.g., hemopoiesis, immune cell development, tissue repair, stem cell maintenance, apoptosis, and adipogenesis [48]. It is known that JAK/STAT is a highly conserved pathway of signal transduction, and dysregulation of this signaling is associated with various diseases, including MPNs, Hodgkin lymphoma, and hepatocellular carcinoma [48–50]. As mentioned before, MPN-related molecular abnormalities play a crucial role in the constitutive activation of JAK/STAT signaling. A few in vitro studies have also analyzed the impact of the mutated *CALR* on the activation of this signaling pathway [10,34,51–53]. Increased activation of JAK/STAT signaling has been reported, but it is important to note that this activation is unique due to the capability of the novel C-terminus of the *CALR* mutant to bind directly to MPL [10,51,52,54]. This statement was clarified in vivo, where *c-mpl*-deficient mice were protected from MPN disease with the *CALR* phenotype [55,56]. Moreover, *CALR*-mutated PMF patients responded to JAK2 inhibition, and control of the symptoms and quality of life were improved, which also shows CALR involvement in JAK/STAT signaling [55,57,58]. Contrary to the mentioned results, other studies' molecular analysis showed no association between mutated calreticulin and JAK/STAT but represented the increased activity of ERK1/2, MAPK, and PI3K/Akt/mTOR [36,37,53,56,59,60]. Furthermore, it has recently been suggested that the consequences of *CALR* mutations on megakaryopoiesis are likely to be mediated not only by MAPK but also by STAT5 signaling, which is accompanied by MPL-dependent activation [34]. Based on the conflicting results of the mentioned studies, there is a need for further research and elucidation of the effect of the mutated *CALR* on JAK/STAT signaling pathway activation.

The PI3K/Akt/mTOR (phosphatidylinositol 3-kinase/Protein kinase B/mammalian target of rapamycin) signaling pathway is involved in most cellular processes, e.g., cell proliferation, adhesion, cell death, migration, and invasion. It was noticed that PIK3/Akt/mTOR is commonly activated in human cancers [61–63]. The constitutive activation of the PI3K/Akt/mTOR signaling pathway was determined to be central to MPN pathogenesis. In addition, it was suggested that the PI3K/Akt/mTOR cascade regulates cell growth and proliferation signals downstream of the JAK/STAT signaling pathway [60]. Preclinical studies have shown that this signaling pathway inhibitor alone and in combination with JAK/STAT inhibitors reduced proliferation and induced apoptosis in cells carrying *JAK2* or *MPL* mutations [60,64–67]. However, there is little data that represent mutated calreticulin's impact on the PI3K/Akt/mTOR signaling pathway. Independent research groups have determined that *CALR* mutants induce the phosphorylation of JAK2, STAT1, STAT3, and STAT5, while PIK3/Akt/mTOR and MAPK signaling systems are weakly activated [51,55]. However, it is important to note that this kind of signaling activation is also dependent on human *MPL* expression. Kollman et al. (2017) revealed that *CALR*-mutant murine 32D cell line without exogenous MPL showed increased Akt phosphorylation [36]. Considering the controversial and limited results of the mentioned studies, it is necessary to fully elucidate the mechanism that determines crosstalk between mutated *CALR* and the PI3K/Akt/mTOR signaling pathway.

The Hedgehog (Hh) signaling pathway is a highly conserved pathway of signal transduction from the cell membrane to the nucleus. Hh signaling plays an important role in normal embryonic growth and the development of many tissues and organs. Lately, it has been shown that the Hh pathway plays a role in carcinogenesis in different tumors, as well as in the pathogenesis of hematologic malignancies [68–73]. However, there is little data on the association between the Hh signaling pathway and MPNs [74–76]. Bhagwat and coauthors [74] reported that the expression of *PTCH1* and *GLI1* was increased up to 100-fold in granulocytes derived from patients with MPNs compared with control granulocytes. In addition, it was found that components of the Hh pathway cooperate with other signaling pathways to produce the biological phenotype of PMF [76]. Contrary to these results, it was found that in the *C. elegans* model with initiated *CALR* 52 deletion and *CALR* 5 bp insertion, most of the Hedgehog signaling pathway targets were downregulated [77]. Moreover, these results are reinforced by the Lucijanic et al. (2020) study, in which *GLI1* expression was analyzed in patients with myelofibrosis and healthy controls. The findings of the mentioned study imply that the upregulation of *GLI1* does not appear to be a characteristic of myelofibrosis etiopathogenesis [78]. Therefore, due to inconclusive data, it is necessary to expand the current experiments analyzing mutant calreticulin and Hedgehog signaling pathway association.

Several studies have revealed the importance of reactive oxygen species (ROS) in MPNs: MPN patients demonstrated increased levels of ROS [79], and cellular models exhibited the production of ROS in vitro [80]. In addition, separate research groups have reported that *JAK2, MPL,* and *CALR* variants are associated with other DNA alterations leading to an inflammatory state characterized by excessive production of ROS [81,82]. Apart from the activation of cell signaling pathways, calreticulin, a multifunctional protein, is involved in many cellular processes. The impact of *CALR* 52 bp deletion and 5 bp insertion in the pathogenesis of MPNs has been partly clarified, but there is little data that describes the effects of the mentioned mutations on the physiological functions of calreticulin. Recently, it has been shown that cells overexpressing *CALR* demonstrate increased sensitivity to ER and oxidative stress [40,83]. To our knowledge, only a few studies have analyzed mutated calreticulin's impact on oxidative stress in a cell culture model [40,41]. It was determined that cells expressing mutated *CALR* showed increased ROS intracellular levels and increased levels of DNA damage upon oxidative stress exposure using Melittin and Miltirone. Additionally, CALR mutants were characterized by a decreased ability to reduce intracellular ROS levels and repair oxidative DNA damage. It is known that calreticulin is involved in various biological processes, including cell death. However, only Genovese with colleagues [41] data showed an increase in oxidative stress-induced apoptosis levels in cells carrying *CALR* mutations. Taken together, functional analysis for a deeper understanding of the *CALR* 52 bp deletion and 5 bp insertion on native calreticulin functions is essential.

To sum up, the pathogenesis of MPNs is very complex, and dysregulated signaling pathways and their crosstalk with mutated calreticulin may offer additional therapeutic targets. Therefore, there is a need for further research and elucidation of the mechanism underlying the crosstalk between mutated *CALR* and cell signaling pathways, JAK/STAT, PI3K/Akt/mTOR, and Hedgehog, which are important in MPN pathogenesis. In this study, we explored the potent effect of targeting JAK/STAT, PI3K/Akt/mTOR, and Hedgehog signaling pathways with specific inhibitors in vitro and subsequently carried out target gene expression and protein level analysis in cells carrying the *CALR* 52 bp deletion and 5 bp insertion, as well as in cells with *JAK2* p.V617F and *JAK2*/*CALR* wild-type. This research is unique because most studies analyze mutant *CALR* when *MPL* expression is present, but we performed experiments in a cell culture model lacking *MPL* expression. In this complex study, we also explored how *CALR* 52 bp deletion and 5 bp insertion affect the oxidative stress response and whether aberrant response could indicate a pathogenic mechanism in mutant *CALR*-mediated cellular transformation. Subsequently, we tested the effect of the *CALR* mutation on the capacity of cells to respond to oxidative stress-induced DNA damage. Data on the role of mutant calreticulin in oxidative stress-induced apoptosis are limited; therefore, we intended to analyze whether the impaired ability to reduce oxidative stress entails a different ability to induce apoptosis. The cell cycle involvement in malignant processes is determined; unfortunately, to the extent of our knowledge, no data shows the impact of mutated calreticulin on cell cycle progression in the context of oxidative stress. Thus, we also aimed to evaluate cell cycle distribution after oxidative stress induction in *CALR*-mutated cells.

2. Results

2.1. The Dependence of CALR Del52, CALR Ins5 Cells on JAK/STAT, PI3K/Akt/mTOR, and Hedgehog Signaling

Herein, we demonstrated the dependence of different cellular models on the JAK/STAT, PI3K/Akt/mTOR, and Hedgehog signaling pathways. Firstly, we evaluated the effect of RAD001 (against mTOR), CYT387 (against JAK1/2), and HPI-1 (against Hedgehog signaling) inhibitors as a single agent. A reduction in cell viability was observed in all tested cell lines using alamarBlue and trypan exclusion assays. Our study results indicate that inhibitors progressively reduced cell viability as the concentration and exposure duration increased. The dose−response study demonstrated that agents targeting JAK/STAT, PI3K/Akt/mTOR, and Hedgehog signaling pathways exert significant inhibition of *CALR*-mutated cells (Figures 1–6). It is important to mention that the results related to SET-2 and UT-7 cells' antiproliferative response to specific inhibitors were published previously in our article [84].

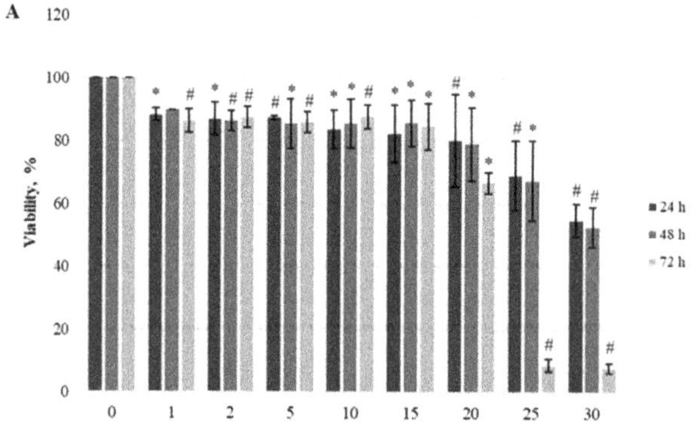

Figure 1. *Cont.*

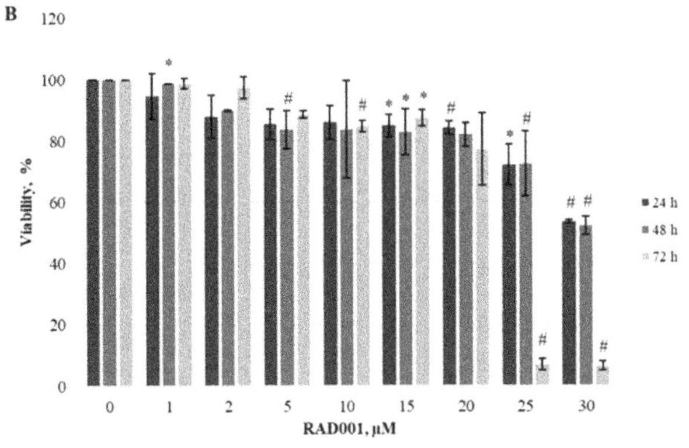

Figure 1. *CALR* Del52 cell line viability reduction by RAD001 treatment. *CALR* Del52 cells were treated with varying concentrations of RAD001 for 24, 48, and 72 h before alamarBlue (**A**) and trypan exclusion assays (**B**) were performed. * $p < 0.05$ vs. DMSO-treated control. # $p < 0.01$ vs. DMSO-treated control.

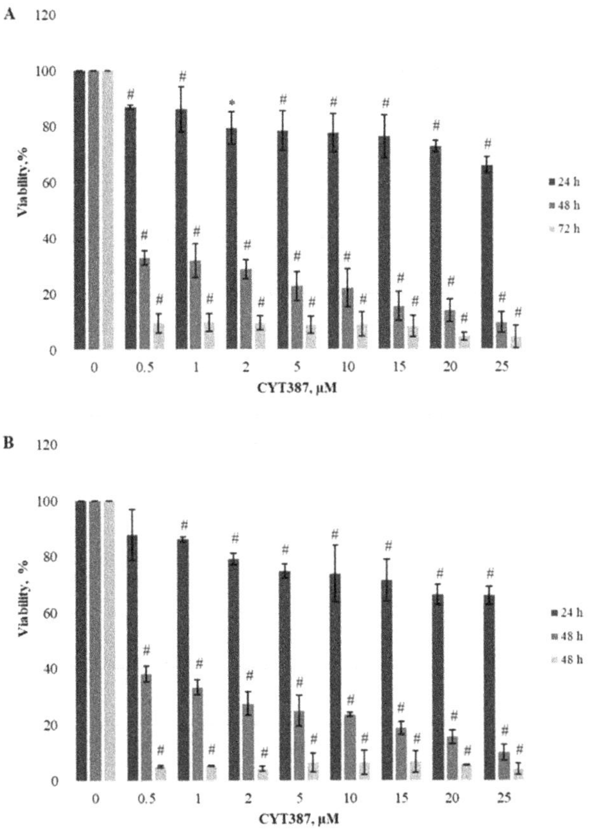

Figure 2. Reduction of *CALR* Del52 cell line viability by CYT387 treatment. *CALR* Del52 cells were treated with varying concentrations of CYT387 for 24, 48, and 72 h before alamarBlue (**A**) and trypan exclusion assays (**B**) were performed. * $p < 0.05$ vs. DMSO-treated control. # $p < 0.01$ vs. DMSO-treated control.

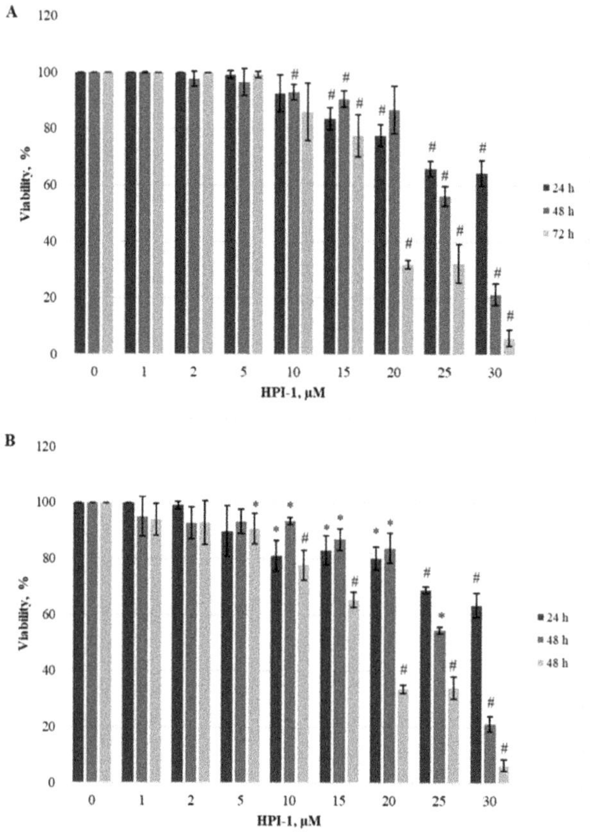

Figure 3. Reduction of *CALR* Del52 cell line viability by HPI-1 treatment. *CALR* Del52 cells were treated with varying concentrations of HPI-1 for 24, 48, and 72 h before alamarBlue (**A**) and trypan exclusion assays (**B**) were performed. * $p < 0.05$ vs. DMSO-treated control. # $p < 0.01$ vs. DMSO-treated control.

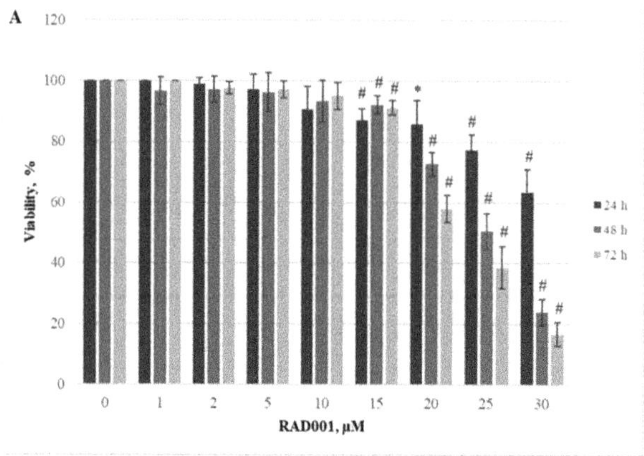

Figure 4. *Cont.*

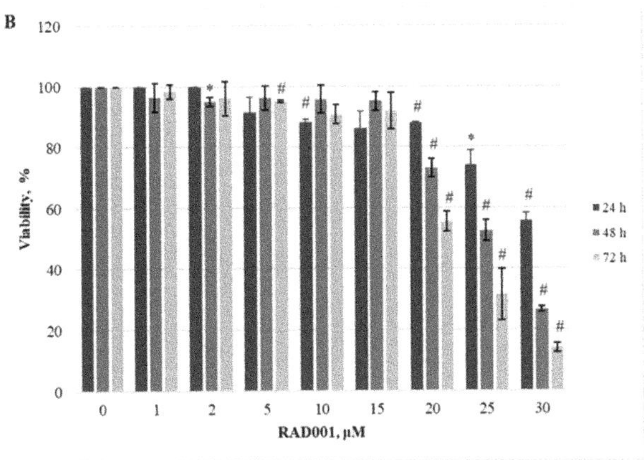

Figure 4. *CALR* Ins5 cell line viability reduction by RAD001 treatment. *CALR* Ins5 cells were treated with varying concentrations of RAD001 for 24, 48, and 72 h before alamarBlue (**A**) and trypan exclusion assays (**B**) were performed. * $p < 0.05$ vs. DMSO-treated control. # $p < 0.01$ vs. DMSO-treated control.

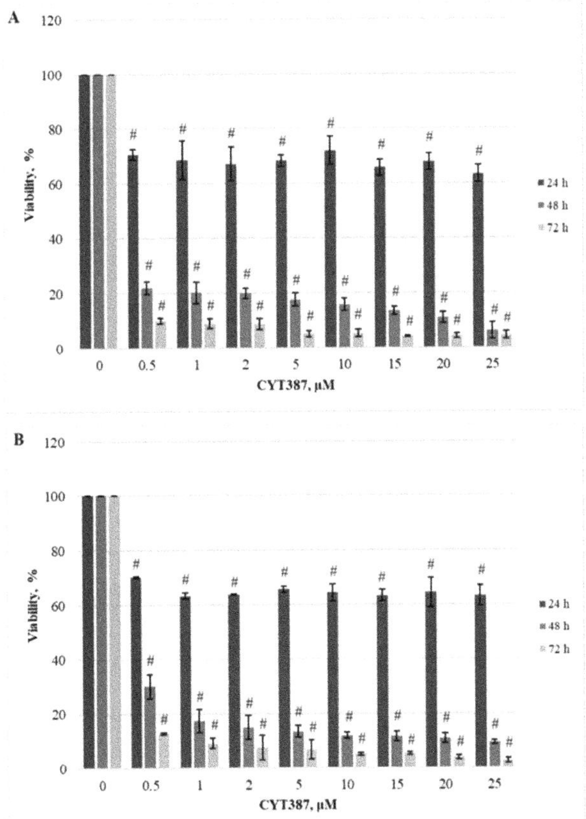

Figure 5. Reduction of *CALR* Ins5 cell line viability by CYT387 treatment. *CALR* Ins5 cells were treated with varying concentrations of CYT387 for 24, 48, and 72 h before alamarBlue (**A**) and trypan exclusion assays (**B**) were performed. # $p < 0.01$ vs. DMSO-treated control.

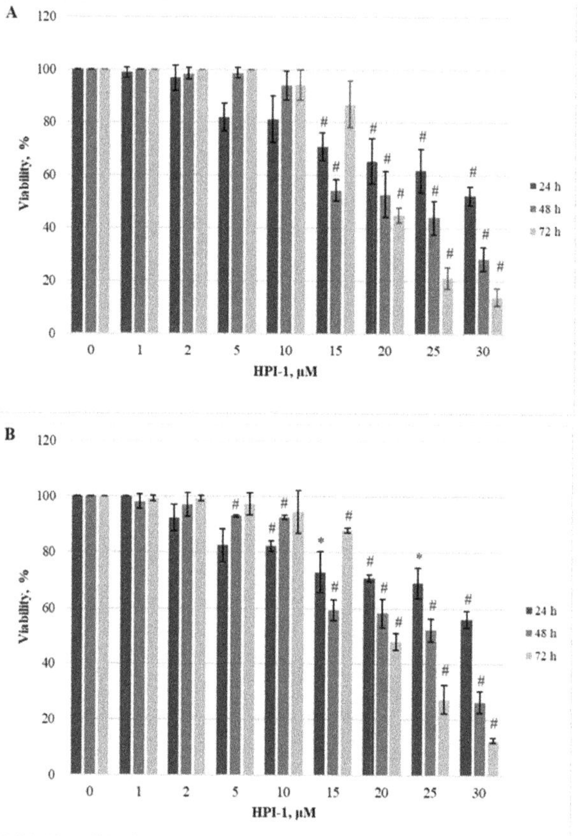

Figure 6. Reduction of *CALR* Ins5 cell line viability by HPI-1 treatment. *CALR* Ins5 cells were treated with varying concentrations of HPI-1 for 24, 48, and 72 h before alamarBlue (**A**) and trypan exclusion assays (**B**) were performed. * $p < 0.05$ vs. DMSO-treated control. # $p < 0.01$ vs. DMSO-treated control.

No statistically significant differences were found between the IC50 values of the inhibitors when *CALR* Del52 cells were treated for 24 h ($p > 0.05$). However, *CALR*-mutated cells were extremely sensitive, demonstrating low IC50 values for JAK/STAT inhibitor CYT387 compared to RAD001 after 48 h and 72 h exposure (0.84 vs. 41.05, p = 0.0001 and 0.34 vs. 19.32, p = 0.0001, respectively) when cell viability was assessed with trypan blue exclusion assay. This difference was confirmed by the alamarBlue test (2.71 vs. 42.32, p = 0.001, and 0.39 vs. 18.58, p = 0.0001). *CALR*-mutated cells were less sensitive to HPI-1 inhibitor compared to CYT387 after 48 and 72 h treatment (26.93 vs. 0.84, p = 0.0001 and 17.44 vs. 0.34, p = 0.0001) (according to trypan blue assay results). The results were confirmed by the alamarBlue test, where IC50 values were 27.66 vs. 2.71 (p = 0.012) and 18.36 vs. 0.39 (p = 0.0001). Moreover, a statistically significant difference was found between the RAD001 and HPI-1 treatments. The trypan blue exclusion assay data showed that cells harboring the *CALR* 52 bp deletion were more sensitive to HPI-1 compared to RAD001 (26.93 vs. 41.05, p = 0.02 (48 h) and 17.44 vs. 19.32, p = 0.002 (72 h)). However, this difference was not confirmed by the alamaBlue test ($p > 0.05$) (Table S1, Supplementary Material). No statistically significant differences were found between CYT387, RAD001, and HPI-1 inhibitors' IC50 values when *CALR* Ins5 cells were treated for 24 h ($p > 0.05$). However, dose-response studies with trypan blue exclusion assay showed that *CALR* Ins5 cells were more sensitive to CYT387 after 48 and 72 h exposure, compared to RAD001 treatment (0.47

vs. 27.01, $p = 0.0001$ and 0.32 vs. 21.01, $p = 0.0001$, respectively). The difference was also confirmed by the alamarBlue test (0.80 vs. 25.92, $p = 0.0001$, and 0.61 vs. 22.31, $p = 0.0001$). Furthermore, a statistically significant difference was found between the CYT387 and HPI-1 treatments. The Hedgehog signaling inhibitor HPI-1 had less inhibitory potential than CYT387, as a trypan blue exclusion assay data showed. After 48 and 72 h of treatment, IC50 values were as follows: 22.94 vs. 0.47, $p = 0.0001$, and 20.09 vs. 0.32, $p = 0.0001$, respectively. The alamarBlue test demonstrated similar results: 21.72 vs. 0.80, $p = 0.0001$, and 19.61 vs. 0.61, $p = 0.0001$. A statistically significant difference was found between RAD001 and HPI-1 treatments, but only in the data obtained from the alamarBlue assay. The data showed that cells harboring the *CALR* 5 bp insertion were more sensitive to HPI-1 after 48 and 72 h exposure, compared to RAD001 (21.72 vs. 25.92, $p = 0.004$ and 19.61 vs. 22.31, $p = 0.010$) (Table S1, Supplementary Material). Assessing agent sensitivity among cell lines, data from this and a previously published study [84] show that cells with *CALR* mutations are more sensitive to the tested inhibitors than the control UT-7 cell line.

Briefly, our previous study provided a broad overview of MPN-related signaling pathways and conducted a dose-response analysis of RAD001, CYT387, and HPI-1 in SET-2 and UT-7 cells. We found that SET-2 cells expressing the *JAK2* p. V617F mutation showed increased sensitivity toward the tested agents compared to the control UT-7 cells. Our data indicate that the cell line expressing *JAK2* p.V617F is exquisitely sensitive to CYT387 as a single agent, showing proliferation arrest. We found that *JAK2* mutated cells were more sensitive to inhibition of the PI3K/Akt/mTOR and Hh pathways than the wild-type counterpart UT-7 cell line. CYT387 presented lower IC50 values compared to RAD001 and HPI-1 in the UT-7 cell line after 24, 48, and 72 h of treatment [84].

To sum up, our data indicate that the cells expressing *CALR* mutations were exquisitely sensitive to CYT387 as a single agent, showing proliferation arrest. Moreover, we found that the SET-2 cell line, *CALR* Del52, and *CALR* Ins5 cells were more sensitive to the inhibition of PI3K/Akt/mTOR and Hedgehog signaling pathways than the wild-type counterpart UT-7 cell line.

2.2. The Expression of JAK/STAT, PI3K/Akt/mTOR, and Hedgehog Signaling Pathways-Related Genes in CALR Del52, CALR Ins5, SET-2 and UT-7 Cells

In the next step of our study, we aimed to analyze the expression of JAK/STAT, PI3K/Akt, and Hedgehog signaling-related genes, which are the main components of these signaling pathways. *STAT1* and *STAT5* are related to JAK/STAT signaling, *EIF4EBP1* and *RPS6KB1* are the main components of the PI3K/Akt/mTOR pathway, and *PTCH1* expression is associated with Hedgehog signaling. To assess the changes in gene expression, the RT-qPCR method was applied.

It was found that there were significant differences in target gene expression between *CALR* Del52, *CALR* Ins5, SET-2, and UT-7 cells, which served as control cells with wild-type *JAK2* and *CALR*. *RPS6KB1* gene was found to be increased in the *JAK2* mutated SET-2 cell line by 2.390-fold ($p = 0.046$) compared to that in the UT-7 cell line (Figure 7B). *RPS6KB1* gene was also upregulated in *CALR* Del52 and *CALR* Ins5 cells (1.510-fold, $p = 0.048$ and 1.382-fold, $p = 0.022$, respectively) (Figure 7B). Moreover, *STAT5A* gene expression was found to be increased by 1.775-fold ($p = 0.050$) in SET-2 and by 1.466-fold ($p = 0.037$) in *CALR* Del52 cells compared to the UT-7 cell line (Figure 7C). The expression of the *STAT1* gene was significantly increased by 11.985-fold ($p = 0.026$) in the SET-2 cell line compared to that in wild-type UT-7 cells (Figure 7D). The *EIF4EBP1* gene showed a tendency for upregulation; however, the change in gene expression did not reach the significance level (Figure 7A). No *PTCH1* expression was detected in any of the tested cell lines.

It can be concluded that the expression of JAK/STAT and PI3K/Akt/mTOR signaling pathways-related genes is increased in *CALR* Del52, *CALR* Ins5, and SET-2 cells.

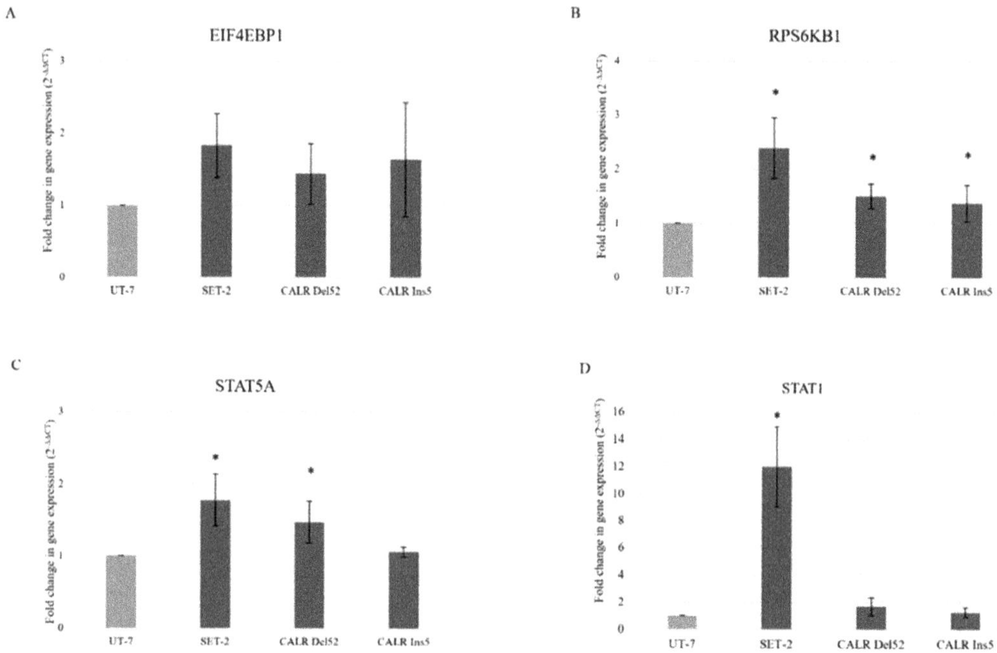

Figure 7. Gene expression in *CALR* Del52, *CALR* Ins5, and SET-2 cells. (**A**) *EIF4EBP1*, (**B**) *RPS6KB1*, (**C**) *STAT5A*, and (**D**) *STAT1* relative expression levels ($2^{-\Delta\Delta Ct}$) were normalized to *ACTB* gene expression as an endogenous control. Bar graphs represent the mean of three independent experiments. Error bars show the standard deviation from the mean. The differences between the UT-7 cell line, which served as a *JAK2* and *CALR* wild-type control, and SET-2 and *CALR*-mutated cells were evaluated using an independent sample *t*-test. Gene expression, which is significantly different from the control at $p < 0.05$, is represented as *.

2.3. Phosphorylation Level of JAK/STAT and PI3K/Akt/mTOR Signaling Pathways-Related Proteins in CALR Del52, CALR Ins5, SET-2, and UT-7 Cells

Here, we aimed to determine whether the increase in mRNA corresponded with elevated total and phosphorylated protein levels in the tested cell lines. Western blot and densitometry analyses were performed to evaluate the change in protein level.

We focused on molecules that are the main targets of mTORC1, i.e., *EIF4EBP1* and *RPS6KB1*, and mRNA analysis showed significantly increased expression of *RPS6KB1*. However, Western blot and densitometry analysis revealed that *CALR* Del52, *CALR* Ins5, SET-2, and UT-7 cells lack total and phosphorylated S6K1 protein (encoded by the *RPS6KB1* gene) expression levels (data not presented). Therefore, for further analysis, only phosphorylated 4E-BP1 was used as a marker of mTORC1 activity. It was determined that SET-2 cells harboring *JAK2* mutation, *CALR* Del52, and *CALR* Ins5 cells had upregulated levels of total 4E-BP1 protein (Figure 8).

Western blot data revealed a significant 2.445-fold ($p = 0.005$) and 3.581-fold ($p = 0.001$) increase in phosphorylation of 4E-BP1 in SET-2 and *CALR* Ins5 cells (compared to control UT-7 cell line), respectively (Figure 9).

Further, we aimed to analyze whether the JAK/STAT signaling pathway targets, STAT5 and STAT1, are affected in cells harboring *CALR* and *JAK2* mutations. The total STAT5A protein level (Figure 10) was significantly reduced in SET-2 cells (3.704-fold, $p = 0.010$), whereas STAT5A expression in *CALR*-mutated cells did not differ from that in the UT-7 control cell line.

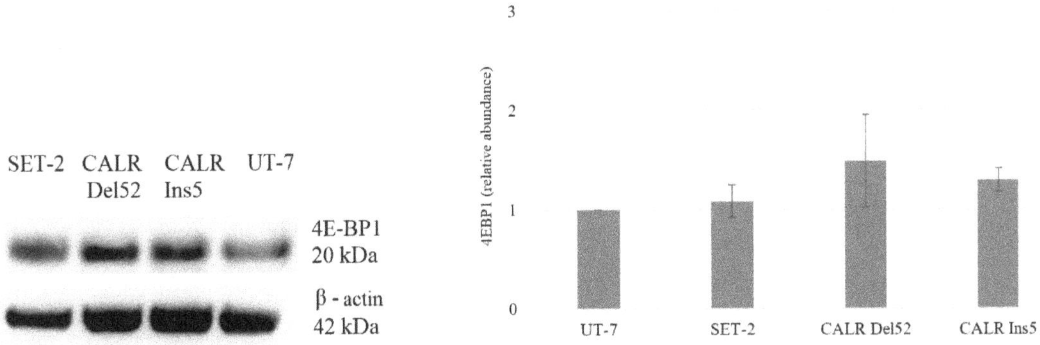

Figure 8. Changes in 4E-BP1 protein levels in *CALR* Del52, *CALR* Ins5, and SET-2 cell lines. Representative pictures of protein bands on the left of the figure are obtained from Western blot membranes and show protein expression levels. Densitometric quantification of total 4E-BP1 levels was normalized to that of β-actin for fold-change calculations. Bar graphs represent the mean of at least three independent experiments. Error bars show the standard deviation from the mean. The differences in protein expression between the UT-7 cell line, which served as a *JAK2* and *CALR* wild-type control, and SET-2 and *CALR*-mutated cells, were evaluated using an independent sample *t*-test.

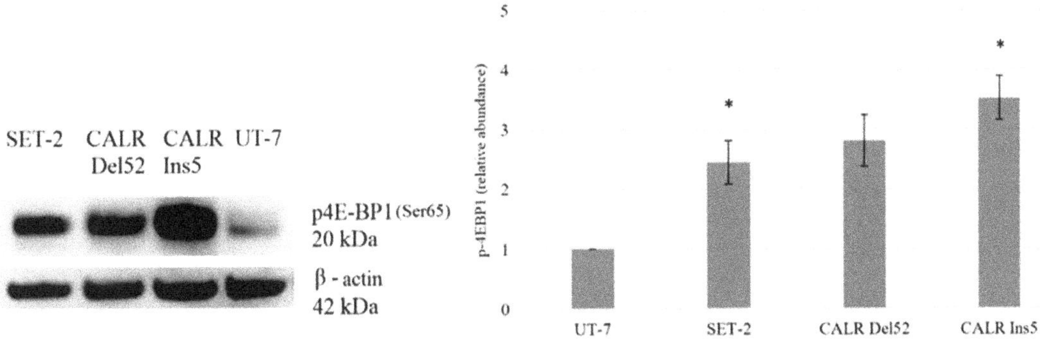

Figure 9. Induction of the phosphorylation of 4E-BP1 in *CALR* Del52, *CALR* Ins5, and SET-2 cell lines. Representative pictures of protein bands on the left of the figure are obtained from Western blot membranes and show induced activation of 4E-BP1. Densitometric quantification of phosphorylated 4E-BP1 levels was normalized to total 4E-BP1 for fold-change calculations. The bar graphs represent the mean of at least three independent experiments. Error bars show the standard deviation from the mean. The differences in protein levels between the UT-7 cell line, which served as a *JAK2* and *CALR* wild-type control, and SET-2 and *CALR*-mutated cells, were evaluated using an independent sample *t*-test. Protein levels significantly different from the control ($p < 0.05$) are represented as *.

Next, we evaluated the phosphorylated STAT5A protein levels. Our data revealed that the phosphorylation of STAT5A was increased in cells carrying mutated *CALR*. Western blot analysis indicated a 3.30-fold ($p = 0.050$) increase in STAT5A phosphorylation in *CALR* Del52 cells. Moreover, *CALR* Ins5 cells showed a 5.677-fold ($p = 0.046$) increase in STAT5 phosphorylation (Figure 11).

The upregulated total STAT1 levels were found only in SET-2 and *CALR* Ins5 cells (9.773-fold, $p = 0.002$ and 3.429-fold, $p = 0.030$, respectively) (Figure 12).

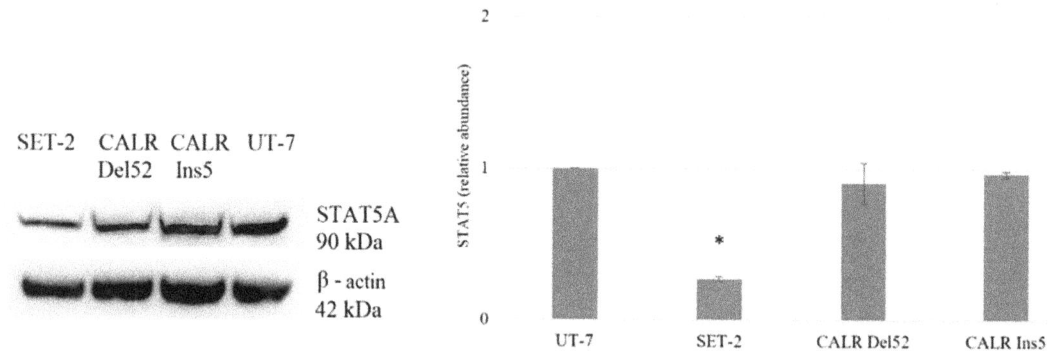

Figure 10. Changes in STAT5A protein levels in *CALR* Del52, *CALR* Ins5, and SET-2 cell lines. Representative pictures of protein bands on the left of the figure are obtained from Western blot membranes and show protein expression. Densitometric quantification of total STAT5A levels was normalized to that of β-actin for fold-change calculations. The bar graphs represent the mean of at least three independent experiments. Error bars show the standard deviation from the mean. The differences in protein levels between the UT-7 cell line, which served as a *JAK2* and *CALR* wild-type control, and SET-2 and *CALR*-mutated cells, were evaluated using an independent sample *t*-test. Protein level significantly different from the control at $p < 0.05$ is represented as *.

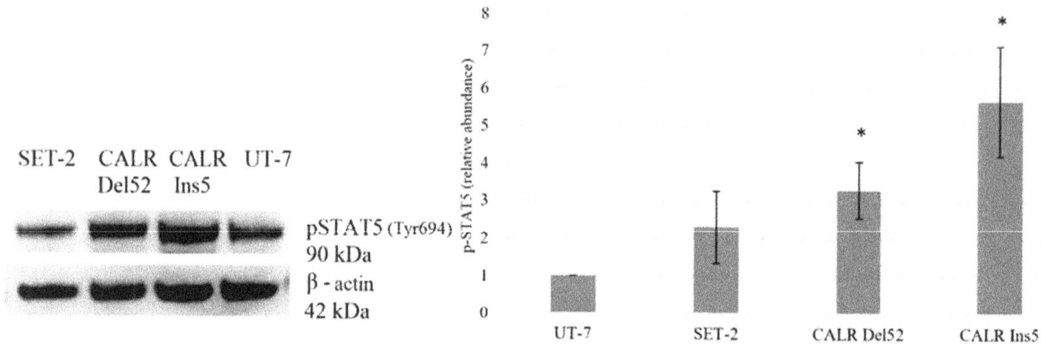

Figure 11. Induction of the phosphorylation of STAT5A in *CALR* Del52, *CALR* Ins5, and SET-2 cell lines. Representative pictures of protein bands on the left of the figure are obtained from Western blot membranes and show induced activation of STAT5A. Densitometric quantification of phosphorylated STAT5A levels was normalized to total STAT5A for fold-change calculations. The bar graphs represent the mean of at least three independent experiments. Error bars show the standard deviation from the mean. The differences in protein levels between the UT-7 cell line, which served as a *JAK2* and *CALR* wild-type control, and SET-2 as well, as *CALR*-mutated cells, were evaluated using an independent sample *t*-test. Protein level significantly different from the control at $p < 0.05$ is represented as *.

Lastly, the expression level of phosphorylated STAT1 was evaluated. Western blot revealed a detectable reduction in STAT1 phosphorylation in SET-2 cells. However, no detectable phosphorylation of STAT1 protein was found in *CALR* Del52 and *CARL* Ins5 cells (Figure 13).

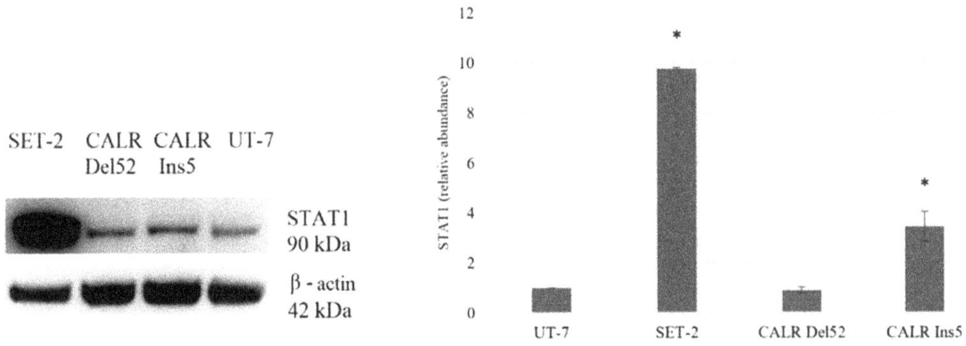

Figure 12. Changes in STAT1 protein levels in *CALR* Del52, *CALR* Ins5, and SET-2 cell lines. Representative pictures of protein bands on the left of the figure are obtained from Western blot membranes and show protein expression. Densitometric quantification of total STAT1 levels was normalized to β-actin levels for fold-change calculations. The bar graphs represent the mean of at least three independent experiments. Error bars show the standard deviation from the mean. Differences in protein levels between the UT-7 control cell line and SET-2, as well as *CALR*-mutated cells, were evaluated using an independent sample *t*-test. Protein level significantly different from the control at $p < 0.05$ is represented as *.

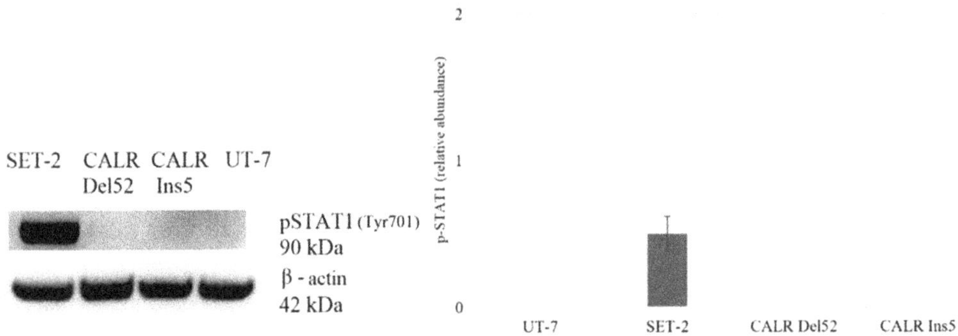

Figure 13. Changes in STAT1 protein phosphorylation in *CALR* Del52, *CALR* Ins5, and SET-2 cell lines. Representative pictures of protein bands on the left of the figure are obtained from Western blot membranes and show induced activation of STAT1. Densitometric quantification of phosphorylated STAT1 levels was normalized to total STAT1 for fold-change calculations. The bar graphs represent the mean of at least three independent experiments. The protein level differences between the UT-7 cell line, which served as a *JAK2* and *CALR* wild-type control, and SET-2 as well, as *CALR*-mutated cells, were evaluated using an independent sample *t*-test. Error bars show the standard deviation from the mean.

2.4. *Effect of CALR Mutations on the Physiological Calreticulin Functions*

As mentioned before, calreticulin is a major chaperone in the ER and plays a role in several cellular processes, e.g., control of protein folding, calcium homeostasis, and cellular stress response. However, there is little data that describes the effects of *CALR* mutations on the physiological function of calreticulin. It has been demonstrated that cells overexpressing *CALR* show increased sensitivity to ER and oxidative stress [40,83]. Thus, we aimed to determine how *CALR* 52 bp deletion and 5 bp insertion affect the oxidative stress response and whether an abnormal response could indicate a pathogenic mechanism in mutant *CALR*-mediated cellular transformation. To analyze the effect of common *CALR* mutations on the response to oxidative stress, all tested cells were exposed to hydrogen peroxide (H_2O_2) for 24 h. Subsequently, the cells were incubated for an additional 24 h to reduce the ROS accumulation induced by H_2O_2.

The quantitative measurement of cells undergoing oxidative stress was performed using the cell analyzer Muse with the corresponding kit, according to the manufacturer's protocol.

It was revealed that after H_2O_2 treatment, *CALR* Del52 cells showed elevated levels of ROS compared to the UT-7 cell line harboring wild-type *CALR* (50.8 ± 3.3% vs. 36.7 ± 2.3%, $p = 0.005$). Contrary, *JAK2* p.V617F positive SET-2 cell line showed relatively low ROS levels compared to the control UT-7 cells (24.4 ± 2.0% vs. 36.7 ± 2.3%, $p = 0.0001$) (Figure 14). We showed that these differences are more remarkable after 24 h of repair. *CALR* Del52 and *CALR* Ins5 cells could not reduce intracellular ROS levels, while the control UT-7 cells were able to counteract ROS accumulation (53.7 ± 6.8% vs. 29.5 ± 1.6%, $p = 0.009$ and 45.1 ± 3.2% vs. 29.5 ± 1.6%, $p = 0.006$, respectively). The SET-2 cell line efficiently decreased the percentage of ROS-positive cells compared to the control (16.2 ± 5.3% vs. 29.5 ± 1.6%, $p = 0.038$) (Figure 14).

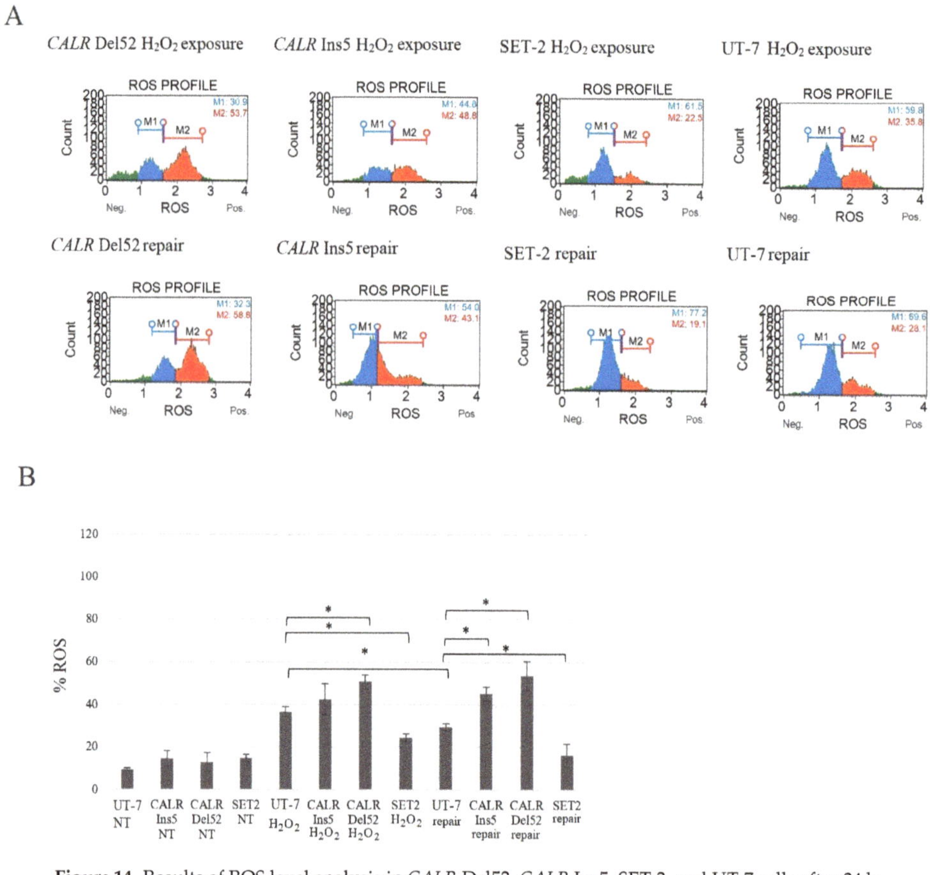

Figure 14. Results of ROS level analysis in *CALR* Del52, *CALR* Ins5, SET-2, and UT-7 cells after 24 h of exposure to H_2O_2 and 24 h of repair. (**A**) Representative ROS profile histograms are shown. (**B**) The graph represents the percentage of positive ROS in different cell lines. Values represent the mean and a standard deviation of at least three experiments performed in triplicate. An asterisk represents $p < 0.05$ vs. control.

Next, we aimed to study whether *CALR* 52 bp deletion and 5 bp insertion can affect the efficiency of repairing the DNA damage induced by oxidative stress. The cells expressing the wild-type *CALR* and *JAK2*, as well as mutated cells, were exposed to H_2O_2 for 24 h. Subsequently, the cells were given an additional 24 h to repair the DNA damage induced by H_2O_2 treatment. pATM and pH2AX were measured using cytometry and the Muse Multi-Color

DNA Damage Kit. The phosphorylation of ATM and H2AX was taken together to analyze the results.

Our study demonstrated that *CALR* Del52 cells are characterized by statistically significant higher levels of DNA damage compared to the control UT-7 cell line (65.2 ± 2.8% vs. 42.3 ± 3.5%, $p = 0.037$). Moreover, *CALR* Ins5 cells showed a higher level of phosphorylated ATM and H2AX compared to *CALR* wild-type cells (87.6 ± 1.2% vs. 42.3 ± 3.5%, $p = 0.032$). These differences were exceptional after cells were given an additional 24 h to repair oxidative stress-induced DNA damage. After 24 h of repair, the control UT-7 cell line was able to repair DNA damage induced by H_2O_2 treatment. On the contrary, *CALR* Del52 and *CALR* Ins5 cells were not able to repair DNA damage, as evidenced by the pATM and pH2AX levels (66.3 ± 1.5% vs. 31.2 ± 0.5%, $p = 0.011$ and 90.5 ± 0.9% vs. 31.2 ± 0.5%, $p = 0.001$, respectively). The SET-2 cell line with *JAK2* mutation showed moderate DNA damage after H_2O_2 treatment and was able to repair it (13.1 ± 0.9% vs. 31.2 ± 0.5%, $p = 0.006$). According to our study results, cells carrying *CALR* 52 bp deletion and 5 bp insertion had a lower capability to repair DNA damage induced by oxidative stress (Figure 15).

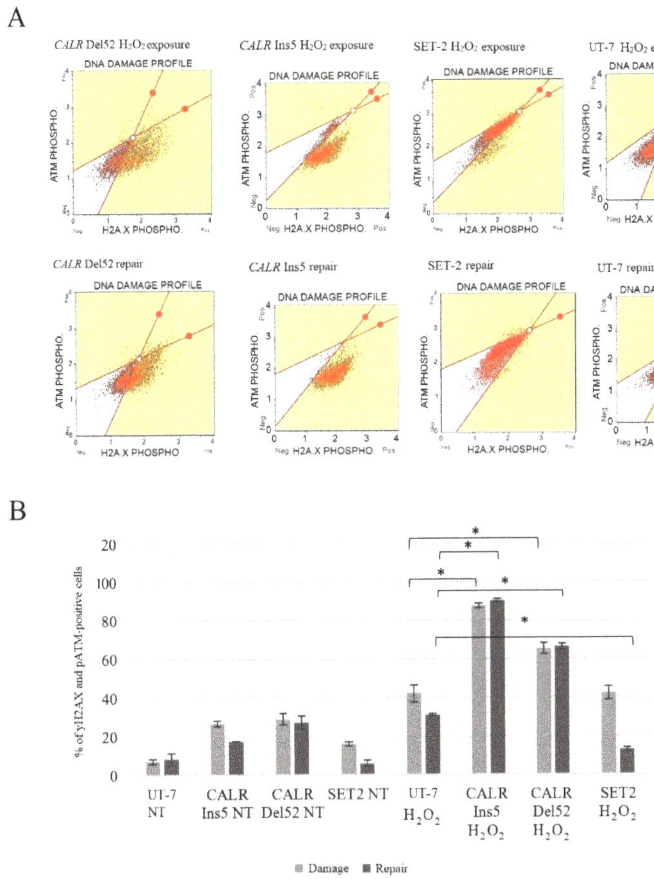

Figure 15. *CALR* mutations impair oxidative stress-induced DNA damage repair. DNA damage in SET-2, *CALR* Del52, *CALR* Ins5, and UT-7 was detected after 24 h of exposure to H_2O_2 and 24 h of repair using the Muse Multi-Color DNA Damage Kit. (**A**) Representative scatterplots of pATM and

pH2AX profiles in *JAK2*-mutated, *CALR*-mutated, and wild-type cells. (**B**) The graph shows the percentage of cells expressing phosphorylated ATM and H2AX. Values show the mean with a standard deviation of at least three experiments performed in triplicate. An asterisk represents $p < 0.05$ vs. control.

Calreticulin plays a role in a variety of biological processes, including cell death. Nevertheless, data on the effects of mutant calreticulin on oxidative stress-induced apoptosis are limited. Therefore, we intended to analyze whether the impaired ability to reduce oxidative stress entails a different ability to induce cell death. Apoptosis was assessed using the Muse Annexin V and Dead Cell Kit.

It was determined that apoptosis was significantly increased in cells harboring the *CALR* 5 bp insertion (78.0 ± 16.4% vs. 50.9 ± 1.4%, $p = 0.012$). In addition, the apoptosis level was higher (53.8 ± 5.9%, $p = 0.063$) in *CALR* Del52 cells, even though it was not statistically significant. On the contrary, SET-2 cells showed a lower level of apoptosis compared to the control UT-7 cell line; however, the difference was not statistically significant (50.0 ± 10.4%, $p = 0.887$ vs. 50.9 ± 1.4%, $p = 0.667$) (Figure 16).

A

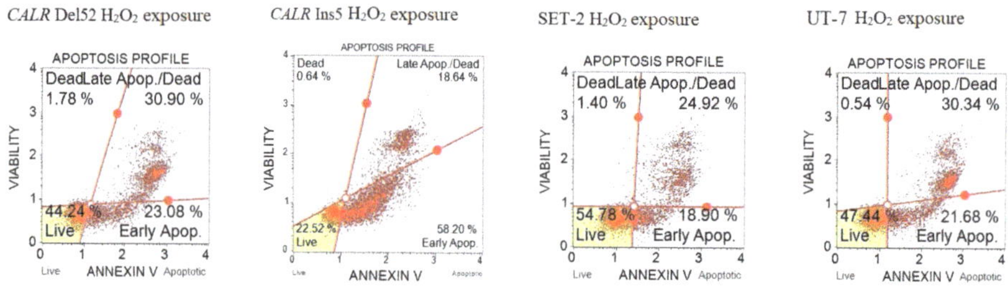

B

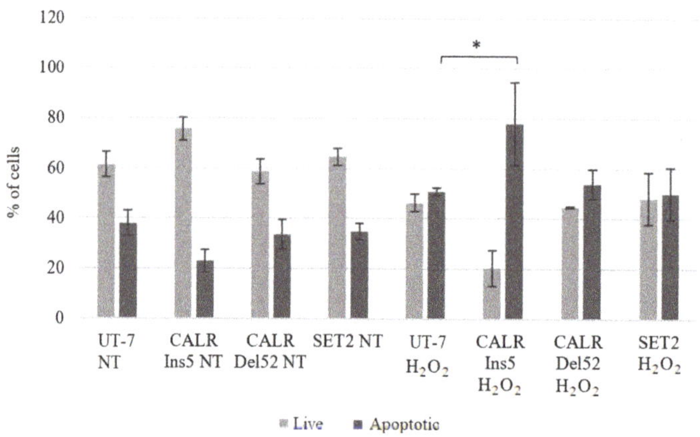

Figure 16. An increase in apoptosis level in *CALR* Ins5 cells after H_2O_2-induced oxidative stress. The evaluation of apoptosis levels in the tested cells was performed after 24 h of exposure to H_2O_2 using the Muse Annexin V and Dead Cell Kit. (**A**) Representative scatter plots of the apoptosis profile are shown. (**B**) The graph shows the percentage of apoptotic cells. Values show the mean with a standard deviation of at least three experiments performed in triplicate. An asterisk represents $p < 0.05$ vs. control.

Lastly, we aimed to analyze the cell cycle distribution after oxidative stress induction in *CALR*-mutated and *JAK2*-mutated cells. Cell cycle machinery is seen in essentially all tumor types and represents a driving force of tumorigenesis; however, to the best of our knowledge, no data show the impact of mutated *CALR* on cell cycle progression in the context of oxidative stress. The analysis of the cell cycle distribution was carried out after 24 h of exposure to H_2O_2 using the Muse Cell Cycle Kit.

It was determined that cells harboring *CALR* 52 bp deletion showed cell cycle arrest at the G2/M phase (Figure 17) compared to the control UT-7 cell line after H_2O_2 treatment (38.3 ± 4.2% vs. 27.3 ± 6.3%, p = 0.038). Furthermore, the H_2O_2 exposure was shown to arrest the cell cycle at the G2/M phase in *CALR* Ins5 cells (42.4 ± 0.7% vs. 27.3 ± 6.3%, p = 0.015). Cell cycle changes were not found in the SET-2 cell line carrying the *JAK2* mutation. Our data suggest that the *CALR* mutation affects not only apoptosis levels but also cell cycle arrest at the G2/M phase after H_2O_2-induced oxidative stress. It is important to note that cell cycle arrest at G2/M blocks cell cycle progression, providing the potential for DNA damage repair [85].

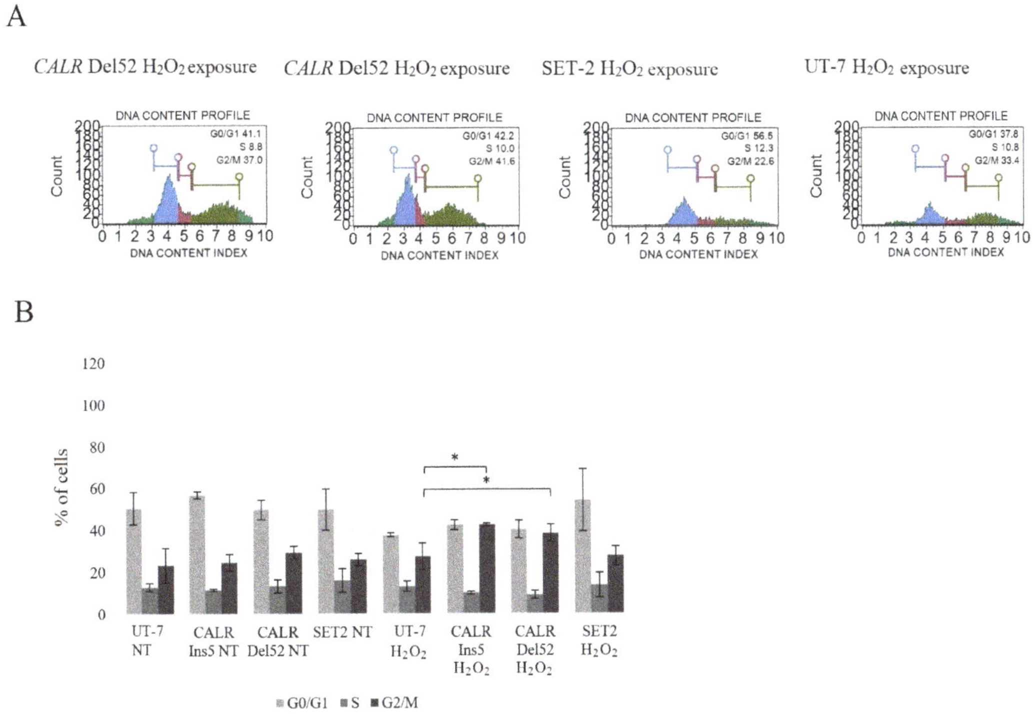

Figure 17. *CALR*-mutated cells cycle arrest at the G2/M phase after H_2O_2-induced oxidative stress. The analysis of the cell cycle was performed after 24 h of exposure to H_2O_2 using a Muse Cell Cycle Kit. (**A**) Representative histograms of cell cycle distribution in the tested cell lines. (**B**) The graph represents the percentage of cell cycle distribution. Values show the mean with a standard deviation of at least three experiments performed in triplicate. An asterisk represents $p < 0.05$ vs. control.

3. Discussion

The role of mutated calreticulin in various biological processes and its association with MPN have recently been analyzed in several studies. However, the involvement of the *CALR* 52 bp deletion and *CALR* 5 bp insertion in the pathogenesis of MPNs has not been fully investigated, and the final conclusions have not been presented. Thus, in our study, we intended to contribute to a deeper analysis of the molecular mechanisms of mutated

CALR. In the first part of our research, we aimed to determine the mutant *CALR* association with JAK/STAT and alternative PI3K/Akt/mTOR and Hedgehog signaling pathways that are related to MPNs.

The dependence of *CALR* Del52, *CALR* Ins5, SET-2, and UT-7 cells on the aforementioned signaling pathways was assessed using the specific inhibitors RAD001 (against mTOR), CYT387 (against JAK1/2), and HPI-1 (against Gli1/2). Subsequently, target gene expression and protein levels of JAK/STAT, PI3K/Akt/mTOR, and Hedgehog signaling pathway components were determined. In more detail, the results that address the antiproliferative effect of inhibitors on SET-2 and UT-7 cell viability have already been published in our previous article [84], but these results are inseparable from our current study research; therefore, a brief discussion and comparison of the previously obtained results is necessary. We found that all specific inhibitors progressively reduced the number of viable cells as the concentration and exposure time increased. It was observed that cells carrying the *CALR* mutation were less resistant to the CYT387 inhibitor than SET-2 cells expressing *JAK2* p.V617F and UT-7 cells with wild-type *JAK2* and *CALR*. Our results indicate that CYT387 inhibited the proliferation of cells harboring *CALR* mutations with the lowest IC50 values compared to RAD001 and HPI-1. Furthermore, *STAT5A* gene expression was elevated in cells with *CALR* 52 bp deletion. Consistent with these data, Western blot analysis showed that phosphorylated STAT5 protein levels were also increased in *CALR* Del52 cells. Although significant *STAT5* and *STAT1* gene expression was not detected, protein quantification revealed that STAT1 and phosphorylated STAT5 levels increased in *CALR* Ins5 cells. Our results agree with those of previous studies showing that the JAK/STAT signaling pathway is activated in cells harboring *CALR* mutations. However, only a few studies have performed dose-response experiments using *CALR*-mutated cells and JAK/STAT inhibitors [10,35,52]. The functional effects of mutated *CALR* were analyzed in murine Ba/F3 and 32D cells [10,52], which were transduced with *CALR* mutations and showed significant accumulation in the absence of interleukin-3. Moreover, transduced cells also demonstrated sensitivity to the JAK2 kinase inhibitor, suggesting that the interleukin-3-independent growth of *CALR*-mutated cells depends on the JAK/STAT pathway. Increased activation of JAK/STAT signaling pathways was also found after analysis of the phosphorylation of STAT5. However, other researchers have reported distinct JAK/STAT signaling signatures in *CALR*-mutated cells. It was determined that MARIMO cells carrying the *CALR* 61 bp deletion were resistant to JAK1/2 inhibitor, compared to *JAK2* p.V617F-mutant cells. The MARIMO cell line independence on JAK/STAT signaling was confirmed with Western blot analysis, where cells showed reduced levels of JAK2, phosphorylated JAK2, STAT5, phosphorylated STAT5, STAT1, phosphorylated STAT1, STAT3, and phosphorylated STAT3. Nevertheless, *JAK2* transcript levels in MARIMO cells were similar to those in *JAK2*-mutated cells, suggesting decreased translation or increased degradation of JAK2 protein [35]. Recently, it has been suggested that the consequences of *CALR* 52 bp deletion and 5 bp insertion for megakaryopoiesis are likely to be mediated by the MAPK and STAT5 pathways accompanied by MPL-dependent activation. The mentioned results were obtained in a complex analysis with $CD34^+$ cells infected with lentiviral constructs expressing mutant *CALR*, MARIMO, and murine cells, Ba/F3 and 32D harboring *CARL* 52 bp deletion and 5 bp insertion [34]. Such differences in the described results could be due to the different cell types used for the experiments, their mutational status, cultivation conditions, and assays that were carried out. For example, the origin of Ba/F3 and 32D cells is different from that of cells that carry *CALR* mutations in humans, i.e., the mentioned suspension cells originated from mice. *CALR* expression and mutations are associated with megakaryocytic cells. Murine Ba/F3 and 32D cells are not characterized by megakaryocytic features associated with *CALR*-mutated MPNs. It is well known that distinct types of cells act differently; therefore, the obtained results can also vary because of the chosen cellular model's additional mutational spectrum, as in the case of the MARIMO cell line where a 61 bp deletion is present. Here, we intended to replicate the cellular model, which is more like the *CALR*-mutated cells found in humans, so we focused on a cell line with megakaryocytic features, i.e., UT-7 cells in which common *CALR* mutations were initiated. Only a few studies have analyzed *CALR's* role of *CALR* in MPN pathogenesis using circulating CD34$^+$ cells or cells cultured from blood or bone marrow samples of patients with MPN [38,44–47]. In agreement with our results, Abba et al. [44] found constitutive phosphorylation of STAT5 in circulating CD34$^+$ cells harboring *CALR* mutations compared to cells with non-mutated *CALR*. Unfortunately, the limited amount of research related to patient cell samples, as well as the distinct types of performed experiments and their targets, leads to the inability to perform an in-depth comparison between our study and others. We have to accept that the 'clinical' cell model is desirable for analyzing MPNs' biological processes and would allow us to find the differences in cell signaling system activation between patient-based and genome-modified cells.

It has been reported that *CALR* mutants are associated with MPL, which leads to the activation of JAK/STAT, PI3K/Akt/mTOR, and MAPK [51,55,56,59,60,86]. We must admit that we performed experiments with cells lacking *MPL* expression, i.e., genome-edited UT-7 cells harboring *CALR* 52 bp deletion or 5 bp insertion. Thus, it can be hypothesized that the JAK/STAT signaling pathway in *CALR*-mutated cells may also be activated in an MPL-independent manner.

The activated PI3K/Akt/mTOR signaling pathway plays one of the main roles in MPN pathogenesis [60]. However, there is little data that shows the impact of mutated *CALR* on PI3K/Akt/mTOR signaling cascade activation. It was found that *CALR* mutants induced phosphorylation of JAK2, STAT1, STAT3, and STAT5, but the PI3K/Akt/mTOR and MAPK pathways were weakly activated [51,55] in the Ba/F3 cell line expressing human *MPL*. Meanwhile, *CALR*-mutant 32D cells without exogenous MPL showed increased activation of AKT [36]. Here, in our study, the association of mutated *CALR* with the PI3K/Akt/mTOR system was assessed, and this complex analysis showed that cells with a *CALR* 52 bp deletion and *CALR* 5 bp insertion are characterized by activated PI3K/Akt/mTOR. *CALR*-mutated cells were more sensitive to RAD001 inhibitors compared to cells with wild-type *CALR*. Moreover, gene expression analysis revealed increased expression of the *RPS6KB1* gene in both *CALR*-mutated cell lines. Although after Western blot analysis, the S6K1 protein levels were not detected in all tested cell lines, significantly increased levels of phosphorylated 4E-BP1 were observed in *CALR* Ins5 cells. These observations indicate that the PI3K/Akt/mTOR signaling pathway might be a new potential target for the treatment of *CALR*-mutated MPN. It is important to note that these are the very first results indicating PI3K/Akt/mTOR signaling activation through mutant *CALR* (together with the lack of MPL expression), so the need arises for further research regarding the association between CALR and the PI3K/Akt/mTOR pathway.

It is necessary to identify alternative cell signaling pathways that might be involved in the pathogenesis of MPN mutant clones, and this could be targeted alone or in combination with JAK/STAT for improved therapeutic benefit [67,87,88]. Several studies have shown that the Hedgehog signaling pathway plays important roles in normal hemopoiesis and the pathogenesis of myeloid malignancies [74,78,87,88]. An increase in the expression of Hh target genes, including *GLI1* and *PTCH1*, was observed by quantitative PCR in granulocytes isolated from MPN patients compared to normal controls. The Hh pathway activity was also found in a murine bone marrow model of PMF [74]. It has been suggested that components of the Hh pathway cooperate with TGFβ, p53, and mTOR-related genes to produce the biological phenotype of PMF [76]. The most recent study was performed using the *C. elegans* model that naturally lacks *JAK2* and *MPL* expression [77]. *CALR* 52 bp deletion and 5 bp insertion were introduced into nematodes using CRISPR/Cas9 methodology. It was found that *CALR*-mutant worms were characterized by the aberrant expression of signal transducers and receptors in the Hh signaling pathway. It was concluded that most of the target genes were downregulated in the *C. elegans* model with *CALR* mutation; mutant calreticulin alone, without JAK2/MPL intervention, can affect transcriptional alterations in Hh signaling. Contrary to these results, a preclinical model showed that granulocytes from MPN patients had elevated Hh target gene expression compared to controls [74], but the *CALR* mutational status was not mentioned in this study. Moreover, Hedgehog ligand inhibitors fully targeted the Hh pathway in murine *JAK2* p.V617F positive cells [89]. Here, we revealed that *CALR*-mutated cells were more sensitive to the Hedgehog inhibitor, HPI-1, compared to the UT-7 cell line used as a control. However, the expression of the *PTCH1* gene, which encodes the target of the Hh signaling pathway, was not detected, and subsequently, the analysis of protein levels was omitted. Therefore, it is important to note that due to inconclusive data, there is a need to expand current experiments analyzing mutant *CALR* and Hedgehog association.

In our previous study, we found that SET-2 cells expressing *JAK2* p. V617F mutation showed increased sensitivity toward the tested agents compared to control UT-7 cells [84]. CYT387 inhibited the proliferation of SET-2 cells with the lowest IC50 compared to RAD001 and HPI-1 inhibitors. In this study, gene expression and Western blot analysis confirmed JAK/STAT signaling pathway activation in SET-2 cells. Elevated STAT1 and STAT5 gene expression and higher STAT1 and STAT5 protein levels were observed. Our findings acknowledged other study results where the rate of *JAK2* mutation-positive cell proliferation, gene expression, and protein levels after JAK/STAT inhibitors exposure, were analyzed [3,64,90–92]. Moreover, the results of our study confirm those of previous reports, suggesting that cells harbor *JAK2* p. The V617F mutation is sensitive to mTOR inhibitors such as RAD001 [3,64]. The IC50 value was greater compared to other studies, but this could be due to different cell cultivation conditions, types of plastics, and assays used for cell viability determination [64]. Nevertheless, the activation of PI3K/Akt/mTOR in SET-2 cells was confirmed by gene expression and protein level analyses, in which elevated *RPS6KB1* gene expression and significant phosphorylation of 4E-BP1 were observed. To date, preclinical data on the potential role of the Hh signaling pathway in MPN with mutated *JAK2* are limited. Only one study showed that the expression of Hh signaling molecules increased up to 100-fold in granulocytes isolated from patients with MPNs [74]. Therefore, cell-based in vitro studies on the effects of Hh pathway inhibitors on MPN cells are warranted. Our previous study was the first to address the antiproliferative effect of HPI-1 on cells carrying *JAK2* mutations. We found that SET-2 cells were significantly more sensitive to HPI-1 inhibitors compared to the wild-type *JAK2* cell line [84]. However, no *PTCH1* gene, which encodes one of the Hh signaling targets, was expressed in SET-2 cells, and subsequently, analysis of protein levels was omitted.

Finally, in our study, we conducted a mutated calreticulin functional analysis. It is known that oxidative stress induces the pathological accumulation of ROS that damages membrane lipids, proteins, and DNA [40,41,81,82,92–94]. As mentioned before, several studies have shown the importance of ROS in MPN pathogenesis; e.g., ROS has one of the major roles in disease progression, as ROS is a mediator of *JAK2* p.V617F-induced DNA damage [79–81]. However, calreticulin plays multiple roles in a variety of cell processes, including responses to oxidative stress [95–97]. It has been determined that *CALR* overexpression increased cell sensitivity to H_2O_2-induced cytotoxicity and played a critical role in oxidative stress-induced apoptosis [97]. Only a few studies have analyzed the effect of mutated *CALR* on oxidative stress in vitro, where *CALR* mutants were expressed in K562 and $CD34^+$ cells [40,41]. Although K562 cells lack *MPL* expression, these cells express the *BCL-ABL1*, and this is the main limitation of using K562 cells as an MPN disease model. Nevertheless, naturally, in MPNs, *CALR* mutations do not occur together with *BCR-ABL1*. Therefore, more accurate conclusions about the association between mutated *CALR* and oxidative stress would be made if *BCR-ABL1* signaling was blocked (e.g., with Imatinib) in the K562 cell line. However, K562 cells expressing mutated *CALR* showed increased ROS levels and increased levels of DNA damage upon oxidative stress exposure to Melittin and Miltirone. In addition, *CALR* mutants were characterized by a decreased ability to reduce intracellular ROS levels and repair oxidative DNA damage compared to *CALR* wild-type K562 cells. Genovese et al. data described how *JAK2* and *CALR* mutations affect oxidative response in $CD34^+$ cells from patients PMF patients and healthy donors [41]. It was determined that ROS increased significantly in both *JAK2*- and *CALR*-mutated cells compared to CD34 + cells from healthy donors. It is important to note that *CALR*-mutated cells showed higher ROS levels than *JAK2*-mutated cells. Moreover, *CALR*-mutated $CD34^+$ cells were unable to reduce ROS levels, while other tested cells efficiently counteracted intracellular ROS accumulation. The results also showed an increase in apoptosis and a greater oxidative stress effect on DNA damage in *CALR*-mutated cells [41]. Here, our study results agreed with the previously mentioned results and showed an association between increased levels of intracellular ROS and mutated *CALR*. Our data indicate higher levels of ROS, apoptosis, and DNA damage compared to the results of Salati et al. and Genovese et al. [40,41]. Moreover, we analyzed cell cycle distribution after H_2O_2-induced oxidative stress, and cell cycle arrest at the G2/M phase in *CALR* Del52 and *CALR* Ins5 cells was determined. This has not been analyzed in previous studies, and our data suggest that the accumulation of G2/M-*CALR*-mutated cells indicates that oxidative stress-induced DNA damage is difficult to repair. The differences in ROS levels, DNA damage, and apoptosis induction may be because of the different cells used in the analysis, as well as the agents used for oxidative stress induction. Salati et al. experiments were carried out using K562 cells carrying *CALR* 52 bp deletion or 5 bp insertion as well as the *BCR-ABL1* variant [40]. Furthermore, the mutation, whether *CALR* 52 bp deletion or *CALR* 5 bp insertion was identified in PMF patients, was not specified in the Genovese et al. study [41]. Therefore, it is not clear which *CALR* mutation has a higher impact on ROS accumulation, apoptosis induction, and oxidative stress-induced DNA damage. In our study, we tried to replicate an MPN cellular model with UT-7 cells after the introduction of *CALR* 52 bp deletion and *CALR* 5 bp insertion. UT-7 cells are not characterized by the expression of activating *BCR-ABL1* signaling or typical mutations that are found to significantly initiate cell proliferation and the pathophysiological state. In the mentioned studies, two main agents were used as oxidative stress inducers, namely H_2O_2 [97] and Melittin [40,41]. Here, we used a well-known and approved oxidative stress inducer H_2O_2, while Melittin is quite a new agent inducing oxidative stress in human suspension cells [98]. Despite differences between the studies that were conducted, the tendency for *CALR* 52 bp deletion and 5 bp insertion to impair native calreticulin function is still present. To sum up, *CALR*-mutated cells are more sensitive to oxidative stress, which leads to increased DNA damage.

Our study provides a broad description of the molecular mechanisms that are activated in cells carrying *CALR* mutations. However, this study has certain limitations that need to be acknowledged. First, analysis related to the presence of a double mutation when both *JAK2* and *CALR* mutations occur could be carried out. Although there are a few cases of MPNs with double mutations, it is still not clear how this affects the pathogenesis of these diseases. Moreover, as with most studies of this type, more signaling pathways with corresponding molecules involved in pathogenic processes can always be investigated. Therefore, it would be useful to investigate the activity of other signaling pathways (e.g., MAPK, Aurora A) in cells with *CALR* 52 bp deletion and 5 bp insertion. In addition, because increased activity of JAK/STAT and PI3K/Akt/mTOR signaling pathways was found in *CALR*-mutated cells, it would be possible to study the response of cells with mutated *CALR* to drugs (e.g., ruxolitinib and anagrelide) that are currently used in the treatment of MPN (here, we used specific inhibitors that are still only at the preclinical stage but effective against targets in the tested signaling pathways). Despite the limitations mentioned, the discussed findings provide a more detailed understanding of the complex biology of mutated calreticulin, which might be used to create new molecularly targeted therapeutic strategies for MPNs in the future.

4. Materials and Methods

4.1. Cell Culture

Cell lines. Suspension cell lines, SET-2 and UT-7, were obtained from The German Collection of Microorganisms and Cell Cultures (DSMZ, Braunschweig, Germany). DSMZ carried out the mentioned cell line authentication. The *JAK2* p.V617F mutation and wild-type *CALR* are characteristics of the SET-2 cell line. SET-2 cells were grown in RPMI-1640 medium (Gibco, Gaithersburg, MD, USA) supplemented with 20% fetal bovine serum (FBS), 100 U/mL penicillin, 100 µg/mL streptomycin, and 2 mM L-glutamine (Gibco, Gaithersburg, MD, USA). The UT-7 cell line exhibited wild-type *CALR*, *JAK2*, and *EPOR*. In addition, UT-7 cells lack *MPL* expression [99,100]. The UT-7 cell line was cultured in α-MEM medium (Gibco, Gaithersburg, MD, USA) supplemented with 20% FBS, 100 U/mL penicillin, 100 µg/mL streptomycin, 2 mM L-glutamine (Gibco, Gaithersburg, MD, USA), and recombinant human granulocyte macrophage-colony stimulating factor (Sigma-Aldrich, St. Louis, MO, USA) at a final concentration of 5 ng/mL in the prepared medium.

DNA constructs and *CALR* gene targeting. CRISPR/Cas9 system was utilized to initiate *CALR* 52 bp deletion and 5 bp insertion in the UT-7 cell line. Megakaryocytes play a central role in the pathogenesis of ET and PMF; therefore, we focused on a cell line with megakaryocytic features, i.e., UT-7 cells. The UT-7 cell line is a good model for examining MPL-independent molecular pathways behind the effect of the *CALR* 52 bp deletion and *CALR* 5 bp insertion [99,100].

The *CALR* gene sequence was obtained from the GenBank sequence collection of the National Center for Biotechnology Information (National Biosciences, Inc., Bethesda, MD, USA). The CRISPR specially developed design tools, *CRISPR* Design from Zhang Lab (https://www.zlab.bio/) and SnapGene (GSL Biotech LLC, Boston, MA, USA), were used to generate single guide RNA (sgRNA) patterns targeting distinct portions of the *CALR* gene.

For the establishment of sgRNA, two targets in the *CALR* gene were chosen, i.e., for each common *CALR* gene mutation, and, subsequently, nucleotide sequences with the sgRNA generating region were produced. Briefly, the nucleotide sequences with the sgRNA encoding pattern were produced, annealed, phosphorylated, and cloned into a human codon-optimized *S. pyogenous* Cas9-sgRNA vector (pSpCas9(BB)-2A-Puro (pX459) V2.0 (#62988) plasmid (Addgene, Teddington, UK). Constructs were introduced by chemical transformation into competent *E. coli* DH5α for cloning purposes using a selectable marker of Ampicillin. Finally, plasmid construct amplification in *E. coli* DH5α was accomplished, and plasmid DNA was extracted and validated.

In parallel, single-stranded oligodeoxynucleotide donor templates were prepared for each *CALR* gene mutation. Single-stranded oligodeoxynucleotide donor templates were used for the endogenous cellular repair pathway, homology-directed repair (HDR), which was employed to repair CRISPR/Cas9-generated double-stranded DNA breaks and subsequently led to precise alterations at the specified genomic location.

Electroporation was applied for UT-7 cell line co-transfection of the generated CRISPR/Cas9 plasmid and HDR donor template. The UT-7 cell line was cultured in T75 flasks (TPP; Trasadingen, Switzerland) and pelleted by centrifugation at 300× *g* for 5 min. It is known that inhibiting non-homologous end joining (NHEJ) or promoting HDR, either genetically or pharmacologically, leads to increased knock-in efficiency. Here, we chose cell cycle synchronization at the S and G2/M phases that are necessary for HDR, using serum-depleted medium because the serum starvation-re-feeding method had no impact on UT-7 cell proliferation. Therefore, UT-7 cells were serum-deprived for 24 h and restimulated to enter the S and G2/M phases by re-feeding cells with 20% serum for 24 h before electroporation. The cell cycle distribution was analyzed using a Muse Cell Cycle Kit (protocol is presented in Section 4.7) at the end of each period. Further, the cells were pelleted and counted using a Neubauer hemocytometer (Weber Scientific, Hamilton, OH, USA) under an optical microscope. UT-7 cells were suspended in laboratory made electroporation medium at a concentration of 16.875 × 10^6 cells/mL. Next, a volume of 50 µL (0.54 × 10^6 cells) was transferred between stainless steel plate electrodes separated by a 2 mm gap. The final concentration of the pRJ1-del52 and pRJ3-ins5 plasmid constructs was 0.295 µg/mL, whereas the *CALR* mutation-specific HDR template concentration was 4 µM. A BTX T820 electroporator (Harvard Apparatus) (Artisan Technology Group, Champaign, IL, USA) was used for pulsing and changing the voltage and pulse duration. A square wave 1 HV (i.e., high voltage) pulse, 1400 V/cm pulse strength, and 250 µs pulse duration were applied. The electroporation regimen was carried out at room temperature. After pulsing, the cells were transferred into 24-well (TPP; Trasadingen, Switzerland) plates and left for 20 min for recovery. After the recovery period, UT-7 cells were seeded into a 24-well plate, which was supplemented with a culture medium of up to 450 μL. Afterward, the plates were placed in a cell culture incubator for 48 h.

Thereafter, the transfection medium was replaced with a selective medium containing 1 μg/mL puromycin (Gibco, Gaithersburg, MD, USA), and a single clone isolation method was used to select each cell that carried a *CALR* 52 bp deletion and *CALR* 5 bp insertion. A fresh puromycin-containing medium was changed every other day, and stable cell colonies with initiated specific *CALR* mutations were selected and grown to the amounts needed for further applications.

A PCR-based amplicon length differentiation assay was applied to confirm the presence of the *CALR* 52 bp deletion and *CALR* 5 bp insertion in the genome of a putative genome-modified cell line [101].

All tested cell lines were grown in a standard cell culture incubator maintained at 37 °C, 100% relative humidity, and 5% CO_2. Cell morphology and number were routinely checked using an Olympus CK40 phase contrast microscope (Olympus Corporation, Tokyo, Japan).

4.2. Cell Viability Assays

Signaling system inhibitors. The mTOR signaling inhibitor RAD001 (Everolimus) (targeting TORC1) was purchased from Alfa Aesar (Alfa Aesar, Haverhill, MA, USA). CYT387 (Momelotinib), an ATP-competitive JAK1/JAK2 inhibitor (Abcam, Cambridge, UK), was also used in this study. Hedgehog signaling pathway inhibitor-1 (HPI-1) (active against Gli1/Gli2) was purchased from Sigma-Aldrich (Sigma-Aldrich, St. Louis, MO, USA). All the mentioned inhibitors were diluted at room temperature with 100% dimethylsulfoxide (DMSO) (Sigma-Aldrich, St. Louis, MO, USA,) to a concentration of 10 mM. The prepared inhibitor solutions were stored at −20 °C and used only once in the experiments.

AlamarBlue test. Cell proliferation was analyzed by the colorimetric alamarBlue cell viability assay (Thermo Fisher Scientific, Waltham, MA, USA) using a Tecan Sunrise™ plate reader (Tecan, Manedorf, Switzerland). 24 h before the experiment, 5000 cells were seeded into a 96-well plate (Greiner CELSTAR®, Kremsmünster, Germany). Cells were exposed to specific inhibitors (or an appropriate amount of the inhibitor solvent DMSO) for 24, 48, and 72 h. Following the inhibitor incubation, 10% of the well's volume of alamarBlue reagent was added, and the plates were then placed in the incubator, which was maintained at 37 °C with 5% CO_2 and 100% relative humidity. Absorbance was measured at wavelengths of 550 nm and 620 nm, and subsequently, cell viability was assessed using the formula provided in the manufacturer's protocol. Three independent experiments were performed with five replicates per experiment. Cell viability was normalized to that of the control cells.

Trypan exclusion assay. A trypan dye solution (Gibco, Gaithersburg, MD, USA) was utilized to assess the viability of the cells. 2×10^5 cells were seeded into 35 mm diameter Petri plates (TPP; Trasadingen, Switzerland) 24 h before the experiment. The cells were treated with suitable doses of inhibitors of particular signaling systems (or inhibitor solvent DMSO) at 24, 48, and 72 h. Following incubation, the cells were collected by centrifugation (300 × *g* for 5 min) and 90 μL of 0.4% trypan blue dye was added to 10 μL of the cell suspension. Using an Olympus CK40 microscope (Olympus Corporation, Tokyo, Japan) and a Neubauer hemocytometer chamber, the viability of the cells was evaluated. Three separate experiments were carried out. For every experiment, three replicates were performed. Cell viability was normalized to control cells.

The concentration at which 50% inhibition (IC50) of cell proliferation occurred was calculated using Excel add-in ED50V10.

4.3. RNA Extraction and Reverse Transcription-Quantitative PCR

The JAK/STAT, PI3K/Akt/mTOR, and Hedgehog signaling components *EIF4EBP1*, *RPS6KB1*, *STAT1*, *STAT5A*, and *PTCH1* genes were included in the gene expression analysis.

The expression of target genes in SET-2, *CALR* Del52, and *CALR* Ins5 cells was evaluated using reverse transcription-quantitative PCR (RT-qPCR). The UT-7 cell line was used as a control. RNA isolation was performed with the RNeasy Mini Kit (Qiagen, Hilden, Germany) using 1×10^6 cells, following the manufacturer's recommendations. RNA quantity was assessed using a Thermo Scientific™ Multiskan Sky™ Microplate Spectrophotometer (Thermo Fisher Scientific, Waltham, MA, USA). RNA integrity was analyzed by agarose gel electrophoresis before cDNA synthesis. RNA samples were stored at −80 °C until use.

Two micrograms of RNA was used for cDNA synthesis using the High-Capacity cDNA Reverse Transcription Kit (Applied Biosystems, Foster City, CA, USA), and gene expression was measured using TaqMan Expression Assays (*EIF4EBP1* Hs00607050_m1, *RPS6KB1* Hs00356367_m1, *STAT1* Hs01013996_m1, *STAT5A* Hs00234181_m1, and *PTCH1* Hs00181117_m1) (Invitrogen, Waltham, MA, USA). According to the manufacturers' recommendations, RT-qPCR was performed using a 7500 Fast Real-time PCR system (Applied Biosystems, Foster City, CA, USA). Utilizing the comparative Ct method, expression data were evaluated after being normalized to the expression levels of the *ACTB* (Invitrogen, Waltham, MA, USA) gene.

4.4. Protein Extraction and Western Blot Analysis

1×10^6 cells/well were seeded into 6-well (TPP; Trasadingen, Switzerland) plates for protein level analysis. The cells were lysed using RIPA lysis buffer (Abcam, Cambridge, UK) with proteinase (Sigma-Aldrich, St. Louis, MO, USA) and phosphatase (Sigma-Aldrich, St. Louis, MO, USA) inhibitors. After removal of the cell culture medium by centrifugation at 300× *g* for 5 min, the cells were washed twice with cold 1X PBS, collected by centrifugation, and further incubated with 100 μL RIPA buffer for 20 min. After incubation, the cell lysate was centrifuged at 10,000× *g* for 20 min at 4 °C to pellet the cell debris. The supernatant was collected, and protein concentration was measured using the Pierce™ BCA Protein Assay Kit (Thermo Fisher Scientific, Waltham, MA, USA) and Thermo Scientific™ Multiskan Sky™ Microplate Spectrophotometer (Thermo Fisher Scientific, Waltham, MA, USA) at 570 nm according to the manufacturer's recommendations. Protein samples were stored at −20 °C until use.

After denaturing the samples at +70 °C, 40 μg of protein was loaded onto NuPage™ 4–12% Bis-Tris Plus Gels (Invitrogen, Waltham, MA, USA) for vertical protein electrophoresis. After electrophoresis, the proteins were transferred to a PVDF membrane (Invitrolon™ PVDF/Filter Paper Sandwich, Invitrogen, Waltham, MA, USA) using a semi-wet transfer unit Mini Blot module (Invitrogen, Waltham, MA, USA). Further, the membrane was blocked with a blocking buffer and incubated overnight at +4 °C with a primary antibody against phospho-STAT1 Tyr701 (#33-3400, Invitrogen, Waltham, MA, USA), STAT1 (#SC-464, Santa Cruz Biotechnology, Dallas, TX, USA), phospho-STAT5 Tyr694 (#71-6900, Invitrogen, Waltham, MA, USA), STAT5 (#44-368G, Invitrogen, Waltham, MA, USA), phospho-4E-BP1 Ser65 (#MA-14948, Invitrogen, Waltham, MA, USA), 4E-BP1 (#9644, Cell signaling Technology, Danvers, MA, USA), phospho-S6K1 Thr389 (#9205, Cell signaling Technology, Danvers, MA, USA), phospho-S6K1 Thr389 (#9234S, Cell signaling Technology, Danvers, MA, USA) and S6K1 (#2708S, Cell signaling Technology, Danvers, MA, USA), and β-actin (#AM-4302, Invitrogen, Waltham, MA, USA). After washing with 1X Pierce™ TBS Tween20 buffer (Thermo Fisher Scientific, Waltham, MA, USA), the blots were incubated with the relevant Anti-Rabbit HRP-conjugated, Anti-Mouse HRP-conjugated, or Anti-Mouse Alkaline-Phosphatase-conjugated secondary antibody solution (Invitrogen, Waltham, MA, USA). Before detection, the blots were washed with 1X Pierce™ TBS Tween20 buffer and distilled water. The proteins were detected with Super Signal™ West Pico PLUS Chemiluminescent Substrate, SuperSignal™ West Atto Ultimate Sensitivity Substrate (Thermo Fisher Scientific, Waltham, MA, USA), or Novex™ AP Chemiluminescent Substrate (CDPStar™) (Invitrogen, Waltham, MA, USA) for the detection of horseradish peroxidase (HRP) and alkaline phosphatase (AP), respectively, according to the manufacturer's recommendations. Chemiluminescent images were visualized using the ChemiDoc™ XRS+ system (Bio-Rad

Laboratories, Hercules, CA, USA) and analyzed with ImageLab 6.0.1 Software (Bio-Rad Laboratories, Hercules, CA, USA). β-actin protein was used as a loading control for the normalization of the target protein expression level.

4.5. Detection of Intracellular Reactive Oxygen Species

Hydrogen peroxide (H_2O_2) was added to the cell culture to induce oxidative stress. Intracellular reactive oxygen species (ROS) were evaluated using a flow cytometry-based method. 24 h before the experiment, 1×10^6 cells were seeded in a 6-well plate. For 24 h, the cells were subjected to an H_2O_2 solution (concentration 400 μM and 0 μM). The cells subjected to 500 μM H_2O_2 solution served as a positive control to calibrate the instrument parameters. The Muse Oxidative Stress Kit (Merck Millipore, Burlington, MA, USA) was used to assess cell populations under oxidative stress, following the manufacturer's instructions. Subsequently, cell analysis was performed, and the signal was detected using a Muse Cell Analyzer (Merck Millipore, Burlington, MA, USA).

The ability of the cells to reduce oxidative stress after H_2O_2 exposure was also evaluated. Cells exposed to H_2O_2 were transferred to a medium without hydrogen peroxide and incubated for 24 h. ROS levels were determined according to a previously described protocol. The software package Muse 1.4 was utilized to ascertain the percentage of cells experiencing oxidative stress.

4.6. Apoptosis Level Analysis

24 h before the experiment, 2×10^5 cells were seeded in a 6-well plate. Cells were exposed to H_2O_2 (concentration 0 and 400 μM) solution for 24 h. After exposure, cell apoptosis analysis was performed using the Muse Annexin V and Dead Cell Kit (Merck Millipore, Burlington, MA, USA) according to the manufacturer's recommended protocol. Cell analysis was performed, and the signal was detected using a Muse Cell Analyzer (Merck Millipore, Burlington, MA, USA). The obtained data were analyzed using the Muse 1.4 software package.

4.7. Cell Cycle Assay

The changes in cell cycle distribution were assessed with the Muse Cell Analyzer using the Muse Cell Cycle Kit (Merck Millipore, Burlington, MA, USA). Cells were seeded in a 6-well plate 24 h before the experiment (1×10^6 cells per well). The cells were exposed to H_2O_2 (concentration 0 and 400 μM) solution for 24 h. Next, the analysis of the cell cycle was performed according to the manufacturer's protocol. The signal was detected with a cell analyzer, and the results were analyzed using the Muse 1.4 software package.

4.8. DNA Damage Measurement

The Muse Multi-Color DNA Damage Kit (Merck Millipore, Burlington, MA, USA) was used for DNA damage assessment. 24 h before the experiment, 1.5×10^6 cells were seeded in a 6-well plate. Cells were exposed to H_2O_2 (concentration 0 and 400 μM) solution for 24 h. Cells exposed to 10 μM etoposide were used as a positive DNA damage control. After exposure, analysis of DNA damage was performed according to the manufacturer's protocol. The signal was detected using the Muse Cell Analyzer, and the results were analyzed using the Muse 1.4 software package.

The ability of cells to repair DNA damage caused by oxidative stress was also assessed. The cells that were exposed to H_2O_2 were transferred to a medium without the addition of hydrogen peroxide and incubated for an additional 24 h, and DNA lesions were assessed according to a previously described protocol.

4.9. Statistical Analysis

IBM SPSS Statistics 22.0 (IBM Corp., Armonk, NY, USA) software was used to perform statistical analysis. Results were determined to be normally distributed using the Shapiro–Wilk test for normality. Data were analyzed using an independent sample *t*-test and one-way analysis of variance (ANOVA), followed by a post-hoc Tukey's multiple comparison test when appropriate. All experiments were repeated at least three times, with three to five replicates. All data are shown as the means with standard deviation (S.D.), while the $p < 0.05$ value was considered statistically significant.

5. Conclusions

Our research provides novel evidence on *CALR*'s association with JAK/STAT, PI3K/Akt/mTOR, and Hedgehog signaling pathways that are important in MPN pathogenesis. Our data indicate that the JAK/STAT and PI3K/Akt/mTOR signaling pathways are activated in cells carrying the *CALR* 52 bp deletion and *CALR* 5 bp insertion. To unravel the MPL-independent mechanisms underlying the effect of *CALR* mutations, we performed experiments in a cell culture model lacking MPL expression. This research is unique because most studies have analyzed mutant calreticulin when *MPL* expression is present. We determined that the activation of the mentioned signaling pathways does not necessarily depend on the interaction between CALR and MPL. We also showed that *CALR* gene mutations impair physiological calreticulin function, leading to reduced responses to oxidative stress and DNA damage. Functional analysis revealed that the accumulation of G2/M-*CALR*-mutated cells indicates that oxidative stress-induced DNA damage is difficult to repair. The mentioned cell cycle delay has not been shown in other studies analyzing mutated calreticulin. Taken together, this study contributes to a deeper understanding of the specific molecular mechanisms underlying *CALR*-mutated myeloproliferative neoplasms.

Supplementary Materials: The following supporting information can be downloaded at https://www.mdpi.com/article/10.3390/ijms25189873/s1.

Author Contributions: Conceptualization, R.V., B.J., D.L., S.Š., E.J. and R.U. Methodology, R.V. and B.J.; Formal analysis, R.V. Investigation, R.V., B.J. and D.L.; Resources, R.V., B.J., D.L., S.Š., E.J. and R.U. Data Curation, R.V. Writing—Original draft preparation, R.V. Writing—Review and Editing, B.J., D.L., S.Š., E.J. and R.U. Visualization, R.V.; Supervision, S.Š., E.J. and R.U. Project Administration, S.Š., E.J. and R.U. Funding Acquisition, S.Š, E.J. and R.U. All authors have read and agreed to the published version of the manuscript.

Funding: This research received no external funding.

Institutional Review Board Statement: Not applicable.

Informed Consent Statement: Not applicable.

Data Availability Statement: The data are contained in the article or Supplementary Material. Further inquiries can be directed to the corresponding author.

Acknowledgments: We would like to express our gratitude to Virginijus Šikšnys and Tautvydas Karvelis from Vilnius University for introducing us to the CRISPR/Cas9 genome editing system and allowing us to perform our experiments in their laboratory.

Conflicts of Interest: The authors declare no conflicts of interest.

References

1. Thapa, B.; Fazal, S.; Parsi, M.; Rogers, H.J. *Myeloproliferative Neoplasms*; StatPearls Publishing: Treasure Island, FL, USA, 2024.
2. Greenfield, G.; McMullin, M.F.; Mills, K. Molecular pathogenesis of the myeloproliferative neoplasms. *J. Hematol. Oncol.* **2021**, *14*, 103. [CrossRef] [PubMed]
3. Bartalucci, N.; Tozzi, L.; Bogani, C.; Martinelli, S.; Rotunno, G.; Villeval, J.; Vannucchi, A.M. Co-targeting the PI3K/mTOR and JAK2 signalling pathways produces synergistic activity against myeloproliferative neoplasms. *J. Cell Mol. Med.* **2013**, *17*, 1385–1396. [CrossRef] [PubMed]
4. Grinfeld, J.; Nangalia, J.; Green, A.R. Molecular determinants of pathogenesis and clinical phenotype in myeloproliferative neoplasms. *Haematologica* **2017**, *102*, 7–17. [CrossRef] [PubMed]
5. Allahverdi, N.; Yassin, M.; Ibrahim, M. Environmental Factors, Lifestyle Risk Factors, and Host Characteristics Associated with Philadelphia Negative Myeloproliferative Neoplasm: A Systematic Review. *Cancer Control* **2021**, *28*, 10732748211046802. [CrossRef]

6. James, C.; Ugo, V.; Le Couédic, J.; Staerk, J.; Delhommeau, F.; Lacout, C.; Garçon, L.; Raslova, H.; Berger, R.; Bennaceur-Griscelli, A.; et al. A unique clonal JAK2 mutation leading to constitutive signalling causes polycythaemia vera. *Nature* **2005**, *434*, 1144–1148. [CrossRef]
7. Pietra, D.; Li, S.; Brisci, A.; Passamonti, F.; Rumi, E.; Theocharides, A.; Ferrari, M.; Gisslinger, H.; Kralovics, R.; Cremonesi, L.; et al. Somatic mutations of JAK2 exon 12 in patients with JAK2 (V617F)-negative myeloproliferative disorders. *Blood* **2008**, *111*, 1686–1689. [CrossRef]
8. Scott, L.M.; Tong, W.; Levine, R.L.; Scott, M.A.; Beer, P.A.; Stratton, M.R.; Futreal, P.A.; Erber, W.N.; McMullin, M.F.; Harrison, C.N.; et al. JAK2 exon 12 mutations in polycythemia vera and idiopathic erythrocytosis. *N. Engl. J. Med.* **2007**, *356*, 459–468. [CrossRef]
9. Barbui, T.; Barosi, G.; Birgegard, G.; Cervantes, F.; Finazzi, G.; Griesshammer, M.; Harrison, C.; Hasselbalch, H.C.; Hehlmann, R.; Hoffman, R.; et al. Philadelphia-negative classical myeloproliferative neoplasms: Critical concepts and management recommendations from European LeukemiaNet. *J. Clin. Oncol.* **2011**, *29*, 761–770. [CrossRef]
10. Klampfl, T.; Gisslinger, H.; Harutyunyan, A.S.; Nivarthi, H.; Rumi, E.; Milosevic, J.D.; Them, N.C.C.; Berg, T.; Gisslinger, B.; Pietra, D.; et al. Somatic mutations of calreticulin in myeloproliferative neoplasms. *N. Engl. J. Med.* **2013**, *369*, 2379–2390. [CrossRef]
11. Kralovics, R.; Passamonti, F.; Buser, A.S.; Teo, S.; Tiedt, R.; Passweg, J.R.; Tichelli, A.; Cazzola, M.; Skoda, R.C. A gain-of-function mutation of JAK2 in myeloproliferative disorders. *N. Engl. J. Med.* **2005**, *352*, 1779–1790. [CrossRef]
12. Pardanani, A.D.; Levine, R.L.; Lasho, T.; Pikman, Y.; Mesa, R.A.; Wadleigh, M.; Steensma, D.P.; Elliott, M.A.; Wolanskyj, A.P.; Hogan, W.J.; et al. MPL515 mutations in myeloproliferative and other myeloid disorders: A study of 1182 patients. *Blood* **2006**, *108*, 3472–3476. [CrossRef] [PubMed]
13. Barbui, T.; Thiele, J.; Gisslinger, H.; Kvasnicka, H.M.; Vannucchi, A.M.; Guglielmelli, P.; Orazi, A.; Tefferi, A. The 2016 WHO classification and diagnostic criteria for myeloproliferative neoplasms: Document summary and in-depth discussion. *Blood Cancer J.* **2018**, *8*, 15. [CrossRef] [PubMed]
14. Lu, X.; Chang, R. *Polycythemia Vera*; StatPearls Publishing: Treasure Island, FL, USA, 2024.
15. Tefferi, A.; Barbui, T. Polycythemia vera and essential thrombocythemia: 2017 update on diagnosis, risk-stratification, and management. *Am. J. Hematol.* **2017**, *92*, 94–108. [CrossRef] [PubMed]
16. Pardanani, A.; Tefferi, A. Definition and management of ruxolitinib treatment failure in myelofibrosis. *Blood Cancer J.* **2014**, *4*, e268. [CrossRef]
17. Araki, M.; Komatsu, N. The role of calreticulin mutations in myeloproliferative neoplasms. *Int. J. Hematol.* **2020**, *111*, 200–205. [CrossRef]
18. Nangalia, J.; Massie, C.E.; Baxter, E.J.; Nice, F.L.; Gundem, G.; Wedge, D.C.; Avezov, E.; Li, J.; Kollmann, K.; Kent, D.G.; et al. Somatic CALR mutations in myeloproliferative neoplasms with nonmutated JAK2. *N. Engl. J. Med.* **2013**, *369*, 2391–2405. [CrossRef]
19. Mansier, O.; Luque Paz, D.; Ianotto, J.; Le Bris, Y.; Chauveau, A.; Boyer, F.; Conejero, C.; Fitoussi, O.; Riou, J.; Adiko, D.; et al. Clinical and biological characterization of MPN patients harboring two driver mutations, a French intergroup of myeloproliferative neoplasms (FIM) study. *Am. J. Hematol.* **2018**, *93*, E84–E86. [CrossRef]
20. Merlinsky, T.R.; Levine, R.L.; Pronier, E. Unfolding the Role of Calreticulin in Myeloproliferative Neoplasm Pathogenesis. *Clin. Cancer Res.* **2019**, *25*, 2956–2962. [CrossRef]
21. Hammarén, H.M.; Virtanen, A.T.; Raivola, J.; Silvennoinen, O. The regulation of JAKs in cytokine signaling and its breakdown in disease. *Cytokine* **2019**, *118*, 48–63. [CrossRef]
22. Tsutsumi, N.; Masoumi, Z.; James, S.C.; Tucker, J.A.; Winkelmann, H.; Grey, W.; Picton, L.K.; Moss, L.; Wilson, S.C.; Caveney, N.A.; et al. Structure of the thrombopoietin-MPL receptor complex is a blueprint for biasing hematopoiesis. *Cell* **2023**, *186*, 4189–4203.e22. [CrossRef]
23. Amarante-Mendes, G.P.; Rana, A.; Datoguia, T.S.; Hamerschlak, N.; Brumatti, G. BCR-ABL1 Tyrosine Kinase Complex Signaling Transduction: Challenges to Overcome Resistance in Chronic Myeloid Leukemia. *Pharmaceutics* **2022**, *14*, 215. [CrossRef] [PubMed]
24. Lu, Y.; Weng, W.; Lee, H. Functional roles of calreticulin in cancer biology. *Biomed Res. Int.* **2015**, *2015*, 526524. [CrossRef] [PubMed]
25. Jiang, Y.; Dey, S.; Matsunami, H. Calreticulin: Roles in cell-surface protein expression. *Membranes* **2014**, *4*, 630–641. [CrossRef] [PubMed]
26. Langabeer, S.E. CALR mutations in myeloproliferative neoplasms: An unfolding story. *EXCLI J.* **2020**, *19*, 1399–1400.
27. Lasho, T.L.; Elliott, M.A.; Pardanani, A.; Tefferi, A. CALR mutation studies in chronic neutrophilic leukemia. *Am. J. Hematol.* **2014**, *89*, 450. [CrossRef]
28. Aleem, A.; Algahtani, A.; Alshaman, L.; Aldawsari, N.; Algahtani, F.; Alzahrani, M.; Alotaibi, G.; Alturki, S.; Iqbal, Z. Clinical and Pathologic Characteristics of Essential Thrombocythemia (ET) Patients Harboring Calreticulin (CALR) Mutations. *Blood* **2022**, *140*, 12282–12283. [CrossRef]
29. Rumi, E.; Pietra, D.; Ferretti, V.; Klampfl, T.; Harutyunyan, A.S.; Milosevic, J.D.; Them, N.C.C.; Berg, T.; Elena, C.; Casetti, I.C.; et al. JAK2 or CALR mutation status defines subtypes of essential thrombocythemia with substantially different clinical course and outcomes. *Blood* **2014**, *123*, 1544–1551. [CrossRef]

30. Andrikovics, H.; Krahling, T.; Balassa, K.; Halm, G.; Bors, A.; Koszarska, M.; Batai, A.; Dolgos, J.; Csomor, J.; Egyed, M.; et al. Distinct clinical characteristics of myeloproliferative neoplasms with calreticulin mutations. *Haematologica* **2014**, *99*, 1184–1190. [CrossRef]
31. How, J.; Hobbs, G.S.; Mullally, A. Mutant calreticulin in myeloproliferative neoplasms. *Blood* **2019**, *134*, 2242–2248. [CrossRef]
32. Leonard, W.J.; O'Shea, J.J. Jaks and STATs: Biological implications. *Annu. Rev. Immunol.* **1998**, *16*, 293–322. [CrossRef]
33. Morales-Herrejón, R.; Pérez-Contreras, V.A.; Cortés-Penagos, C. Mutations in CALR gene and its role in the diagnosis and prognosis of chronic myeloproliferative neoplasms. *Rev. Hematol. Mex.* **2021**, *22*, 88–96.
34. Yoshida, H.; Kondo, M.; Ichihashi, T.; Hashimoto, N.; Inazawa, J.; Ohno, R.; Naoe, T. A novel myeloid cell line, Marimo, derived from therapy-related acute myeloid leukemia during treatment of essential thrombocythemia: Consistent chromosomal abnormalities and temporary C-MYC gene amplification. *Cancer Genet. Cytogenet.* **1998**, *100*, 21–24. [CrossRef] [PubMed]
35. Kollmann, K.; Nangalia, J.; Warsch, W.; Quentmeier, H.; Bench, A.; Boyd, E.; Scott, M.; Drexler, H.G.; Green, A.R. MARIMO cells harbor a CALR mutation but are not dependent on JAK2/STAT5 signaling. *Leukemia* **2015**, *29*, 494–497. [CrossRef]
36. Kollmann, K.; Warsch, W.; Gonzalez-Arias, C.; Nice, F.L.; Avezov, E.; Milburn, J.; Li, J.; Dimitropoulou, D.; Biddie, S.; Wang, M.; et al. A novel signalling screen demonstrates that CALR mutations activate essential MAPK signalling and facilitate megakaryocyte differentiation. *Leukemia* **2017**, *31*, 934–944. [CrossRef] [PubMed]
37. Han, L.; Czech, J.; Maurer, A.; Brümmendorf, T.H.; Chatain, N.; Koschmieder, S. Mutant NRAS Q61K is responsible for MAPK pathway activation in the MARIMO cell line and renders these cells independent of the CALR-MPL-JAK2-STAT5 pathway. *Leukemia* **2018**, *32*, 2087–2090. [CrossRef] [PubMed]
38. Ibarra, J.; Elbanna, Y.A.; Kurylowicz, K.; Ciboddo, M.; Greenbaum, H.S.; Arellano, N.S.; Rodriguez, D.; Evers, M.; Bock-Hughes, A.; Liu, C.; et al. Type I but Not Type II Calreticulin Mutations Activate the IRE1α/XBP1 Pathway of the Unfolded Protein Response to Drive Myeloproliferative Neoplasms. *Blood Cancer Discov.* **2022**, *3*, 298–315. [CrossRef]
39. Stein, H.; Bob, R.; Dürkop, H.; Erck, C.; Kämpfe, D.; Kvasnicka, H.M.; Martens, H.; Roth, A.; Streubel, A. A new monoclonal antibody (CAL2) detects CALRETICULIN mutations in formalin-fixed and paraffin-embedded bone marrow biopsies. *Leukemia* **2016**, *30*, 131–135. [CrossRef]
40. Salati, S.; Genovese, E.; Carretta, C.; Zini, R.; Bartalucci, N.; Prudente, Z.; Pennucci, V.; Ruberti, S.; Rossi, C.; Rontauroli, S.; et al. Calreticulin Ins5 and Del52 mutations impair unfolded protein and oxidative stress responses in K562 cells expressing CALR mutants. *Sci. Rep.* **2019**, *9*, 10558. [CrossRef]
41. Genovese, E.; Mirabile, M.; Rontauroli, S.; Sartini, S.; Fantini, S.; Tavernari, L.; Maccaferri, M.; Guglielmelli, P.; Bianchi, E.; Parenti, S.; et al. On Behalf Of The Mynerva MYeloid NEoplasms Research Venture Airc, null The Response to Oxidative Damage Correlates with Driver Mutations and Clinical Outcome in Patients with Myelofibrosis. *Antioxidants* **2022**, *11*, 113. [CrossRef]
42. Baty, R.S. Protective effect of Bosutinib with caspase inhibitors on human K562 cells. *Saudi J. Biol. Sci.* **2022**, *29*, 2323–2328. [CrossRef]
43. Yin, H.; Kanasty, R.L.; Eltoukhy, A.A.; Vegas, A.J.; Dorkin, J.R.; Anderson, D.G. Non-viral vectors for gene-based therapy. *Nat. Rev. Genet.* **2014**, *15*, 541–555. [CrossRef] [PubMed]
44. Abbà, C.; Campanelli, R.; Catarsi, P.; Villani, L.; Abbonante, V.; Sesta, M.A.; Barosi, G.; Rosti, V.; Massa, M. Constitutive STAT5 phosphorylation in CD34+ cells of patients with primary myelofibrosis: Correlation with driver mutation status and disease severity. *PLoS ONE* **2019**, *14*, e0220189. [CrossRef] [PubMed]
45. Feldman, T.; Bercovich, A.; Moskovitz, Y.; Chapal-Ilani, N.; Mitchell, A.; Medeiros, J.J.F.; Biezuner, T.; Kaushansky, N.; Minden, M.D.; Gupta, V.; et al. Recurrent deletions in clonal hematopoiesis are driven by microhomology-mediated end joining. *Nat. Commun.* **2021**, *12*, 2455. [CrossRef] [PubMed]
46. Jia, R.; Kutzner, L.; Koren, A.; Runggatscher, K.; Májek, P.; Müller, A.C.; Schuster, M.; Bock, C.; Loizou, J.I.; Kubicek, S.; et al. High-throughput drug screening identifies the ATR-CHK1 pathway as a therapeutic vulnerability of CALR mutated hematopoietic cells. *Blood Cancer J.* **2021**, *11*, 137. [CrossRef]
47. Anonymous. Abstract Book for the 27th Congress of the European Hematology Association. *HemaSphere* **2022**, *6*, 1. [CrossRef]
48. Owen, K.L.; Brockwell, N.K.; Parker, B.S. JAK-STAT Signaling: A Double-Edged Sword of Immune Regulation and Cancer Progression. *Cancers* **2019**, *11*, 2002. [CrossRef]
49. Küppers, R. New insights in the biology of Hodgkin lymphoma. *Hematol. Am. Soc. Hematol. Educ. Program* **2012**, *2012*, 328–334. [CrossRef]
50. Baxter, E.J.; Scott, L.M.; Campbell, P.J.; East, C.; Fourouclas, N.; Swanton, S.; Vassiliou, G.S.; Bench, A.J.; Boyd, E.M.; Curtin, N.; et al. Acquired mutation of the tyrosine kinase JAK2 in human myeloproliferative disorders. *Lancet* **2005**, *365*, 1054–1061. [CrossRef]
51. Chachoua, I.; Pecquet, C.; El-Khoury, M.; Nivarthi, H.; Albu, R.; Marty, C.; Gryshkova, V.; Defour, J.; Vertenoeil, G.; Ngo, A.; et al. Thrombopoietin receptor activation by myeloproliferative neoplasm associated calreticulin mutants. *Blood* **2016**, *127*, 1325–1335. [CrossRef]
52. Han, L.; Schubert, C.; Köhler, J.; Schemionek, M.; Isfort, S.; Brümmendorf, T.H.; Koschmieder, S.; Chatain, N. Calreticulin-mutant proteins induce megakaryocytic signaling to transform hematopoietic cells and undergo accelerated degradation and Golgi-mediated secretion. *J. Hematol. Oncol.* **2016**, *9*, 45. [CrossRef]
53. Baur, J.A.; Sinclair, D.A. Therapeutic potential of resveratrol: The in vivo evidence. *Nat. Rev. Drug Discov.* **2006**, *5*, 493–506. [CrossRef] [PubMed]

54. Elf, S.; Abdelfattah, N.S.; Chen, E.; Perales-Patón, J.; Rosen, E.A.; Ko, A.; Peisker, F.; Florescu, N.; Giannini, S.; Wolach, O.; et al. Mutant Calreticulin Requires Both Its Mutant C-terminus and the Thrombopoietin Receptor for Oncogenic Transformation. *Cancer Discov.* **2016**, *6*, 368–381. [CrossRef] [PubMed]
55. Marty, C.; Pecquet, C.; Nivarthi, H.; El-Khoury, M.; Chachoua, I.; Tulliez, M.; Villeval, J.; Raslova, H.; Kralovics, R.; Constantinescu, S.N.; et al. Calreticulin mutants in mice induce an MPL-dependent thrombocytosis with frequent progression to myelofibrosis. *Blood* **2016**, *127*, 1317–1324. [CrossRef] [PubMed]
56. Schieber, M.; Crispino, J.D.; Stein, B. Myelofibrosis in 2019: Moving beyond JAK2 inhibition. *Blood Cancer J* **2019**, *9*, 74. [CrossRef] [PubMed]
57. Passamonti, F.; Caramazza, D.; Maffioli, M. JAK inhibitor in CALR-mutant myelofibrosis. *N. Engl. J. Med.* **2014**, *370*, 1168–1169.
58. Morsia, E.; Torre, E.; Poloni, A.; Olivieri, A.; Rupoli, S. Molecular Pathogenesis of Myeloproliferative Neoplasms: From Molecular Landscape to Therapeutic Implications. *Int. J. Mol. Sci.* **2022**, *23*, 4573. [CrossRef]
59. Vainchenker, W.; Constantinescu, S.N. JAK/STAT signaling in hematological malignancies. *Oncogene* **2013**, *32*, 2601–2613. [CrossRef]
60. Khan, I.; Huang, Z.; Wen, Q.; Stankiewicz, M.J.; Gilles, L.; Goldenson, B.; Schultz, R.; Diebold, L.; Gurbuxani, S.; Finke, C.M.; et al. AKT is a therapeutic target in myeloproliferative neoplasms. *Leukemia* **2013**, *27*, 1882–1890. [CrossRef]
61. Sun, P.; Meng, L. Emerging roles of class I PI3K inhibitors in modulating tumor microenvironment and immunity. *Acta Pharmacol. Sin.* **2020**, *41*, 1395–1402. [CrossRef]
62. Tian, T.; Li, X.; Zhang, J. mTOR Signaling in Cancer and mTOR Inhibitors in Solid Tumor Targeting Therapy. *Int. J. Mol. Sci.* **2019**, *20*, 755. [CrossRef]
63. Donahue, T.R.; Tran, L.M.; Hill, R.; Li, Y.; Kovochich, A.; Calvopina, J.H.; Patel, S.G.; Wu, N.; Hindoyan, A.; Farrell, J.J.; et al. Integrative survival-based molecular profiling of human pancreatic cancer. *Clin. Cancer Res.* **2012**, *18*, 1352–1363. [CrossRef]
64. Bogani, C.; Bartalucci, N.; Martinelli, S.; Tozzi, L.; Guglielmelli, P.; Bosi, A.; Vannucchi, A.M. mTOR inhibitors alone and in combination with JAK2 inhibitors effectively inhibit cells of myeloproliferative neoplasms. *PLoS ONE* **2013**, *8*, e54826. [CrossRef] [PubMed]
65. Fiskus, W.; Verstovsek, S.; Manshouri, T.; Smith, J.E.; Peth, K.; Abhyankar, S.; McGuirk, J.; Bhalla, K.N. Dual PI3K/AKT/mTOR inhibitor BEZ235 synergistically enhances the activity of JAK2 inhibitor against cultured and primary human myeloproliferative neoplasm cells. *Mol. Cancer Ther.* **2013**, *12*, 577–588. [CrossRef] [PubMed]
66. Schneider, R.K.; Mullally, A.; Dugourd, A.; Peisker, F.; Hoogenboezem, R.; Van Strien, P.M.H.; Bindels, E.M.; Heckl, D.; Büsche, G.; Fleck, D.; et al. Gli1+ Mesenchymal Stromal Cells Are a Key Driver of Bone Marrow Fibrosis and an Important Cellular Therapeutic Target. *Cell Stem. Cell* **2017**, *20*, 785–800.e8. [CrossRef] [PubMed]
67. Sasaki, K.; Gotlib, J.R.; Mesa, R.A.; Newberry, K.J.; Ravandi, F.; Cortes, J.E.; Kelly, P.; Kutok, J.L.; Kantarjian, H.M.; Verstovsek, S. Phase II evaluation of IPI-926, an oral Hedgehog inhibitor, in patients with myelofibrosis. *Leuk. Lymphoma* **2015**, *56*, 2092–2097. [CrossRef]
68. Bailey, J.M.; Mohr, A.M.; Hollingsworth, M.A. Sonic hedgehog paracrine signaling regulates metastasis and lymphangiogenesis in pancreatic cancer. *Oncogene* **2009**, *28*, 3513–3525. [CrossRef]
69. Ma, X.; Sheng, T.; Zhang, Y.; Zhang, X.; He, J.; Huang, S.; Chen, K.; Sultz, J.; Adegboyega, P.A.; Zhang, H.; et al. Hedgehog signaling is activated in subsets of esophageal cancers. *Int. J. Cancer* **2006**, *118*, 139–148. [CrossRef]
70. Sheng, T.; Li, C.; Zhang, X.; Chi, S.; He, N.; Chen, K.; McCormick, F.; Gatalica, Z.; Xie, J. Activation of the hedgehog pathway in advanced prostate cancer. *Mol. Cancer* **2004**, *3*, 29. [CrossRef]
71. Skoda, A.M.; Simovic, D.; Karin, V.; Kardum, V.; Vranic, S.; Serman, L. The role of the Hedgehog signaling pathway in cancer: A comprehensive review. *Bosn. J. Basic Med. Sci.* **2018**, *18*, 8–20. [CrossRef]
72. Dierks, C.; Grbic, J.; Zirlik, K.; Beigi, R.; Englund, N.P.; Guo, G.; Veelken, H.; Engelhardt, M.; Mertelsmann, R.; Kelleher, J.F.; et al. Essential role of stromally induced hedgehog signaling in B-cell malignancies. *Nat. Med.* **2007**, *13*, 944–951. [CrossRef]
73. Merchant, A.A.; Matsui, W. Targeting Hedgehog-a cancer stem cell pathway. *Clin. Cancer Res.* **2010**, *16*, 3130–3140. [CrossRef] [PubMed]
74. Bhagwat, N.; Keller, M.; Rampal, R.; Shank, K.; Stanchina, E.; Rose, K.; Amakye, D.; Levine, R. Improved Efficacy of Combination of JAK2 and Hedgehog Inhibitors in Myelofibrosis. *Blood* **2013**, *122*, 666. [CrossRef]
75. Zingariello, M.; Martelli, F.; Ciaffoni, F.; Masiello, F.; Ghinassi, B.; D'Amore, E.; Massa, M.; Barosi, G.; Sancillo, L.; Li, X.; et al. Characterization of the TGF-β1 signaling abnormalities in the Gata1low mouse model of myelofibrosis. *Blood* **2013**, *121*, 3345–3363. [CrossRef] [PubMed]
76. Astorga, J.; Carlsson, P. Hedgehog induction of murine vasculogenesis is mediated by Foxf1 and Bmp4. *Development* **2007**, *134*, 3753–3761. [CrossRef] [PubMed]
77. Guijarro-Hernández, A.; Eder-Azanza, L.; Hurtado, C.; Navarro-Herrera, D.; Ezcurra, B.; Novo, F.J.; Cabello, J.; Vizmanos, J.L. Transcriptomic Analysis Reveals JAK2/MPL-Independent Effects of Calreticulin Mutations in a C. elegans Model. *Cells* **2023**, *12*, 186. [CrossRef]
78. Lucijanic, M.; Livun, A.; Tupek, K.M.; Stoos-Veic, T.; Pejsa, V.; Jonjic, Z.; Dzankic, A.F.; Ivic, M.; Kusec, R. Neutral effect of Glioma-associated oncogene-1 expression on survival in myelofibrosis. *Wien. Klin. Wochenschr.* **2020**, *132*, 464–466. [CrossRef]

79. Vener, C.; Novembrino, C.; Catena, F.B.; Fracchiolla, N.S.; Gianelli, U.; Savi, F.; Radaelli, F.; Fermo, E.; Cortelezzi, A.; Lonati, S.; et al. Oxidative stress is increased in primary and post-polycythemia vera myelofibrosis. *Exp. Hematol.* **2010**, *38*, 1058–1065. [CrossRef]
80. Marty, C.; Lacout, C.; Droin, N.; Le Couédic, J.P.; Ribrag, V.; Solary, E.; Vainchenker, W.; Villeval, J.L.; Plo, I. A role for reactive oxygen species in JAK2 V617F myeloproliferative neoplasm progression. *Leukemia* **2013**, *27*, 2187–2195. [CrossRef]
81. Bjørn, M.E.; Hasselbalch, H.C. The Role of Reactive Oxygen Species in Myelofibrosis and Related Neoplasms. *Mediat. Inflamm.* **2015**, *2015*, 648090. [CrossRef]
82. Tefferi, A.; Vaidya, R.; Caramazza, D.; Finke, C.; Lasho, T.; Pardanani, A. Circulating interleukin (IL)-8, IL-2R, IL-12, and IL-15 levels are independently prognostic in primary myelofibrosis: A comprehensive cytokine profiling study. *J. Clin. Oncol.* **2011**, *29*, 1356–1363. [CrossRef]
83. Wu, X.; Liu, X.; Zhu, X.; Tang, C. Hypoxic preconditioning induces delayed cardioprotection through p38 MAPK-mediated calreticulin upregulation. *Shock* **2007**, *27*, 572–577. [CrossRef] [PubMed]
84. Vadeikiene, R.; Savukaitytė, A.; Laukaitienė, D.; Ugenskiene, R.; Juozaitytė, E. Investigation of mTOR, JAK/STAT, and Hedgehog pathways inhibitor effect on the proliferation of haematological cancer cell lines. *Biologija* **2021**, *67*, 122–133. [CrossRef]
85. Stark, G.R.; Taylor, W.R. Analyzing the G2/M checkpoint. *Methods Mol. Biol.* **2004**, *280*, 51–82. [PubMed]
86. Araki, M.; Yang, Y.; Masubuchi, N.; Hironaka, Y.; Takei, H.; Morishita, S.; Mizukami, Y.; Kan, S.; Shirane, S.; Edahiro, Y.; et al. Activation of the thrombopoietin receptor by mutant calreticulin in CALR-mutant myeloproliferative neoplasms. *Blood* **2016**, *127*, 1307–1316. [CrossRef] [PubMed]
87. Campbell, V.; Copland, M. Hedgehog signaling in cancer stem cells: A focus on hematological cancers. *Stem Cells Cloning* **2015**, *8*, 27–38.
88. Tibes, R.; Mesa, R.A. Targeting hedgehog signaling in myelofibrosis and other hematologic malignancies. *J. Hematol. Oncol.* **2014**, *7*, 18. [CrossRef]
89. Klein, C.; Zwick, A.; Kissel, S.; Forster, C.U.; Pfeifer, D.; Follo, M.; Illert, A.L.; Decker, S.; Benkler, T.; Pahl, H.; et al. Ptch2 loss drives myeloproliferation and myeloproliferative neoplasm progression. *J. Exp. Med.* **2016**, *213*, 273–290. [CrossRef]
90. Pardanani, A.; Lasho, T.; Smith, G.; Burns, C.J.; Fantino, E.; Tefferi, A. CYT387, a selective JAK1/JAK2 inhibitor: In vitro assessment of kinase selectivity and preclinical studies using cell lines and primary cells from polycythemia vera patients. *Leukemia* **2009**, *23*, 1441–1445. [CrossRef]
91. Quintás-Cardama, A.; Vaddi, K.; Liu, P.; Manshouri, T.; Li, J.; Scherle, P.A.; Caulder, E.; Wen, X.; Li, Y.; Waeltz, P.; et al. Preclinical characterization of the selective JAK1/2 inhibitor INCB018424: Therapeutic implications for the treatment of myeloproliferative neoplasms. *Blood* **2010**, *115*, 3109–3117. [CrossRef]
92. Vannucchi, A.; Bogani, C.; Bartalucci, N.; Tozzi, L.; Martinelli, S.; Guglielmelli, P.; Paoli, C.; Pieri, L.; Bosi, A. Inhibitors of PI3K/Akt and/or mTOR Inhibit the Growth of Cells of Myeloproliferative Neoplasms and Synergize with JAK2 Inhibitor and Interferon. *Blood* **2011**, *118*, 3835. [CrossRef]
93. Sies, H. Oxidative stress: A concept in redox biology and medicine. *Redox Biol.* **2015**, *4*, 180–183. [CrossRef] [PubMed]
94. Allegra, A.; Pioggia, G.; Tonacci, A.; Casciaro, M.; Musolino, C.; Gangemi, S. Synergic Crosstalk between Inflammation, Oxidative Stress, and Genomic Alterations in BCR-ABL-Negative Myeloproliferative Neoplasm. *Antioxidants* **2020**, *9*, 1037. [CrossRef] [PubMed]
95. Xu, C.; Bailly-Maitre, B.; Reed, J.C. Endoplasmic reticulum stress: Cell life and death decisions. *J. Clin. Investig.* **2005**, *115*, 2656–2664. [CrossRef] [PubMed]
96. Zhang, Y.; Liu, L.; Jin, L.; Yi, X.; Dang, E.; Yang, Y.; Li, C.; Gao, T. Oxidative stress-induced calreticulin expression and translocation: New insights into the destruction of melanocytes. *J. Investig. Dermatol.* **2014**, *134*, 183–191. [CrossRef] [PubMed]
97. Ihara, Y.; Urata, Y.; Goto, S.; Kondo, T. Role of calreticulin in the sensitivity of myocardiac H9c2 cells to oxidative stress caused by hydrogen peroxide. *Am. J. Physiol. Cell Physiol.* **2006**, *290*, 208. [CrossRef]
98. Gajski, G.; Domijan, A.; Žegura, B.; Štern, A.; Gerić, M.; Novak Jovanović, I.; Vrhovac, I.; Madunić, J.; Breljak, D.; Filipič, M.; et al. Melittin induced cytogenetic damage, oxidative stress and changes in gene expression in human peripheral blood lymphocytes. *Toxicon* **2016**, *110*, 56–67. [CrossRef]
99. Komatsu, N.; Kunitama, M.; Yamada, M.; Hagiwara, T.; Kato, T.; Miyazaki, H.; Eguchi, M.; Yamamoto, M.; Miura, Y. Establishment and characterization of the thrombopoietin-dependent megakaryocytic cell line, UT-7/TPO. *Blood* **1996**, *87*, 4552–4560. [CrossRef]
100. Komatsu, N.; Yamamoto, M.; Fujita, H.; Miwa, A.; Hatake, K.; Endo, T.; Okano, H.; Katsube, T.; Fukumaki, Y.; Sassa, S. Establishment and characterization of an erythropoietin-dependent subline, UT-7/Epo, derived from human leukemia cell line, UT-7. *Blood* **1993**, *82*, 456–464. [CrossRef]
101. Trung, N.T.; Quyen, D.T.; Hoan, N.X.; Giang, D.P.; Trang, T.T.H.; Velavan, T.P.; Bang, M.H.; Song, L.H. Rapid, low cost and sensitive detection of Calreticulin mutations by a PCR based amplicon length differentiation assay for diagnosis of myeloproliferative neoplasms. *BMC Med. Genet.* **2019**, *20*, 115. [CrossRef]

International Journal of
Molecular Sciences

MDPI

Article

Loss of Heterozygosity and Mutations in the RAS-ERK Pathway Genes in Tumor Cells of Various Loci in Multiple Myeloma

Maiia Soloveva *, Maksim Solovev, Natalya Risinskaya, Elena Nikulina, Igor Yakutik, Bella Biderman, Tatiana Obukhova, Yulia Chabaeva, Sergej Kulikov, Andrey Sudarikov and Larisa Mendeleeva

National Medical Research Center for Hematology, Novy Zykovski Lane, 4a, 125167 Moscow, Russia; risinska@gmail.com (N.R.); igorya90@list.ru (I.Y.); bella_biderman@mail.ru (B.B.); uchabaeva@gmail.com (Y.C.); dusha@blood.ru (A.S.)
* Correspondence: firs-maia@yandex.ru; Tel.: +7-905-751-30-21

Abstract: Multiple myeloma (MM) is a disease characterized by spatiotemporal heterogeneity of tumor clones. Different genetic aberrations can be observed simultaneously in tumor cells from different loci, and as the disease progresses, new subclones may appear. The role of liquid biopsy, which is based on the analysis of tumor DNA circulating in the blood plasma, continues to be explored in MM. Here, we present an analysis of the STR profiles and mutation status of the *KRAS*, *NRAS*, and *BRAF* genes, evaluated in plasma free circulating tumor DNA (ctDNA), CD138+ bone marrow cells, and plasmacytomas. The prospective single-center study included 97 patients, with a median age of 55 years. Of these, 94 had newly diagnosed symptomatic MM, and three had primary plasma cell leukemia. It should be noted that if mutations were detected only in ctDNA, "non-classical" codons were more often affected. A variety of adverse laboratory and clinical factors have been associated with the detection of rare *KRAS* or *NRAS* gene mutations in bone marrow or ctDNA, suggesting that these mutations may be factors of an unfavorable prognosis for MM. Liquid biopsy studies provide undeniable fundamental information about tumor heterogeneity and clonal evolution in MM. Moreover, we focus on using liquid biopsy to identify new high-risk factors for MM.

Keywords: multiple myeloma; liquid biopsy; plasmacytoma; STR profile; loss of heterozygosity; free circulating tumor DNA in plasma; *NRAS*; *KRAS*; *BRAF* genes

1. Introduction

Multiple myeloma (MM) is a complex disease of the blood system, with an aberrant plasma cell as its substrate. The complexity of the genetic structure of MM is reflected in the phenomenon of spatiotemporal heterogeneity of tumor clones [1–3]. This means that different genetic abnormalities can be observed simultaneously in tumors of different locations in the same patient. As the disease progresses, more mutations are acquired, and subclones that differ from the original clone arise. In this regard, two areas are of particular importance. Firstly, relying solely on a bone marrow sample to assess the risk of myeloma may lead to inaccurate result, as mentioned in our previous research [4]. In this regard, there is a clear need to develop a new or additional diagnostic tool for better risk assignment. This could be a liquid biopsy, for example. Secondly, the mechanisms behind chemoresistance and plasmacytoma development remain poorly understood. This underscores the need for further research into the evolution of tumor clones. Studying mutations and aberrant signaling pathways that contribute to tumor progression and drug resistance is essential for implementing a personalized approach to MM treatment [5]. Despite significant success in the treatment of MM, which became possible due to the introduction of new classes of drugs in combination with high-dose chemotherapy followed by transplantation of autologous hematopoietic stem cells (auto-HSCT), the disease remains incurable and in most cases steadily progresses [6–8]. If there is an appropriate target, the application of drugs that are not usually used to treat MM becomes justified. Thus, with mutations in the genes of the RAS signaling pathway (*BRAF* V600E), attempts are made to use vemurafenib; with *BCL-2* overexpression in patients with t (11;14), venetoclax is used; and in the case of JAK2 pathway activation, ruxolitinib. Other signaling pathways, such as NF-kB and PI3K/mTOR, are also being actively studied, and the search for new potential targets continues [5]. Since *KRAS/NRAS/BRAF* genes are involved in the MAPK pathway, the use of MAPK inhibitors in combination with immunomodulatory drugs in MM patients with mutations in these genes is being discussed [9].

There are few publications on the use of BRAF inhibitors in MM patients with a mutation in the *BRAF* V600E gene. In 2016, researchers from Switzerland reported a clinical observation of the successful use of a vemurafenib and cobimetinib combination in a young patient with refractory extramedullary MM with a *BRAF* V600E gene mutation [10]. In 2018, the results of a multicenter clinical trial on the effectiveness of vemurafenib in patients with different types of cancer (VE-BASKET) were presented. Nine patients with refractory MM were included in this study. In two of them, vemurafenib therapy proved to be highly effective, and the patients were in long-term remission (more than 20 months) at the end of the study. The authors suggest that the lack of antitumor effect in other patients may be explained by the fact that the *BRAF* V600E gene mutation was not the main tumorogenic event [11]. A prospective multicenter phase 2 trial evaluated the effects of combining BRAF/MEK inhibition with encorafenib and binimetinib in 12 relapsed/refractory MM patients who had a *BRAF* V600E mutation. It is important to note that the patients were heavily pre-treated. The overall response rate was high (83.3%), and the median progression-free survival was 5.6 months, indicating this therapy as a successful targeted approach [12]. Another study examined the development of resistance of tumor plasma cells to treatment with BRAF inhibitors. The authors showed that the adaptation of a tumor cell to targeted therapy is based on transcriptional state changes and epigenetic regulation [13].

Currently, in the pathogenesis of MM, not only the mutation profile of oncogenes and tumor suppressor genes are being studied, but also their interaction in the course of the disease. Oncogenic relationships between primary events (translocations and hyperdiploidy), mutations in driver genes, and areas of copy number variations have been proven. For example, associations were found between t(4;14) and mutations in the *FGFR3*, *DIS3*, and *PRKD2* genes. Two surrogate markers of DNA instability were also identified—the APOBEC mutation signature and loss of heterozygosity (LOH). A correlation was found between the degree of LOH and *TP53* gene lesions. It is expected that identifying further relationships will allow for a personalized approach to patient therapy, thereby improving its effectiveness [14].

The course of MM can vary from slowly progressing to lightning-fast forms. It depends on the degree of evolution of the tumor clone, the magnitude of the tumor load, and the presence of adverse risk factors. The signs of high-risk myeloma are diverse and include a range of laboratory and clinical parameters. The issue of searching for new prognostic factors, as well as tools for their detection, is especially relevant due to the existence of patients who, despite the absence of known high-risk factors, failed to achieve a deep antitumor response. Proteomic and genomic studies are currently being conducted to identify additional diagnostic and/or prognostic parameters of MM. Biomarkers determined noninvasively in the circulating bloodstream (microRNA and extracellular DNA) are being studied [15]. The efficacy for detecting markers missing in bone marrow while present in ctDNA for MM monitoring are being investigated [16–18].

The question of why in some MM patients a tumor plasma cell is able to exist outside bone marrow, forming plasmacytomas in other organs and tissues, is extremely interesting. The genetic parameters of plasmacytomas are less studied due to the lack of opportunity to analyze a large number of samples—plasmacytoma biopsy is not a mandatory procedure for MM diagnosis. The invasive nature of plasmacytoma biopsy is another incentive for the use of liquid biopsy.

Here we present a study of MM tumor clones' heterogeneity assessed at disease onset by a wide range of methods in attempt to clarify the potential role of liquid biopsy as a diagnostic and risk stratification tool for MM. The LOH in various loci was studied by multiplex STR-PCR. The mutation status of the *KRAS*, *KRAS*, and *BRAF* genes in ctDNA, CD138+ bone marrow cells, and plasmacytomas was analyzed by AS-PCR and NGS.

2. Results

Table 1 shows the clinical and laboratory parameters of patients at the onset of multiple myeloma. The majority of patients (60%) were diagnosed with stage IIIA of the disease according to Durie–Salmon. Plasmacytomas were detected in 59% of patients (n = 57) at the onset of MM. The vast majority of patients had bone plasmacytomas (n = 51), in 3% of cases (n = 2)—extramedullary, and in 7% of cases (n = 4) both bone and extramedullary plasmacytomas were simultaneously detected. Cytogenetic examination by the FISH method was performed in all patients. In 46% of cases, the cytogenetic risk was determined as standard, in 51% of observations, high-risk cytogenetic aberrations were present, and in another 3% of the cases, the study could not be performed for technical reasons.

Table 1. General characteristics of the patient sample.

Parameters	Patients with MM (n = 97)
Age, years, median and range	55 (29–83)
Males/females	43/54
Type of secretion	
G	59 (61%)
A	19 (20%)
BJ	15 (15%)
D	4 (4%)
Type of FLC	
κ	58 (60%)
λ	39 (40%)
D-S stage	
IA	5 (5%)
IB	2 (2%)
IIA	16 (17%)
IIIA	58 (60%)
IIIB	15 (15%)
Not available	1 (1%)
ISS stage	
I	29 (30%)
II	20 (21%)
III	17(17%)
Not available	31 (32%)
Hemoglobin (g/L), median and range	109 (66–156)
LDH (U/L), median and range	170 (65–694)
% plasma cells in bone marrow aspiration, median and range	16 (2.4–92)
FISH	
Standard risk	45 (46%)
High risk	49 (51%)
Not available	3 (3%)
Plasmacytomas	
Yes	57 (59%)
No	40 (41%)
	n = 57
bone	51 (90%)
extramedullary	2 (3%)
bone and extramedullary	4 (7%)

Table S1 shows the spectrum of high-risk cytogenetic aberrations detected in patients with MM. In 20.4% of cases, two high-risk anomalies were detected simultaneously in various combinations (double-hit myeloma), and three aberrations (triple-hit myeloma) were found in one observation.

STR profile of paired tumor samples (ctDNA and bone marrow) of 93 patients with MM was analyzed. In nine patients, LOH was studied in three localizations: ctDNA, bone marrow, and plasmacytoma. LOH was detected in the MM substrate with different frequency depending on the tumor location. Thus, in 55% of patients (n = 51), aberrant STR loci with LOH were detected in ctDNA. In CD138+ bone marrow cells, the frequency of detection was higher—loci with LOH were found in 64% of patients (n = 60) (Figure 1).

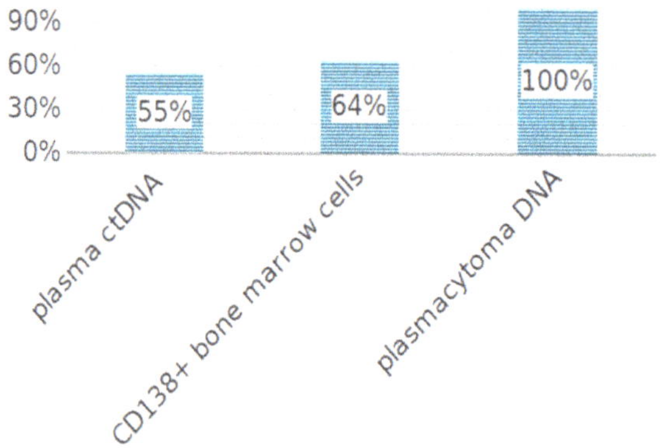

Figure 1. LOH frequency in tumor cells from different loci.

Figure 2 shows the frequency of detection of a different number of aberrant STR loci with LOH in MM. In the majority of patients (51%, n = 48), one to three aberrant STR loci were found in the bone marrow or ctDNA. There was no LOH in either bone marrow or ctDNA in 15% of MM patients (n = 14). In 18% of patients (n = 17), four aberrant STR loci were found in the tumor substrate. Five or more loci with LOH were identified in another 16% of patients (n = 15).

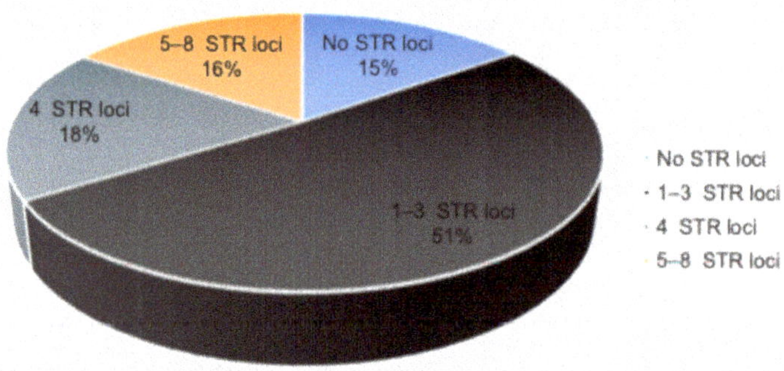

Figure 2. The frequency of LOH detection in ctDNA or bone marrow.

We hypothesized that patients with a large number of LOH loci would be more likely to have high-risk cytogenetic aberrations as a reflection of a large tumor load and genetic instability. We analyzed the frequency of detection of high-risk cytogenetic anomalies in each subgroup. As can be seen from Figure 3, there was no convincing evidence that with an increase in the number of loci with LOH, high-risk cytogenetic aberrations were more often observed.

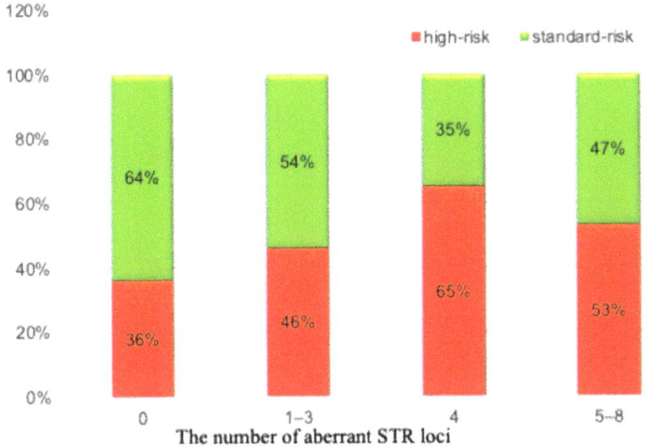

Figure 3. The frequency of detection of high-risk cytogenetic aberrations depending on the number of loci with LOH.

There was also no association found between the number of loci with LOH and the presence of plasmacytomas. Thus, among patients who did not have LOH, 43% had plasmacytomas (6 out of 14). Among patients with one to three aberrant loci, there were 69% of cases of plasmacytomas (33 out of 48). Plasmacytomas were detected in 47% of patients (8 out of 17) with four LOH loci. Finally, among patients with a large number of aberrant loci (five to eight), 60% of cases were with plasmacytomas (9 out of 15).

The analysis of ctDNA in plasma was performed for 93 patients with MM. A concordance analysis was performed for each locus in paired tumor samples from 93 patients with MM (Figure S1). We compared the concentration of free plasma circulating DNA in patients with plasmacytomas (n = 55) and without them (n = 38). There were no differences in values: in patients with plasmacytomas, the concentration was 20 ng/mL (range 2–207), and in patients without plasmacytomas, it was 17 ng/mL (range 2–623).

The length of ctDNA fragments varied from 160 to 450 bp. The Figure S1 shows the distribution of LOH loci depending on the length of ctDNA. Mostly LOH loci were found on ctDNA fragments with a length of 400 bp. It should be noted that when analyzing ctDNA samples with fragment lengths of 160, 170, and 450 bp no LOH loci were detected.

For nine patients, LOH was tested using DNA from three different sources: ctDNA, bone marrow, and plasmacytomas. Additionally, in one patient, two plasmacytomas were analyzed—one from the bone and one extramedullary (Figure 4).

No cases were found with the complete identity of the STR profiles in different tumor locations. Loci with LOH have always been found in plasmacytomas. Plasmacytoma profiles were more similar to that in bone marrow rather than in ctDNA (in six cases). In one interesting observation (#6), seven aberrant STR loci were identified in plasmacytoma DNA, but no LOH was found in bone marrow and ctDNA. Patient #9 with four evaluated sources had the same STR profile in bone marrow, bone and extramedullary plasmacytomas, and two other STR loci with LOH in ctDNA (Figure 5).

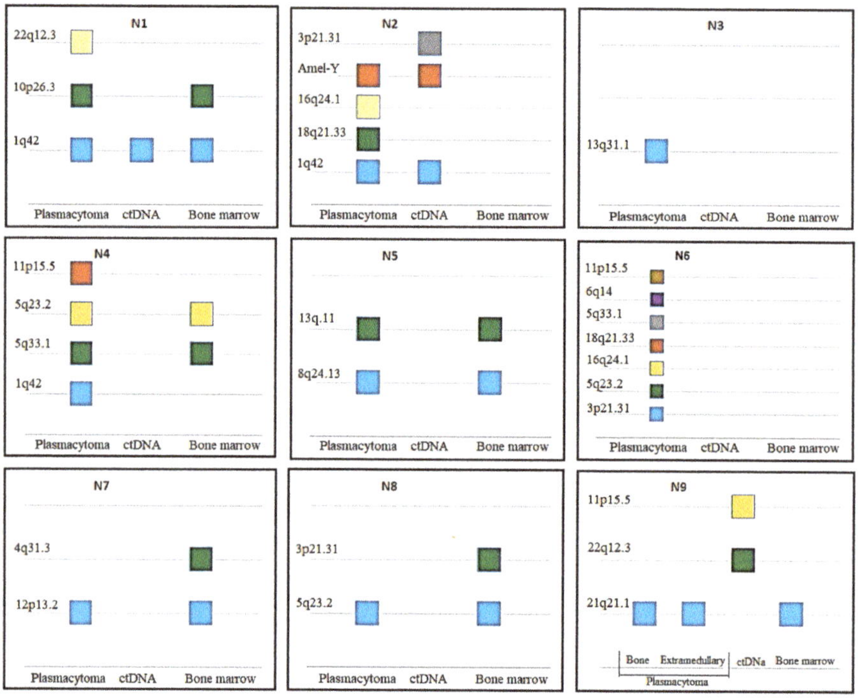

Figure 4. Comparison of STR loci with LOH in plasmacytomas, bone marrow, and ctDNA from nine MM patients.

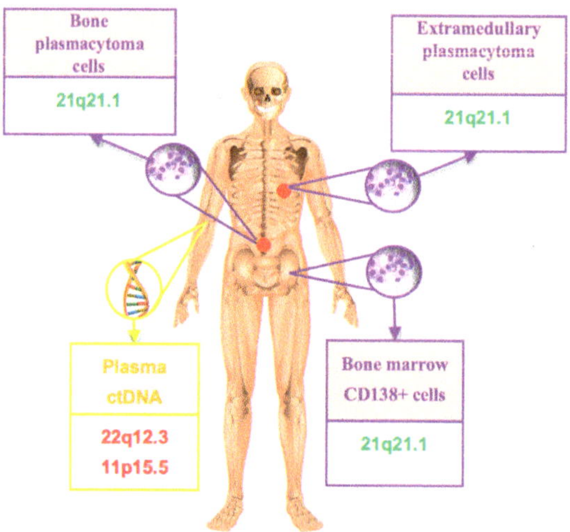

Figure 5. An example of LOH mismatch in DNA from different MM loci. Green highlights the same STR locus in bone marrow and two plasmacytomas, while red marks two different loci found in ctDNA.

Somatic mutations in the *NRAS*, *KRAS*, and *BRAF* genes were evaluated for 91 patients with MM and were found in 44 of these patients (48.5%). Mutations only in the *NRAS* gene were detected in 16.5% of cases (n = 15), only in the *KRAS* gene—in 18.7% of cases (*n* = 17), and only in the *BRAF* gene—in 10% of cases (*n* = 9). In another 3.3% of cases (*n* = 3), two mutations in different genes were detected simultaneously: in two patients, mutations in the *BRAF* (V600E) and *NRAS* (Q61H) genes, and in one case—mutations in the *KRAS* (Q61R) and *NRAS* (Q61R) genes. We also noted two cases with two mutations of the same gene: one patient had two mutations in the *KRAS* gene (G12A, Q61L), and the second patient had two mutations in the *NRAS* gene (Q61K and Q61R).

Most of the *KRAS* and *NRAS* gene mutations we found affected the "classic" codons—12 and 13 for *KRAS*, and 61 for *NRAS*. However, we also found some rare variants (Figure 6).

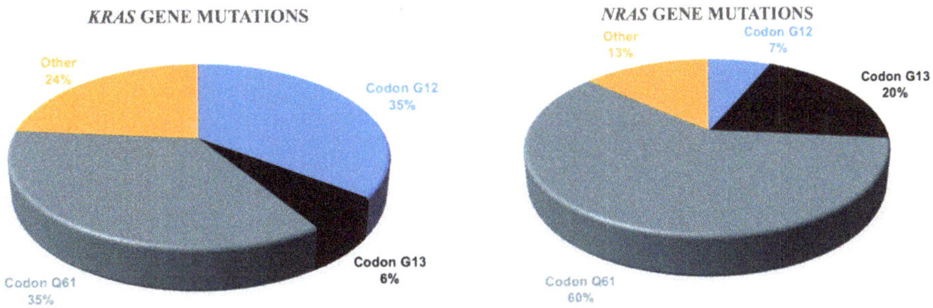

Figure 6. The frequency of *KRAS* and *NRAS* mutations in different codons.

The analysis of paired tumor samples (bone marrow and ctDNA) was performed in 39 MM patients. Mutations in the studied genes were found in 24 patients, while identical patterns in paired tumor samples were detected only in five cases (21%). Mutations of any of the three genes were found in the bone marrow of 21 patients. Mutations of one of the three genes were detected in the ctDNA of nine patients, while in five cases, the same mutations were found in bone marrow. In the remaining four observations, the mutations detected in ctDNA did not correspond to those found in bone marrow. In one case, different *KRAS* gene mutations were detected in paired tumor samples. In three other cases, *KRAS* and *NRAS* gene mutations detected in ctDNA were absent in bone marrow. Although the number of patients in each group was small, there was a trend towards more frequent detection of high-risk cytogenetic aberrations in patients with MAP kinase gene mutations in ctDNA with the absence of these mutations in the bone marrow. Further analysis in patients with RAS-ERK cascade gene mutations, which were exclusively identified in ctDNA, revealed not only that high-risk cytogenetic aberrations were more frequently detected, but also that other unfavorable prognostic factors were present. In addition, it was noted that in three out of four cases (75%), with mutations detected only in ctDNA, "non-classical" codons were affected.

Table 2 shows the data for four patients whose ctDNA had any mutations in the studied genes, as well as for three patients whose bone marrow had rare mutations. As can be seen from the table, these patients had various unfavorable prognostic factors, which reflects the concept of "high-risk myeloma". Thus, in patient #1, with a single nucleotide deletion (c.286 delT) in the *KRAS* gene in addition to cytogenetic aberrations, high LDH activity, an advanced ISS stage, concomitant AL-amyloidosis was observed, and the course of the disease was refractory and recurrent. Despite the implementation of high-dose chemotherapy and auto-HSCT in some patients (#2, 4, and 6), complete remission was not achieved. In the other two cases with rare *NRAS* and *KRAS* gene mutations (#5 and 7), the aggressive course of the disease precluded the completion of the therapy program, and the patients died during induction treatment. These findings suggest the need for further research in this area.

Table 2. Adverse prognostic factors in MM patients with rare mutation variants in the *KRAS* and *NRAS* genes.

#	Mutations in CD138+ Bone Marrow Cells	Mutations in ctDNA	Disease Features
1	none	*KRAS* c.286 delT	High LDH; ISS stage III; double-HIT: del17p13, 1q21; amyloidosis; Relapse/refractory
2	none	*NRAS* L95P	1q21; only partial remission after HSCT
3	none	*KRAS* G12V	High LDH; 1q21; relapse/refractory
4	*KRAS G12S*	*KRASV29A*	T (4;14); only partial remission after 2 rounds of HSCT
5	*NRAS* Y64N	none	Plasma cell leukemia; high LDH; 1q21; extramedullary plasmacytomas; D-myeloma; death in induction
6	*KRAS* A59G	none	only partial remission after HSCT
7	*KRAS* L19F	none	ISS stage III; double HIT: t(14;16), 1q21; relapse/refractory; death in induction

In four patients, we compared the mutation profiles of the RAS-ERK cascade genes not only in bone marrow and ctDNA, but also in the plasmacytoma. In two patients, there was a mutation in the *KRAS* or *NRAS* gene in plasmacytoma tissue, while the corresponding gene was not mutated in bone marrow or ctDNA. The presence of a mutation in plasmacytoma DNA without a corresponding mutation at a different locus suggests the existence of different tumor clones in MM. Bone marrow clearance and immunochemical remission while maintaining a plasmacytoma are probably due to the clonal heterogeneity of the tumor.

Interesting data were obtained from 86 patients who underwent both STR profiling and gene mutation analysis. In patients with a larger number of LOH loci (5–8), mutations in RAS-ERK cascade genes were detected significantly more frequently compared to patients with a smaller number of LOH loci (0–4). The results showed a significant difference between the two groups (73% vs. 44%, $p = 0.048$), Table S2.

In 19 of the 39 patients with the mutation profile of RAS-ERK cascade genes analyzed in paired tumor samples, a mismatch of mutations in cDNA and bone marrow was noted. We compared the results of STR profiling in two tumor loci in this group of patients (Table 3). In the first five patients, no aberrant loci with LOH were detected in the ctDNA, and the RAS-ERK cascade genes were not mutated. One can speculate that the concentration of tumor ctDNA in these patients may have been insufficient for the detection of aberrations by one method or another. However, this assumption was not confirmed (see the last column of the table). In the remaining 14 cases, we saw not only the different status of MAP kinase genes, but also differences in the loci with LOH in the two tumor locations. Thus, in the case of nine with a mutation in the *NRAS* gene, eight aberrant loci with LOH were detected in bone marrow. At the same time, the mutation was absent in ctDNA, and seven loci with LOH were identified, of which only two were shared between ctDNA and bone marrow. The importance of studying different tumor locations to obtain a more complete picture of the MM genetic landscape is therefore evident.

Table 3. LOH in 19 patients with mismatch in MAP kinase gene mutations in paired tumor samples.

#	LOH Loci in Bone Marrow	Mutations in Bone Marrow	LOH Loci in ctDNA	Mutations in ctDNA	DNA Concentration (ng/mL)
1	2	*KRAS*	0	none	17.5
2	2	*BRAF*	0	none	11
3	6	2 *KRAS*	0	none	22
4	0	*NRAS*	0	none	13.5
5	2	*KRAS*	0	none	17

Table 3. *Cont.*

#	LOH Loci in Bone Marrow	Mutations in Bone Marrow	LOH Loci in ctDNA	Mutations in ctDNA	DNA Concentration (ng/mL)
6	0	-	3	*KRAS*	45.75
7	3	*KRAS*	4 (shared 1)	none	46.5
8	0	*KRAS*	6	none	32
9	8	*NRAS*	7 (shared 2)	none	8
10	0	*KRAS*	1	none	10
11	0	*NRAS*	1	none	17
12	2	*KRAS*	5 (shared 1)	none	20
13	2	-	3 (shared 1)	*NRAS*	77
14	5	*KRAS G12S*	3 (shared 2)	*KRAS* V29A	17
15	2	*BRAF*	4 (shared none)	none	30
16	6	*NRAS BRAF*	3 (shared 2)	none	17
17	0	-	4	*KRAS*	50
18	5	*NRAS*	2 (shared none)	none	5
19	1	*BRAF*	1 (shared none)	none	10

3. Discussion

According to the relevant criteria developed by the International Myeloma Working Group (IMWG-2014), the diagnosis of the disease requires the detection of a tumor substrate (detection of more than 10% of plasma cells in bone marrow or histologically proven plasmacytoma) in combination with signs of the CRAB symptom complex and/or markers of tumor activity [19]. Therefore, one of the possible criteria for MM is a plasmacytoma, but it does not occur in all patients. To date, there is no unified classification of plasmacytomas, which causes confusion in the terminology. Thus, there are many different terms in the scientific literature: soft tissue component, extramedullary lesion, bone, intraosseous, extraosseous, extramedullary plasmacytoma. Despite the variety of definitions, we are talking about two types of plasmacytomas—anatomically related to bone and arising autonomously in various organs and tissues. Some authors refer to the term "extramedullary lesion" as anatomically disconnected from bone [20–22]. Other experts consider it important to differentiate these two types of plasmacytomas, calling extramedullary only lesions resulting from the hematogenous spread of a tumor cell into organs and tissues [23–25]. In our opinion, it is not correct to combine these two types of plasmacytomas into one concept. Bone plasmacytomas occur in about half of the patients with MM. Modern treatment strategies, high-dose chemotherapy with auto-HSCT can minimize the adverse effect of bone plasmacytomas on patient survival. Extramedullary plasmacytoma is a rarer variant of the lesion (1.7–4.5%) resulting from the spread of a tumor plasma cell outside the bone marrow by a hematogenic pathway. This is a factor of extremely unfavorable prognosis. The course of MM complicated by an extramedullary lesion is characterized, as a rule, by an unstable antitumor response or its absence, and extremely unfavorable survival rates despite the entire spectrum of modern therapy [25,26]. The pathogenesis of plasmacytoma development continues to be studied. The literature presents the results of studies of plasmacytomas on limited samples of patients [27–30]. Given the rare incidence of extramedullary lesions, it becomes obvious that multicenter collaboration is required to accumulate sufficient patient samples and implement an adequate study. LOH is a manifestation of genetic instability, characterized by the loss of one of the alleles in specific regions of the genome. It is promising to study this phenomenon in various myeloma loci. Several methods can be used to study LOH. Comparative genomic hybridization can help identify submicroscopic deletions and duplications. We previously studied the molecular karyotype of an extramedullary plasmacytoma [31]. STR profiling, on the other hand, is not a very informative method, as it only examines selected DNA markers in the genome. However, it has the advantage of being simple to perform and can be applied to the analysis of DNA samples of any quality, even those that are fragmented or have low concentrations, as is typical for ctDNA [32,33]. In this study, STR profiling was used to analyze a large number of tumor samples from different locations, and interesting information about the spatial heterogeneity of MM was obtained. Considering the limitations of this method, we conclude that it could be used for routine screening, as it is relatively inexpensive and widely available.

Liquid biopsy is considered as a non-invasive alternative to traditional tissue biopsy methods. The study of ctDNA in plasma is a promising approach for research in plasmacytoma pathogenesis. In a work published by Chinese authors, the mutation profiles of ctDNA, bone marrow, and plasmacytomas were compared. The researchers showed that the same mutations in genes were more often detected in plasmacytomas and ctDNA than in bone marrow. The authors concluded that a liquid biopsy can provide insight into the genetic structure of a plasmacytoma, and in addition, serves as a predictor of recurrence. Thus, in several patients whose ctDNA was studied in dynamics, a positive correlation was noted with blood immunochemistry data, while a paraprotein was detected later than a mutation in a certain gene [34]. The advantages of a liquid biopsy are obvious: the procedure of taking blood can be repeated multiple times and does not require a special surgical intervention of the patient, unlike a tumor biopsy. A liquid biopsy makes it possible to study the spectrum of mutations in the tumor even if a plasmacytoma biopsy is not available (for example, due to difficulties in surgical access). In this paper, we analyzed LOH in paired tumor samples. Comparing the STR profile of CD138+ bone marrow cells, plasmacytomas, and ctDNA, we noticed that the STR loci affected in plasmacytomas more often shared with those found in bone marrow than with those found in ctDNA. The question of why tumor markers are sometimes present in peripheral blood circulation in MM patients that are not found in bone marrow or in plasmacytomas seems relevant and requires further study.

In addition, we analyzed the mutation status of MAP kinase genes in bone marrow, ctDNA, and plasmacytoma. According to a recent exome-wide sequencing study, mutations in the *KRAS*, *NRAS*, and *BRAF* genes are reported in 21%, 19%, and 7% of patients with newly diagnosed MM [35]. We measured the frequency of mutations at various codons in the *KRAS* and *NRAS* genes in patients with MM. The results obtained are consistent with those presented in the literature [14]. Specifically, we found mutations affecting codon 12 of the *KRAS* gene in 35% of cases, codon 61—in another 35%, and codon 13—in 6%. According to a study published in 2018, these frequencies were 34%, 35%, and 13%, respectively. We report mutations affecting codon 61 in 60% of cases, while Walker et al. report it in 81%. The authors note that mutations in "non-classical" codons such as Q22, Y64, K117, and A146 of the *KRAS* gene appear in 18% of cases [14]. We found rare mutations not only in the *KRAS* gene, but also in the *NRAS* gene in 24% and 13% of cases, respectively. Specifically, L19F, A59G, V29A, and c.286 delT (in the *KRAS* gene), and L95P and Y64N (in the *NRAS* gene) were encountered. In all patients with rare *KRAS* or *NRAS* gene mutations, a variety of different laboratory and clinical adverse factors were noted. Additionally, if the mutation was found only in ctDNA, "non-classical" codons were affected in 75% of cases. These findings clearly require further investigation on a larger sample of patients. However, it can already be assumed that the identification of these rare mutations may be a factor of an unfavorable prognosis for MM.

Mutations in the BRAF gene are present in various types of neoplasia and cause activation of the Ras-Raf-MEK-ERK signaling pathway. Mutations in the *BRAF* gene are detected in 7% of patients with newly diagnosed myeloma [35]. Here we report a *BRAF* V600E gene mutation in 10% of cases. However, *BRAF* mutations in MM can also affect other codons. Thus, in a paper published in 2018, a unique predominance of *BRAF* D594N variants in the t(14;16) subgroup is noted [14]. Further study of *BRAF*-positive myeloma is required to understand the mechanisms of activation of the signaling pathway and determine the role of targeted drugs in treatment. Clarifying which mutation in the BRAF gene is present in the patient is of practical importance, since BRAF inhibitors are selective against the *BRAF* V600E mutation [36]. Due to a different biological mechanism of action, it is impractical to use BRAF inhibitors in patients with a *KRAS*, *NRAS*, and *BRAF* D594N mutation [37].

In 2018, the entire exome of various ctDNA and bone marrow samples was sequenced in patients with MM. The authors noted a high coincidence in the detection of clonal somatic mutations and copy number variations between ctDNA and bone marrow samples. In addition, mutations that occur exclusively at a particular locus have been identified. The researchers conclude that a joint analysis of all localizations is required to assess complete genetic profile of the tumor [38]. Our data clearly demonstrate the presence of diverse tumor clones in MM. We also observed that patients with a high number of abnormal STR loci are significantly more likely to have mutations in the RAS-ERK pathway genes compared to patients with a lower number of LOH loci (73% vs. 44%, $p = 0.048$). This suggests that with increased genetic instability of the tumor, reflected by a greater number of abnormal loci with LOH, there is also an increased level of somatic mutations in the RAS-ERK pathway genes.

The literature mentions such a phenomenon as allele drop out (allele loss) in STR loci at low concentrations of the studied DNA. However, the authors determine small amounts of DNA in the range from 25 to 100 pg of DNA per PCR sample [39]. In the cohort of patients we studied, plasma concentrations of ctDNA were high enough, which allowed us to take 1 ng of ctDNA or more into PCR. Therefore, we assume that the loss of the allele in the STR loci in ctDNA we observed is associated with aberrations in the tumor genome and its heterogeneity, and not with stochastic effects at low DNA concentrations. Our confidence is confirmed by the coincidence of aberrant STR profiles of genomic and ctDNA in some patients, as well as discrepancies in the mutation profile of *KRAS*, *NRAS*, and *BRAF* genes in ctDNA and genomic DNA from selected CD138+ cells in certain patients. According to our data, the concentration of ctDNA did not differ significantly depending on the presence or absence of plasmacytomas in patients. The median concentration of ctDNA in patients with plasmacytomas was 20 nanograms per milliliter (ng/mL), while it was 17 ng/mL for patients without plasmacytomas. These findings contradict the results reported by Chinese authors, who found higher ctDNA levels in patients with plasmacytomas than in those without [34]. However, it is important to note that the patient samples are considerably different. We included 93 patients, 55 with plasmacytomas, while Long et al. analyzed data from 18 patients, eight of whom had plasmacytomas.

The studies of ctDNA as a tool for assessing minimal residual (MRD) disease in MM are ongoing. The small length of the ctDNA fragments limits the applicability of the method. The peculiarities of ctDNA metabolism are also obstacles to its use. The detection of MRD in bone marrow along with plasma MRD negativity indicate that it is necessary to increase the sensitivity of ctDNA detection [40,41]. Further standardization of ctDNA isolation and analysis methods is required. The applicability of full-exome sequencing in routine clinical practice to determine MRD is still not obvious. However, MRD evaluation was not part of this study's objectives. Instead, we used liquid biopsy as a diagnostic tool to identify new high-risk factors for myeloma. Thus, the value of liquid biopsy in fundamental scientific research on MM is undeniable. However, we assume that ctDNA could also be useful for applied purposes.

4. Materials and Methods

The prospective single-center study included 97 patients (43 men, 54 women) aged 29 to 83 years (median 55), 94 with newly diagnosed symptomatic MM, three patients with primary plasma cell leukemia. All patients attended the National Medical Research Center for Hematology (Moscow, Russia) from 21 September 2021 to 21 February 2024. The diagnosis was established in accordance with the criteria of IMWG-2014. To assess the bone system, patients underwent a low-dose CT scan of the entire body.

A positive immunomagnetic selection of CD138+ bone marrow cells was performed using a monoclonal antibody to CD138 (STEMCELL Technologies, Vancouver, BC, Canada) according to the manufacturer's protocol. A FISH study of CD138+ cells was performed using DNA probes to detect translocations 14q32/High, 8q24/*MYC*, deletions 17p13/*TP53*, 13q14, 1p32, amplification 1q21, and multiple trisomies (Wuhan HealthCare Biotechnology, Wuhan, Hubei, China). Upon detection of t(4;14), t(14;16), del17p13, and 1q21 amplification, the patient was classified to a high cytogenetic risk group.

DNAs were isolated from samples of various localization (blood plasma, CD138+ bone marrow cells) for all patients. In addition, plasmacytoma DNA was isolated from a tumor biopsy in 9 patients. The tumor STR DNA profile was examined relative to the STR profile of the control DNA isolated from the buccal epithelium by multiplex STR-PCR (COrDIS Plus kit (Gordiz LLC, Moscow, Russia) followed by fragment analysis as it was described previously [4]. For all patients with a change in the allele balance in heterozygous STR loci of tumor DNA compared to the control one, a relative decrease in the level of the fluorescent signal of the minor allele (in percent) was calculated.

The mutational status of the *KRAS*, *NRAS*, and *BRAF* genes was studied in 91 patients. In all patients, the study was conducted on genomic DNA isolated from bone marrow samples; in 39 patients, plasma ctDNA samples were additionally examined; and in 4 patients, DNA from three localizations (plasma ctDNA, bone marrow, plasmacytoma) was used. Isolation of genomic DNA from bone marrow samples and sections of paraffin embedded plasmacytoma biopsies was performed according the methodologies described earlier [42,43]. CtDNA from blood plasma was isolated with a QIAamp MinElute ccfDNA Mini Kit (QIAGEN, Hilden, Germany). PCR amplification was performed with a C1000 TouchTM PCR thermal cycler ("Bio-Rad", Hercules, CA, USA) using oligonucleotide pairs specific for exons 2 and 3 of *KRAS* (KRAS-E2F: 5′-CTTAAGCGTCGATGGAGGAG-3′; KRAS-E2R: 5′-GAATGGTCCTGCACCAGTAA-3′; KRAS-E3F: 5′-ATAATCCAGACTGTGTTTCTCCC-3′ and KRAS-E3R: 5′-AAAACAGGGATATTACCTACCTCAT-3′) and NRAS (NRAS-E2F: 5′-GCTCGCCAATTAACCCTGA-3′; NRAS-E2R: 5′-ACAGGTTTTAGAAACTTCAGCAG-3′; NRAS-E3F: 5′-AGGGACAAACCAGATAGGCA-3′ and NRAS-E3R: 5′-ACCTCATTTCCCC ATAAAGATTCA-3′) genes. Each PCR reaction was carried out in a volume of 25 μL containing 2.5 μL of (×10) a PCR buffer (Syntol, Moscow, Russia), 0.25 mM of a dNTPs solution (Syntol, Russia), 0.25 mM of $MgCl_2$ solution (Syntol, Russia), 5 pmol of each primer, 200 ng of genomic DNA, and 1E of SynTaq DNA-polymerase (Syntol, Russia). PCR was carried for 40 cycles with 30 s ofdenaturation at 92 °C and 20 s of annealing at 57 °C followed by a 30 s extension at 72 °C. Cycling was started by 2 min of denaturation at 92 °C and terminated by 10 min of incubation at 72 °C.

Mutations in *KRAS* and *NRAS* genes were identified by high-throughput sequencing (MiSeq, Illumina, San Diego, CA, USA), with confirmation of the findings by Sanger sequencing (Nanophor 05, Institute of Analytical Instrumentation of RAS, Moscow, Russia).

Sequencing libraries were prepared from the accumulated amplicons using the «Nextera XT DNA Library Prep» and «Nextera XT Index Kit v2» (Illumina, USA) according to the manufacturers recommendations. Sequencing was performed with a MiSeq genetic analyzer (Illumina, USA) using the «MiSeq Reagent Micro Kit v2 300-cycles» («Illumina», USA). Data filtration, service sequence deletion, mapping of readings, and search and annotation of variants was carried out with the Trimmomatic [44], BWA [45], SAMtools [46], Vardict [47], and Annovar [48] utilities. The information about clinical significance of the mutations was obtained from open sources (COSMIC and DB SNP).

Sanger sequencing was carried out with a BigDye Terminator v1.1 Cycle Sequencing Kit (Applied Biosystems, Waltham, MA, USA) using a Nanophor 05 genetic analyzer (Institute of Analytical Instrumentation of RAS, Russia).

The *BRAF* V600E mutation was determined by real-time allele-specific PCR (CFX96 Touch, Bio-Rad, USA) according to the methodology described earlier [49].

We used standard methods of descriptive statistics and frequency analysis. To test hypotheses about differences in the distributions of categorical characteristics in comparison groups, we used contingency table analysis and two-sided Fisher's test to assess the level significance. To assess the level of agreement between studies, we used AC1 (Gwet's first-order agreement coefficient).

5. Conclusions

Spatial heterogeneity of tumor clones in MM were assessed using a variety of approaches. Genetic abnormalities in DNA isolated from various sources, including plasma (ctDNA), CD138+ bone marrow cells, and plasmacytomas, were compared. The study of the STR profile in DNA isolated from different tumor localizations demonstrated the anatomical heterogeneity of MM. Future studies are needed to clarify whether the number of STR loci with LOH has prognostic value in MM. The detection of rare mutations in the *KRAS* and *NRAS* genes in MM is associated with a variety of clinical and laboratory adverse factors. Relying solely on a bone marrow sample for risk stratification in MM may lead to an inaccurate result. Given the detection of aberrations in tumor ctDNA that differ from those in bone marrow and plasmacytoma, the issue of practical use of liquid biopsy for risk stratification is being discussed.

Supplementary Materials: The following supporting information can be downloaded at: https://www.mdpi.com/article/10.3390/ijms25179426/s1.

Author Contributions: Conceptualization, M.S. (Maiia Soloveva), N.R., and M.S. (Maksim Solovev); methodology, E.N. and I.Y.; formal analysis, M.S. (Maiia Soloveva), Y.C., and S.K.; investigation, N.R., E.N., I.Y., and B.B.; resources, A.S., T.O., M.S. (Maksim Solovev), and L.M.; data curation, M.S. (Maiia Soloveva) and M.S. (Maksim Solovev); writing—original draft preparation, M.S. (Maiia Soloveva) N.R., and I.Y.; writing—review and editing, A.S.; supervision, A.S. and L.M. All authors have read and agreed to the published version of the manuscript.

Funding: This research received no external funding.

Institutional Review Board Statement: The study was approved by the Ethics Committee of the National Research Center for Hematology (protocol No. 165/June 2021) and conducted in accordance with the Declaration of Helsinki of 1975, as revised in 2008.

Informed Consent Statement: Informed consent was obtained from all subjects involved in the study. Written informed consent has been obtained from the patient(s) to publish this paper.

Data Availability Statement: The data are contained within the article and Supplementary Materials.

Acknowledgments: We thank the doctors of the department (Arutyunyan N., Abakumova A., Irugova E., Krayzman A., Startsev A.) as well as the nursing staff (Gubanova E., Golubeva E.) for their assistance in data collection.

Conflicts of Interest: The authors declare no conflicts of interest.

References

1. Bolli, N.; Avet-Loiseau, H.; Wedge, D.C.; Van Loo, P.; Alexandrov, L.B.; Martincorena, I.; Dawson, K.J.; Iorio, F.; Nik-Zainal, S.; Bignell, G.R.; et al. Heterogeneity of genomic evolution and mutational profiles in multiple myeloma. *Nat. Commun.* **2014**, *5*, 2997. [CrossRef]
2. Melchor, L.; Jones, J.R.; Lenive, O.; Peterson, E.A.; Brioli, A.; Murison, A.; Wardell, C.P.; Kaiser, M.F.; Proszek, P.; Boyle, E.M.; et al. Spatiotemporal Analysis of Intraclonal Heterogeneity in Multiple Myeloma: Unravelling the Impact of Treatment and the Propagating Capacity of Subclones Using Whole Exome Sequencing. *Blood* **2015**, *126*, 371. [CrossRef]
3. Rasche, L.; Chavan, S.S.; Stephens, O.W.; Patel, P.H.; Tytarenko, R.; Ashby, C.; Bauer, M.; Stein, C.; Deshpande, S.; Wardell, C.; et al. Spatial genomic heterogeneity in multiple myeloma revealed by multi-region sequencing. *Nat. Commun.* **2017**, *8*, 268. [CrossRef]
4. Soloveva, M.; Solovev, M.; Nikulina, E.; Risinskaya, N.; Biderman, B.; Yakutik, I.; Obukhova, T.; Mendeleeva, L. Loss of Heterozygosity in the Circulating Tumor DNA and CD138+ Bone Marrow Cells in Multiple Myeloma. *Genes* **2023**, *14*, 351. [CrossRef] [PubMed]

5. Anwer, F.; Gee, K.M.; Iftikhar, A.; Baig, M.; Russ, A.D.; Saeed, S.; Abu Zar, M.; Razzaq, F.; Carew, J.; Nawrocki, S.; et al. Future of Personalized Therapy Targeting Aberrant Signaling Pathways in Multiple Myeloma. *Clin. Lymphoma Myeloma Leuk.* **2019**, *19*, 397–405. [CrossRef]
6. A Dimopoulos, M.; Swern, A.S.; Li, J.S.; Hussein, M.; Weiss, L.; Nagarwala, Y.; Baz, R. Efficacy and safety of long-term treatment with lenalidomide and dexamethasone in patients with relapsed/refractory multiple myeloma. *Blood Cancer J.* **2014**, *4*, e257. [CrossRef]
7. Richardson, P.G.; Sonneveld, P.; Schuster, M.W.; Irwin, D.; Stadtmauer, E.A.; Facon, T.; Harousseau, J.-L.; Ben-Yehuda, D.; Lonial, S.; Goldschmidt, H.; et al. Bortezomib or high-dose dexamethasone for relapsed multiple myeloma. *N. Engl. J. Med.* **2005**, *352*, 2487–2498. [CrossRef] [PubMed]
8. Kumar, S.K.; Lee, J.H.; Lahuerta, J.J.; Morgan, G.; Richardson, P.G.; Crowley, J.; Haessler, J.; Feather, J.; Hoering, A.; Moreau, P.; et al. Risk of progression and survival in multiple myeloma relapsing after therapy with IMiDs and bortezomib: A multicenter international myeloma working group study. *Leukemia* **2012**, *26*, 149–157. [CrossRef]
9. Pasca, S.; Tomuleasa, C.; Teodorescu, P.; Ghiaur, G.; Dima, D.; Moisoiu, V.; Berce, C.; Stefan, C.; Ciechanover, A.; Einsele, H. KRAS/NRAS/BRAF Mutations as Potential Targets in Multiple Myeloma. *Front. Oncol.* **2019**, *9*, 1137. [CrossRef]
10. Mey, U.J.M.; Renner, C.; Von Moos, R. Vemurafenib in combination with cobimetinib in relapsed and refractory extramedullary multiple myeloma harboring the BRAF V600E mutation. *Hematol. Oncol.* **2017**, *35*, 890–893. [CrossRef]
11. Raje, N.; Chau, I.; Hyman, D.M.; Ribrag, V.; Blay, J.-Y.; Tabernero, J.; Elez, E.; Wolf, J.; Yee, A.J.; Kaiser, M.; et al. Vemurafenib in Patients With Relapsed Refractory Multiple Myeloma Harboring *BRAF*^{V600} Mutations: A Cohort of the Histology-Independent VE-BASKET Study. *JCO Precis. Oncol.* **2018**, *2*, 1–9. [CrossRef] [PubMed]
12. Giesen, N.; Chatterjee, M.; Scheid, C.; Poos, A.M.; Besemer, B.; Miah, K.; Benner, A.; Becker, N.; Moehler, T.; Metzler, I.; et al. A phase 2 clinical trial of combined BRAF/MEK inhibition for *BRAF*V600E-mutated multiple myeloma. *Blood* **2023**, *141*, 1685–1690. [CrossRef] [PubMed]
13. Waldschmidt, J.M.; Kloeber, J.A.; Anand, P.; Frede, J.; Kokkalis, A.; Dimitrova, V.; Potdar, S.; Nair, M.S.; Vijaykumar, T.; Im, N.G.; et al. Single-Cell Profiling Reveals Metabolic Reprogramming as a Resistance Mechanism in*BRAF*-Mutated Multiple Myeloma. *Clin. Cancer Res.* **2021**, *27*, 6432–6444. [CrossRef] [PubMed]
14. Walker, B.A.; Mavrommatis, K.; Wardell, C.P.; Ashby, T.C.; Bauer, M.; Davies, F.E.; Rosenthal, A.; Wang, H.; Qu, P.; Hoering, A.; et al. Identification of novel mutational drivers reveals oncogene dependencies in multiple myeloma. *Blood* **2018**, *132*, 587–597. [CrossRef]
15. Gupta, N.; Sharma, A. Emerging biomarkers in Multiple Myeloma: A review. *Clin. Chim. Acta* **2019**, *503*, 45–53. [CrossRef]
16. Mazzotti, C.; Buisson, L.; Maheo, S.; Perrot, A.; Chretien, M.-L.; Leleu, X.; Hulin, C.; Manier, S.; Hébraud, B.; Roussel, M.; et al. Myeloma MRD by deep sequencing from circulating tumor DNA does not correlate with results obtained in the bone marrow. *Blood Adv.* **2018**, *2*, 2811–2813. [CrossRef]
17. Kis, O.; Kaedbey, R.; Chow, S.; Danesh, A.; Dowar, M.; Li, T.; Li, Z.; Liu, J.; Mansour, M.; Masih-Khan, E.; et al. Circulating tumour DNA sequence analysis as an alternative to multiple myeloma bone marrow aspirates. *Nat. Commun.* **2017**, *8*, 15086. [CrossRef]
18. Mithraprabhu, S.; Khong, T.; Ramachandran, M.; Chow, A.; Klarica, D.; Mai, L.; Walsh, S.; Broemeling, D.; Marziali, A.; Wiggin, M.; et al. Circulating tumour DNA analysis demonstrates spatial mutational heterogeneity that coincides with disease relapse in myeloma. *Leukemia* **2016**, *31*, 1695–1705. [CrossRef]
19. Rajkumar, S.V.; Dimopoulos, M.A.; Palumbo, A.; Blade, J.; Merlini, G.; Mateos, M.-V.; Kumar, S.; Hillengass, J.; Kastritis, E.; Richardson, P.; et al. International Myeloma Working Group updated criteria for the diagnosis of multiple myeloma. *Lancet Oncol.* **2014**, *15*, e538–e548. [CrossRef]
20. Usmani, S.Z.; Heuck, C.; Mitchell, A.; Szymonifka, J.; Nair, B.; Hoering, A.; Alsayed, Y.; Waheed, S.; Haider, S.; Restrepo, A.; et al. Extramedullary disease portends poor prognosis in multiple myeloma and is over-represented in high-risk disease even in the era of novel agents. *Haematologica* **2012**, *97*, 1761–1767. [CrossRef]
21. Varettoni, M.; Corso, A.; Pica, G.; Mangiacavalli, S.; Pascutto, C.; Lazzarino, M. Incidence, presenting features and outcome of extramedullary disease in multiple myeloma: A longitudinal study on 1003 consecutive patients. *Ann. Oncol.* **2010**, *21*, 325–330. [CrossRef] [PubMed]
22. Bladé, J.; de Larrea, C.F.; Rosiñol, L.; Cibeira, M.T.; Jiménez, R.; Powles, R. Soft-Tissue Plasmacytomas in Multiple Myeloma: Incidence, Mechanisms of Extramedullary Spread, and Treatment Approach. *J. Clin. Oncol.* **2011**, *29*, 3805–3812. [CrossRef]
23. Weinstock, M.; Ghobrial, I.M. Extramedullary multiple myeloma. *Leuk. Lymphoma* **2012**, *54*, 1135–1141. [CrossRef] [PubMed]
24. Rasche, L.; Bernard, C.; Topp, M.S.; Kapp, M.; Duell, J.; Wesemeier, C.; Haralambieva, E.; Maeder, U.; Einsele, H.; Knop, S. Features of extramedullary myeloma relapse: High proliferation, minimal marrow involvement, adverse cytogenetics: A retrospective single-center study of 24 cases. *Ann. Hematol.* **2012**, *91*, 1031–1037. [CrossRef]
25. Rosiñol, L.; Beksac, M.; Zamagni, E.; Van de Donk, N.W.C.J.; Anderson, K.C.; Badros, A.; Caers, J.; Cavo, M.; Dimopoulos, M.; Dispenzieri, A.; et al. Expert review on soft-tissue plasmacytomas in multiple myeloma: Definition, disease assessment and treatment considerations. *Br. J. Haematol.* **2021**, *194*, 496–507. [CrossRef] [PubMed]
26. McAvera, R.; Quinn, J.; Murphy, P.; Glavey, S. Genetic Abnormalities in Extramedullary Multiple Myeloma. *Int. J. Mol. Sci.* **2023**, *24*, 11259. [CrossRef]
27. Dahl, I.M.S.; Rasmussen, T.; Kauric, G.; Husebekk, A. Differential expression of CD56 and CD44 in the evolution of extramedullary myeloma. *Br. J. Haematol.* **2002**, *116*, 273–277. [CrossRef]

28. Firsova, M.V.; Mendeleeva, L.P.; Kovrigina, A.M.; Solovev, M.V.; Savchenko, V.G. Plasmacytoma in patients with multiple myeloma: Morphology and immunohistochemistry. *BMC Cancer* **2020**, *20*, 346. [CrossRef] [PubMed]
29. Liu, Y.; Jelloul, F.; Zhang, Y.; Bhavsar, T.; Ho, C.; Rao, M.B.; Lewis, N.E.; Cimera, R.B.; Baik, J.B.; Sigler, A.B.; et al. Genetic Basis of Extramedullary Plasmablastic Transformation of Multiple Myeloma. *Am. J. Surg. Pathol.* **2020**, *44*, 838–848. [CrossRef]
30. Weinstock, M.; Aljawai, Y.; Morgan, E.A.; Laubach, J.; Gannon, M.; Roccaro, A.M.; Varga, C.; Mitsiades, C.S.; Paba-Prada, C.; Schlossman, R.; et al. Incidence and clinical features of extramedullary multiple myeloma in patients who underwent stem cell transplantation. *Br. J. Haematol.* **2015**, *169*, 851–858. [CrossRef]
31. Firsova, M.V.; Risinskaya, N.V.; Solovev, M.V.; Obukhova, T.N.; Kislitsyna, M.A.; Nikulina, E.E.; Yakutik, I.A.; Abramova, T.V.; Sudarikov, A.B.; Kovrigina, A.M.; et al. Multiple myeloma with extramedullary plasmacytoma: Pathogenesis and clinical case. *Oncohematology* **2022**, *17*, 67–80. [CrossRef]
32. Risinskaya, N.; Kozhevnikova, Y.; Gavrilina, O.; Chabaeva, J.; Kotova, E.; Yushkova, A.; Isinova, G.; Zarubina, K.; Obukhova, T.; Kulikov, S.; et al. Loss of Heterozygosity in the Tumor DNA of De Novo Diagnosed Patients Is Associated with Poor Outcome for B-ALL but Not for T-ALL. *Genes* **2022**, *13*, 398. [CrossRef]
33. Risinskaya, N.; Mangasarova, Y.; Nikulina, E.; Kozhevnikova, Y.; Chabaeva, J.; Yushkova, A.; Magomedova, A.; Kulikov, S.; Julhakyan, H.; Kravchenko, S.; et al. STR Profiling Reveals Tumor Genome Instability in Primary Mediastinal B-Cell Lymphoma. *Curr. Oncol.* **2022**, *29*, 3449–3459. [CrossRef]
34. Long, X.; Xu, Q.; Lou, Y.; Li, C.; Gu, J.; Cai, H.; Wang, D.; Xu, J.; Li, T.; Zhou, X.; et al. The utility of non-invasive liquid biopsy for mutational analysis and minimal residual disease assessment in extramedullary multiple myeloma. *Br. J. Haematol.* **2020**, *189*, e45–e48. [CrossRef]
35. Walker, B.A.; Boyle, E.M.; Wardell, C.P.; Murison, A.; Begum, D.B.; Dahir, N.M.; Proszek, P.Z.; Johnson, D.C.; Kaiser, M.F.; Melchor, L.; et al. Mutational Spectrum, Copy Number Changes, and Outcome: Results of a Sequencing Study of Patients With Newly Diagnosed Myeloma. *J. Clin. Oncol.* **2015**, *33*, 3911–3920. [CrossRef]
36. Chapman, P.B.; Hauschild, A.; Robert, C.; Haanen, J.B.; Ascierto, P.; Larkin, J.; Dummer, R.; Garbe, C.; Testori, A.; Maio, M.; et al. Improved survival with vemurafenib in melanoma with BRAF V600E mutation. *N. Engl. J. Med.* **2011**, *364*, 2507–2516. [CrossRef]
37. Heidorn, S.J.; Milagre, C.; Whittaker, S.; Nourry, A.; Niculescu-Duvas, I.; Dhomen, N.; Hussain, J.; Reis-Filho, J.S.; Springer, C.J.; Pritchard, C.; et al. Kinase-Dead BRAF and Oncogenic RAS Cooperate to Drive Tumor Progression through CRAF. *Cell* **2010**, *140*, 209–221. [CrossRef]
38. Manier, S.; Park, J.; Capelletti, M.; Bustoros, M.; Freeman, S.S.; Ha, G.; Rhoades, J.; Liu, C.J.; Huynh, D.; Reed, S.C.; et al. Whole-exome sequencing of cell-free DNA and circulating tumor cells in multiple myeloma. *Nat. Commun.* **2018**, *9*, 1691. [CrossRef]
39. Grisedale, K.S.; van Daal, A. Comparison of STR profiling from low template DNA extracts with and without the consensus profiling method. *Investig. Genet.* **2012**, *3*, 14. [CrossRef]
40. Vij, R.; Mazumder, A.; Klinger, M.; O'Dea, D.; Paasch, J.; Martin, T.; Weng, L.; Park, J.; Fiala, M.; Faham, M.; et al. Deep Sequencing Reveals Myeloma Cells in Peripheral Blood in Majority of Multiple Myeloma Patients. *Clin. Lymphoma Myeloma Leuk.* **2014**, *14*, 131–139.e1. [CrossRef]
41. Gozzetti, A.; Bocchia, M. Liquid biopsy and blood-based minimal residual disease evaluation in multiple myeloma. *Oncol. Res. Featur. Preclin. Clin. Cancer Ther.* **2023**, *31*, 271–274. [CrossRef]
42. Sidorova, J.V.; Sorokina, T.V.; Biderman, B.V.; Nikulina, E.E.; Kisilichina, D.G.; Naumova, E.V.; Pochtar', M.E.; Lugovskaia, S.A.; Ivanova, V.L.; Kovaleva, L.G.; et al. The detection of minimal residual disease in patients with chronic B-cell lymphatic leukemia using patient-specified polymerase chain reaction. *Klin. Lab. Diagn.* **2011**, *12*, 22–24. (In Russian)
43. Sidorova, J.V.; Biderman, B.V.; Nikulina, E.E.; Sudarikov, A.B. A simple and efficient method for DNA extraction from skin and paraffin-embedded tissues applicable to T-cell clonality assays. *Exp. Dermatol.* **2011**, *21*, 57–60. [CrossRef]
44. Bolger, A.M.; Lohse, M.; Usadel, B. Trimmomatic: A flexible trimmer for Illumina sequence data. *Bioinformatics* **2014**, *30*, 2114–2120. [CrossRef] [PubMed]
45. Li, H.; Durbin, R. Fast and accurate long-read alignment with Burrows–Wheeler transform. *Bioinformatics* **2010**, *26*, 589–595. [CrossRef] [PubMed]
46. Li, H.; Handsaker, B.; Wysoker, A.; Fennell, T.; Ruan, J.; Homer, N.; Marth, G.; Abecasis, G.; Durbin, R.; 1000 Genome Project Data Processing Subgroup. The Sequence Alignment/Map format and SAMtools. *Bioinformatics* **2009**, *25*, 2078–2079. [CrossRef]
47. Lai, Z.; Markovets, A.; Ahdesmaki, M.; Chapman, B.; Hofmann, O.; McEwen, R.; Johnson, J.; Dougherty, B.; Barrett, J.C.; Dry, J.R. VarDict: A novel and versatile variant caller for next-generation sequencing in cancer research. *Nucleic Acids Res.* **2016**, *44*, e108. [CrossRef]
48. Wang, K.; Li, M.; Hakonarson, H. ANNOVAR: Functional annotation of genetic variants from high-throughput sequencing data. *Nucleic Acids Res.* **2010**, *38*, e164. [CrossRef] [PubMed]
49. Yakutik, I.A.; Al-Radi, L.S.; Biderman, B.V.; Nikitin, E.A. Detection of BRAF V600E mutation in patients with hairy cell leukemia by allele-specific RT-PCR. *Hematol. Transfusiology* **2014**, *59*, 16–19. (In Russian)

International Journal of
Molecular Sciences

MDPI

Article

An Optimized Peptide Antagonist of CXCR4 Limits Survival of BCR–ABL1-Transformed Cells in Philadelphia-Chromosome-Positive B-Cell Acute Lymphoblastic Leukemia

Johanna Pohl [1], Angela Litz [1], Omar El Ayoubi [1], Armando Rodríguez-Alfonso [2,3], Ludger Ständker [2], Mirja Harms [4], Jan Münch [4], Hassan Jumaa [1,*] and Moumita Datta [1,*]

1 Institute of Immunology, Ulm University Medical Center, 89081 Ulm, Germany; lemir.el-ayoubi@uni-ulm.de (O.E.A.)
2 Core Facility Functional Peptidomics, Ulm University Medical Center, 89081 Ulm, Germany; armando.rodriguez-alfonso@uni-ulm.de (A.R.-A.); ludger.staendker@uni-ulm.de (L.S.)
3 Core Unit Mass Spectrometry and Proteomics, Ulm University Medical Center, 89081 Ulm, Germany
4 Institute of Molecular Virology, Ulm University Medical Center, 89081 Ulm, Germany; mirja.harms@uni-ulm.de (M.H.); jan.muench@uni-ulm.de (J.M.)
* Correspondence: hassan.jumaa@uni-ulm.de (H.J.); moumita.datta@uni-ulm.de (M.D.)

Abstract: Philadelphia-chromosome-positive acute lymphoblastic leukemia (Ph$^+$ ALL) is characterized by reciprocal chromosomal translocation between chromosome 9 and 22, leading to the expression of constitutively active oncogenic BCR–ABL1 fusion protein. CXC chemokine receptor 4 (CXCR4) is essential for the survival of BCR–ABL1-transformed mouse pre-B cells, as the deletion of CXCR4 induces death in these cells. To investigate whether CXCR4 inhibition also effectively blocks BCR–ABL1-transformed cell growth in vitro, in this study, we explored an array of peptide-based inhibitors of CXCR4. The inhibitors were optimized derivatives of EPI-X4, an endogenous peptide antagonist of CXCR4. We observed that among all the candidates, EPI-X4 JM#170 (referred to as JM#170) effectively induced cell death in BCR–ABL1-transformed mouse B cells but had little effect on untransformed wild-type B cells. Importantly, AMD3100, a small molecule inhibitor of CXCR4, did not show this effect. Treatment with JM#170 induced transient JNK phosphorylation in BCR–ABL1-transformed cells, which in turn activated the intrinsic apoptotic pathway by inducing *cJun*, *Bim*, and *Bax* gene expressions. Combinatorial treatment of JM#170 with ABL1 kinase inhibitor Imatinib exerted a stronger killing effect on BCR–ABL1-transformed cells even at a lower dose of Imatinib. Surprisingly, JM#170 actively killed Sup-B15 cells, a BCR–ABL1$^+$ human ALL cell line, but had no effect on the BCR–ABL1$^-$ 697 cell line. This suggests that the inhibitory effect of JM#170 is specific for BCR–ABL1$^+$ ALL. Taken together, JM#170 emerges as a potent novel drug against Ph$^+$ ALL.

Keywords: BCR–ABL1; CXCR4; AMD3100; Imatinib; cell survival; EPI-X4 derivatives

1. Introduction

The expression of the BCR–ABL1 fusion protein is a hallmark of Ph$^+$ ALL, which affects around one-third of adult ALL cases and ~3–5% of pediatric ALL cases [1]. The oncogenic fusion of the breakpoint cluster region (BCR) at chromosome 22 and the tyrosine-protein kinase ABL1 at chromosome 9 results from a reciprocal chromosomal translocation t(9;22)(q34;q11), which leads to constitutive tyrosine kinase activation [2,3]. The prognosis of the disease was very poor until the advent of tyrosine kinase inhibitors (TKIs) such as Imatinib mesylate [4–6]. The current treatment regimen for Ph$^+$ ALL generally involves chemotherapy in combination with TKI, followed by allogeneic hematopoietic stem cell transplantation (allo-HCT) [7]. In some cases, the combination of TKI with chemotherapy can achieve long-term remission without allo-HCT. Although the inclusion of TKIs in frontline therapy has revolutionized the outcome of the disease, the emergence of TKI resistance through acquired mutation(s) in the ABL kinase domain poses a significant threat to the prognosis of the disease. Some of these mutations, e.g., T315I, can now be targeted by the advanced third-generation TKI inhibitor Ponatinib [8]. However, the toxicity associated with some of the advanced therapeutics as well as their limited access in many of the clinics worldwide make it challenging for clinicians, especially those in resource-constrained situations [7]. This therefore necessitates the continuous search for new, improved inhibitors as single or combinatorial therapeutics [9].

Previously, our laboratory showed that the G-protein coupled chemokine receptor CXCR4 promotes the survival of BCR–ABL1-transformed mouse B cells [10]. Deletion of CXCR4 results in rapid cell death and the complete absence of colony formation in vitro by these cells. Mechanistically, CXCR4 associates with the interleukin 7 receptor (IL7R) on the surface of BCR–ABL1 cells. This leads to the recruitment of IL7R-associated proteins such as Janus kinase 3 (JAK3) in close proximity to CXCR4, thereby activating the JAK-STAT pathway and stimulating cell survival. The hyper-phosphorylation of JAK1-3 is observed in BCR–ABL1-transformed cells, which is reduced by the inducible deletion of CXCR4 in these cells. Thus, the association between these two receptors is a prerequirement for BCR–ABL- induced cell transformation [10].

The above observation raises the question as to whether, similar to deletion, the inhibition of CXCR4 also exerts an inhibitory effect on BCR–ABL1-transformed cells. Several small-molecule and peptide inhibitors are available for CXCR4, of which only AMD3100 (Plerixafor) and BL-8040 are FDA-approved drugs, used in stem cell transplantation [11,12]. Owing to the unfavorable side effects of some of these drugs, there is an urgent need to develop novel CXCR4 antagonists. The endogenous peptide inhibitor of CXCR4 (EPI-X4), a 16 mer peptide derived from human serum albumin, exhibits specific binding to CXCR4 and the subsequent blocking of CXCL12-mediated CXCR4 activation [13]. To improve its efficacy and plasma stability, several derivatives of EPI-X4 have been designed using quantitative structure–activity relationship (QSAR) studies [14,15]. For instance, activity-improved derivative EPI-X4 JM#21 has shown therapeutic efficacies in mouse models of inflammatory diseases [14] as well as in oncologic applications [16]. To further improve the stability of optimized EPI-X4 derivatives, they have been conjugated to long-chain fatty acids, leading to increased serum albumin affinity and, thus, to an improved circulation half-life [17]. Previous work from our laboratory have shown that most of these advanced EPI-X4 derivatives potentially block CXCL12-mediated intracellular calcium release in BCR–ABL1-transformed cells in the nanomolar range [14,17]. However, the effect of these advanced derivatives on the survival of BCR–ABL1 cells has not yet been investigated.

Thus, in the current study, we tested an array of advanced EPI-X4 derivatives for their efficacy in inhibiting BCR–ABL1 cell growth and compared the effect with those of the small-molecule CXCR4 antagonist AMD3100 and the ABL1 TKI Imatinib. We also explored the signaling cascade alterations induced by these inhibitors and tested if the combination of the EPI-X4 derivative with Imatinib exerted a superior cell killing effect. Furthermore, we tested whether the inhibitors would be effective in human ALL cell lines and primary xenograft cells to evaluate their therapeutic potential.

2. Results

2.1. Optimized EPI-X4 Derivative JM#170 Potentially Blocks Growth of BCR–ABL1-Transformed Mouse B Cells In Vitro

Previously, we have shown that optimized EPI-X4 derivatives such as the 12-mer peptides WSC02 and JM#21 and fatty-acid-conjugated peptides JM#143, JM#169, JM#170, and JM#192 (Table 1) are potent inhibitors of CXCR4 activation as they block CXCL12-induced calcium signaling in BCR–ABL1-transformed mouse bone marrow (BM) B cells [14,17]. To investigate whether this inhibition of CXCR4 signaling exerts any effect on cell survival in vitro, we treated the BCR–ABL1-transformed cells with increasing concentrations (1, 5, and 10 μM) of the above inhibitors as well as AMD3100, a potent small-molecule CXCR4 antagonist, and measured cell growth using real-time live cell imaging in IncuCyte for 96 h. Imatinib, an ABL1 kinase inhibitor known to kill BCR–ABL1 cells at a concentration of 1 μM, was used as the positive control. BCR–ABL1 cells express intrinsic GFP; thus, the enrichment in GFP-positive cells can be used as a marker of cell growth. As depicted in Figure 1A, treatment with the solvent control DMSO led to the accumulation of GFP^+ cells over time, while treatment with 1 μM Imatinib completely blocked cell growth (Figure 1A, last panel, and Figure 1D). Among the EPI-X4 derivatives, only JM#170 showed a significant reduction in GFP enrichment at 10 μM compared to DMSO (Figure 1A, second panel, and Figure 1B). The remaining inhibitors had no effect on BCR–ABL1 cell growth, except for JM#169, which showed a significant reduction in cell growth only after 72 h (Supplementary Figure S1A,B). Interestingly, JM#170 blocked cell growth as early as 24 h, while the effect of the small-molecule inhibitor AMD3100 was only distinct at later time points (72 and 96 h, Figure 1A,C). Of note, the inhibitory effect of AMD3100 was also detectable at a lower concentration of 5 μM (Figure 1C). Taken together, the inhibition of CXCR4 by JM#170 and AMD3100 led to the inhibition of BCR–ABL1 cell growth in vitro.

Table 1. Sequence of the optimized EPI-X4 derivatives.

EPI-X4 Derivative	Sequence	Molecular Weight (Da)	Reference
Original	LVRYTKKVPQVSTPTL	1832	[13]
WSC02	IVRWSKKVPCVS	1401	[13]
JM#21	ILRWSRKLPCVS	1458	[14]
JM#143	ILRWSRK * (Glu-Pal)LPCVS	1825	Harms et al., 2024 [17]
JM#169	IVRWSKK * (Pal)VPCVS	1640	Harms et al., 2024 [17]
JM#170	ILRWSRK * (Pal)-NH_2	1197	Harms et al., 2024 [17]
JM#192	ILRWSRK * (Glu-Pal)-NH_2	1325	Harms et al., 2024 [17]

* Modified residue—C16 long-chain fatty acid (palmitic acid) linked to the ε-amino side chain of K either directly or via a glutamic acid linker.

To understand whether this inhibition of cell growth in the presence of JM#170 and AMD3100 was due to cell death induced by the inhibitors, we incubated the cells with 10 μM JM#170 and AMD3100 for different durations and stained them with viability dye. Imatinib (1 μM) served as the positive control. The results showed that JM#170 induced strong and rapid cell death in BCR–ABL1 cells, with ~70% of cells dying within 1 h of treatment (Figure 1E and Supplementary Figure S2). Cell viability remained low over time, with a prominent increase at 72 h, which could be explained by the loss of stability of peptide-based inhibitors in the serum-containing media. Imatinib, as previously stated, exerted a strong and persistent killing effect on BCR–ABL1-transformed cells starting from 24 h after treatment.

Surprisingly, AMD3100 did not induce any loss of cell viability within the experimental time period (Figure 1E). Thus, to understand how AMD3100 blocked BCR–ABL1 cell growth as observed before (Figure 1A,C), we labeled the cells with cell trace cell proliferation dye and treated them with 10 μM each of JM#170 and AMD3100. The level of cell proliferation was measured via the dye dilution method. As depicted in Figure 1F,G, AMD3100 significantly reduced the proliferation of BCR–ABL1 cells as compared to DMSO at 48 and 72 h after treatment. This is in line with our previous finding that AMD3100 blocked cell growth only after ~48 h (Figure 1A,C). Interestingly, JM#170 had no effect on proliferation, as cells that survived JM#170 treatment proliferated equally to DMSO-treated ones (Figure 1F). Thus, the mode of action of the two CXCR4 inhibitors are different—while AMD3100 blocks proliferation, JM#170 induces rapid death of BCR–ABL1 cells.

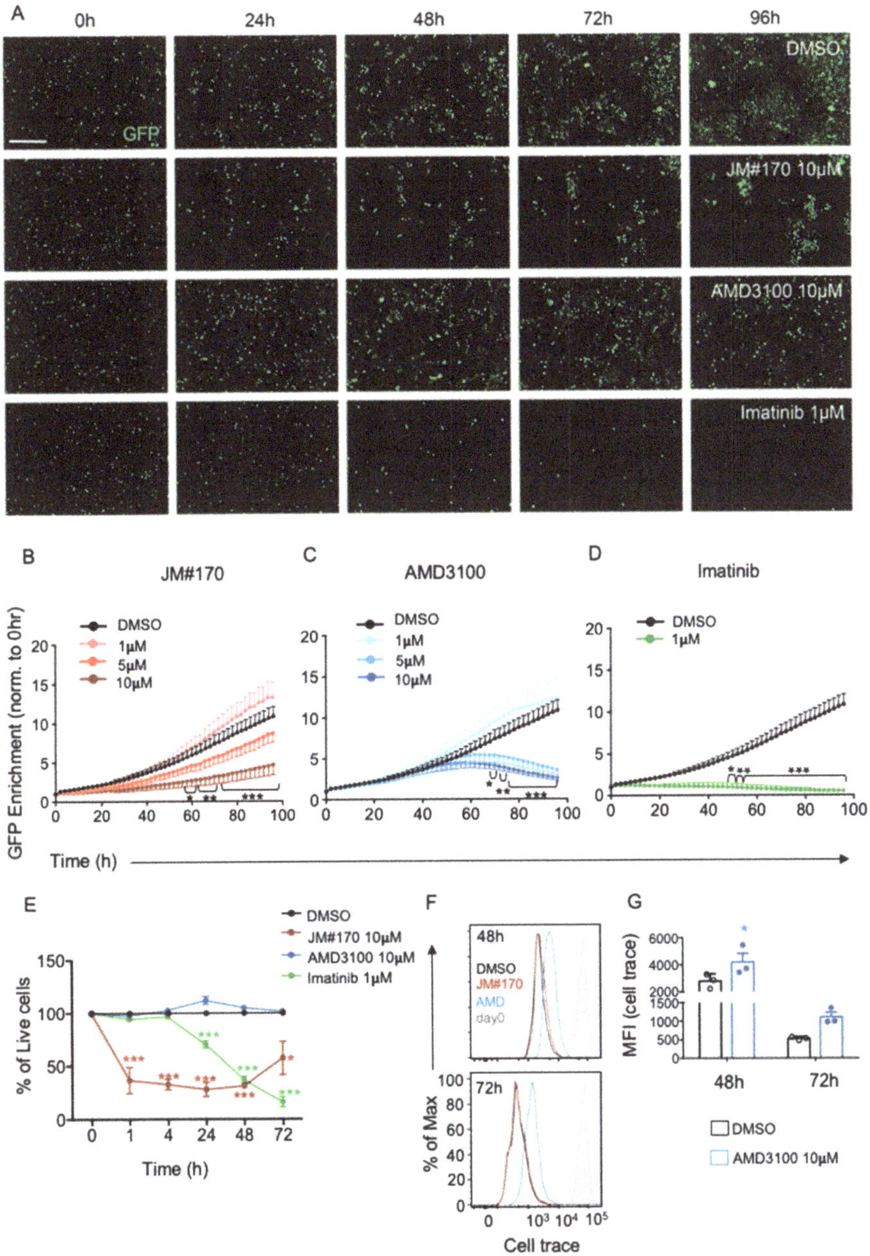

Figure 1. Effect of JM#170 on cellular growth in BCR–ABL1-transformed mouse B cells. (**A**) Real-time imaging of BCR–ABL1-transformed mouse B cells treated with solvent (DMSO), 10 μM JM#170 or AMD3100 or 1 μM Imatinib over 96 h. Images are representative of one experiment out of n = 4–5. Scale bar: 200μm. (**B**,**C**) Quantification of GFP$^+$ cell enrichment as a marker of BCR–ABL1 cell growth in control (DMSO) and different (1, 5, and 10 μM) concentrations of JM#170 (**B**) and AMD3100 (**C**) treated cells over 96 h. The count of GFP$^+$ cells for each time point for each treatment was normalized with respect to the corresponding count at 0 h. Graph represents mean ± SEM, n = 4–5.

(**D**) Similar quantification in control (DMSO) and 1 μM Imatinib-treated cells. Graph represents mean ± SEM, $n = 5$. Statistical analysis—two-way ANOVA with Dunnett's multiple comparison test. * $p < 0.05$, ** $p < 0.01$, *** $p < 0.001$. (**E**) Flow cytometric analysis of viability of BCR–ABL1 cells treated with solvent (DMSO), 10 μM JM#170 or AMD3100, or 1 μM Imatinib over the indicated time period. The live cell count for each treatment for each time point was normalized with the corresponding live cell count for DMSO and is represented as a percentage. Graph represents mean ± SEM, $n = 3$. Statistical analysis—two-way ANOVA with Sidak's multiple comparison test. * $p < 0.05$, *** $p < 0.001$. (**F**) Flow cytometric analysis of proliferation of BCR–ABL1 cells treated with DMSO and 10 μM each of JM#170 and AMD3100 for the indicated time period. (**G**) Quantification of cell trace dye dilution, represented by the median fluorescence intensity (MFI) of the dye in DMSO and AMD3100-treated BCR–ABL1 cells after 48 and 72 h of treatment. Bar represents mean ± SEM, $n = 3$. Statistical analysis—two-way ANOVA with Sidak's multiple comparison test. * $p < 0.05$.

To address the hypothesis that JM#170 specifically targets CXCR4, we performed an anti-CXCR4 antibody competition assay. BCR–ABL1-transformed cells were treated with increasing concentrations of JM#170, AMD3100 and Imatinib in the presence of a fixed concentration of anti-CXCR4 antibody, followed by flow cytometric analysis to measure the amount of bound antibody. Both JM#170 and AMD3100 significantly inhibited the antibody binding to CXCR4 (Supplementary Figure S1C). However, JM#170 was effective at a much lower concentration (~10 nM) than AMD3100 (~1 μM). Imatinib, on the other hand, had no effect on antibody binding to CXCR4 as it did not interact with CXCR4 (Supplementary Figure S1C). This suggests that JM#170 specifically targets CXCR4 in BCR–ABL1-transformed B cells.

2.2. *JM#170 Does Not Affect the Survival of Untransformed B Cells*

To address whether the growth inhibition observed in the presence of JM#170 or AMD3100 was specific for BCR–ABL1 cells or caused by the general toxicity of the molecules, we tested their effects on untransformed mouse BM B cells. Previous reports from our laboratory have demonstrated that BM B cells isolated from $Rag2^{-/-}$ $\lambda5^{-/-}$ $Spl65^{-/-}$ triple knockout (TKO) mice are blocked at the pro-B-cell stage due to lack of V(D)J recombination [18,19]. These cells can be cultured in the presence of IL7. Similar to WT BM B cells, the transformation of TKO cells with BCR–ABL1 led to enhanced cell growth compared to that of untransformed (empty pMIG vector-transfected (TKO-EV)) cells (Supplementary Figure S3A,B), indicating that the TKO mutations do not bring about any unexpected cell phenotype. We therefore used these untransformed TKO-EV cells to investigate the effect of the inhibitors. The cells were similarly treated with increasing concentrations of JM#170 and AMD3100, and 1 μM Imatinib, and they were subjected to real-time imaging in IncuCyte for 96 h. As depicted in Figure 2A–C, neither JM#170 nor AMD3100 had any effect on the survival of TKO-EV cells at any concentration tested. Imatinib, as expected, also had no effect on the TKO-EV cells (Figure 2A,D). It could be argued that CXCR4 surface expression may vary between the cell types, with TKO-EV being low in CXCR4 expression, leading to no effect on CXCR4 inhibition. To address this, we measured the cell surface expression of CXCR4 in BCR–ABL1 and TKO-EV cells. The results indicated that the cells expressed comparable amounts of CXCR4 on the surface (Figure 2E). In addition, we tested the inhibitors in normal WT mouse BM-derived B cells. Neither of the inhibitors had any effect on them (Supplementary Figure S3C). Thus, the growth inhibitory effects of JM#170 and AMD3100 are specific to BCR–ABL1 transformed cells and not due to the general toxicity of the molecules.

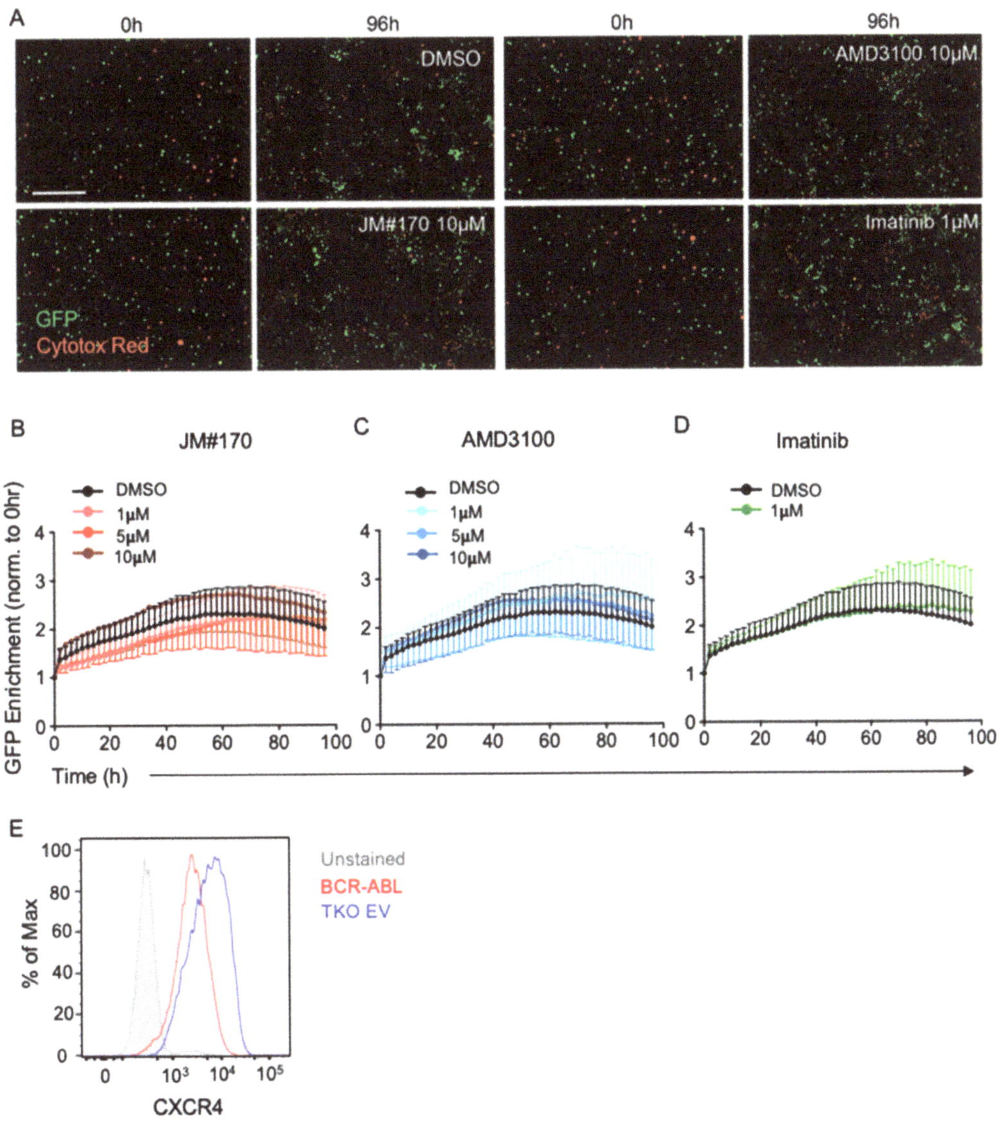

Figure 2. Effect of JM#170 on cellular growth in untransformed mouse bone marrow B cells. (**A**) Real-time imaging of bone marrow B cells derived from *Rag2*$^{-/-}$ $\lambda5^{-/-}$ *Slp65*$^{-/-}$ TKO mice treated with solvent (DMSO), 10 μM of JM#170 or AMD3100, or 1 μM Imatinib over 96 h. Cells expressed intrinsic GFP and were labeled with Cytotox Red dye to measure cell death. Images are representative of one experiment of $n = 3$. Scale bar: 200 μm. (**B**,**C**) Quantification of GFP$^+$ cell enrichment as a marker of TKO cell growth in control (DMSO) and treatments with different (1, 5, and 10 μM) concentrations of JM#170 (**B**)- and AMD3100 (**C**) over 96 h. The count of GFP$^+$ cells for each time point for each treatment was normalized with respect to the corresponding count at 0 h. Graph represents mean ± SEM, $n = 3$. (**D**) Similar quantification in control (DMSO) and 1 μM Imatinib-treated TKO cells. Graph represents mean ± SEM, $n = 3$. (**E**) Histogram showing CXCR4 expression on the surface of BCR–ABL1 (red line) and TKO (blue line) cells. Grey-filled histogram represents unstained sample. Statistical analysis—two-way ANOVA with Dunnett's multiple comparison test.

2.3. JM#170 Blocks CXCL12-Induced ERK1/2 and PI3K Signaling in BCR–ABL1 Cells

From our previous study, we knew that both JM#170 and AMD3100 block the intracellular calcium response upon CXCR4 activation [14,17]. To check if they also block CXCR4-downstream PI3K and MAP kinase (MAPK) activation, we transiently treated the cells with inhibitors and performed Western blotting to detect AKT and ERK1/2 phosphorylation. In the absence of CXCL12 stimulation, the basal level of S473 phosphorylation of AKT remained low, with no changes observed after the addition of the inhibitors (Figure 3A, left panel; Figure 3B; Supplementary Figure S7). Similarly, basal ERK1/2 phosphorylation at T202/Y204 also remained low in the absence of CXCL12, although a slight increase was observed in DMSO-, JM#170-, and AMD3100-treated cells compared to untreated cells (Figure 3A, left panel; Figure 3C; Supplementary Figure S7). This might be expected as DMSO is known to alter cellular homeostasis. However, when stimulated with CXCL12, a strong and rapid increase in AKT and ERK1/2 phosphorylation was observed in DMSO treated cells within 5 min of stimulation, while for both JM#170- and AMD3100-treated cells, this elevation was blocked (Figure 3A, right panel; Figure 3B,C; Supplementary Figure S7). The phosphorylation level for both AKT and ERK decreased over time; however, they remained high in the control compared to that in JM#170- and AMD3100-treated cells. Thirty minutes after stimulation, both signaling pathways seemed to be downregulated. Interestingly, Imatinib did not affect CXCL12-mediated AKT and ERK activation in the initiation phase (5 min), but the signal terminated rapidly especially for ERK (Figure 3A, right panel; Figure 3B,C; Supplementary Figure S7). Collectively, these data clearly suggest that JM#170 and AMD3100 inhibit the PI3K and ERK signaling pathways downstream of CXCR4 activation.

2.4. JM#170 Induces Phosphorylation of JNK and Triggers Intrinsic Apoptotic Pathway in BCR–ABL1 Cells

While analyzing the activation of CXCR4-downstream MAPK pathways in the presence of the inhibitors, we observed that the treatment with JM#170 transiently upregulated basal JNK phosphorylation in BCR–ABL1 cells compared to that in the control DMSO in the absence of any CXCL12 stimulation (Figure 4A,B, Supplementary Figure S8). A small but significant increase in JNK phosphorylation was observed 5 min after stimulation, while such upregulation was not observed in AMD3100-treated cells. Notably, Imatinib treatment significantly reduced basal JNK phosphorylation at 5 and 15 min after treatment (Figure 4A,B, Supplementary Figure S8). JNK is known to be activated under various cellular stress conditions, including treatment with inhibitors, which ultimately leads to cell apoptosis [20]. Therefore, to investigate whether JM#170-mediated JNK activation induced apoptosis in BCR–ABL1 cells, we measured the activation of executioner caspases 3 and 7. As depicted in Figure 4C, a significant increase in caspase 3/7 activation was observed in JM#170-treated cells compared to that in DMSO-treated ones 24 and 48 h after treatment. AMD3100, on the other hand, did not induce any caspase activation. Caspase activation was significantly lower in these cells than in DMSO-treated cells (Figure 4C). Next, we checked caspase 8 activation as a marker of the death-receptor-mediated extrinsic apoptotic pathway. The results suggested that neither JM#170 nor AMD3100 induced caspase 8; rather, they downregulated it in comparison to DMSO (Figure 4D). This indicates that JM#170 triggers the intrinsic apoptosis pathway in BCR–ABL1 cells. This is further corroborated by the observation that the JM#170 treatment led to the significant up-regulation of pro apoptotic genes downstream of JNK activation (Figure 4E). *Jun* and *Bim* were significantly elevated in the presence of JM#170 24 h after treatment, while *Bax* was mildly upregulated. Interestingly, a significant increase in anti-apoptotic *Bcl2* gene expression was also observed in these cells, which could indicate a compensatory effect to balance the induction of apoptosis. Notably, the expression of the other anti-apoptotic gene *Bcl-xl* was not altered at all (Figure 4E). The inactivation of *FasL* in the JM#170-treated cells again supported the noninvolvement of the death-receptor-mediated extrinsic apoptotic pathway. The overall level of gene expression alteration diminished after 48 h, with still significantly elevated levels of *Bax*, *Bim*, and *Bcl2* in JM#170-treated cells (Figure 4F). AMD3100, on the contrary, did not upregulate any gene expression at any time points (Figure 4E,F).

Thus, collectively, these data reflect that JM#170 spontaneously activates the JNK pathway and triggers intrinsic apoptosis in BCR–ABL1-transformed cells—a process not elicited by AMD3100.

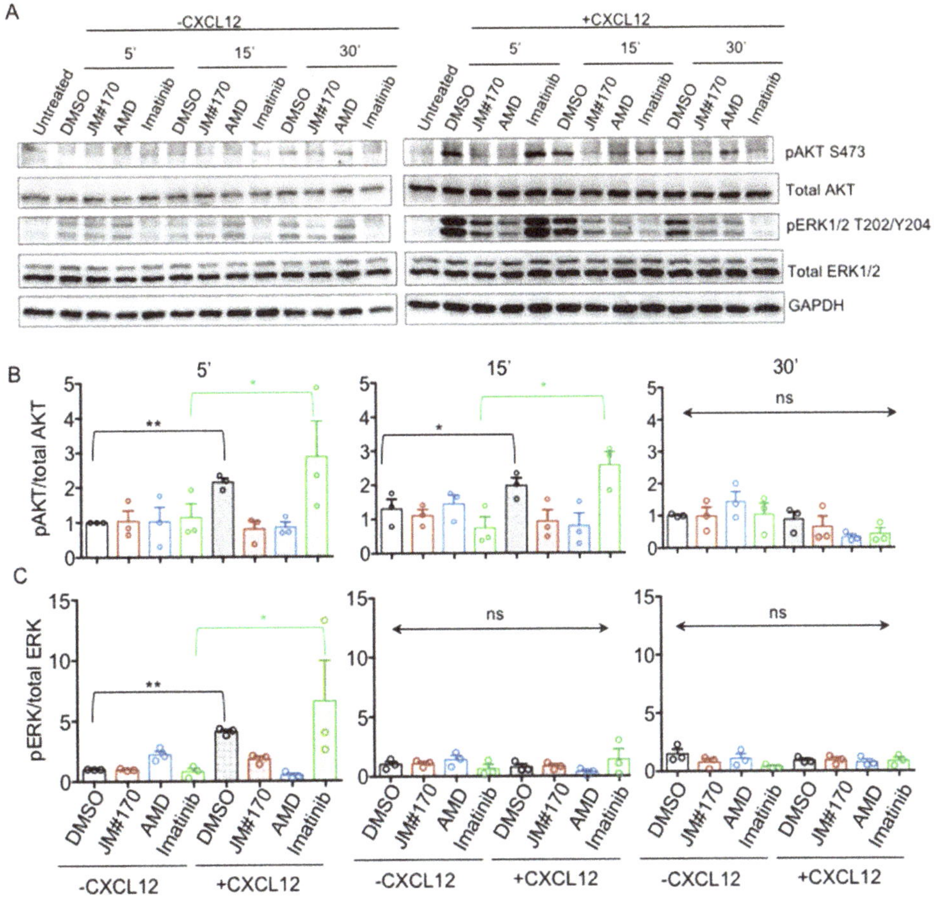

Figure 3. Inhibitory effect of JM#170 on CXCL12-induced CXCR4-downstream signal activation in BCR–ABL1 cells. (**A**) Western blot analysis depicting the level of AKT and ERK1/2 phosphorylation in BCR–ABL1 cells treated with DMSO, 10 μM of JM#170 or AMD3100, and 1 μm Imatinib for the indicated time period in the absence (left panel) and presence (right panel) of CXCL12 stimulation. GAPDH was used as the loading control. Image representative of $n = 3$ independent experiments. (**B**,**C**) Quantification of AKT (**B**) and ERK1/2 (**C**) phosphorylation for the Western blotting presented in (**A**). The band intensity of the phosphoprotein was normalized with respect to the total protein for each treatment and is represented as fold change with respect to 5 min DMSO (considering 5 min DMSO as 1). Bar represents mean ± SEM, $n = 3$. Each circle represents one individual experiment. Statistical analysis—one-way ANOVA with Sidak's multiple comparison test. * $p < 0.05$, ** $p < 0.01$. ns: not significant.

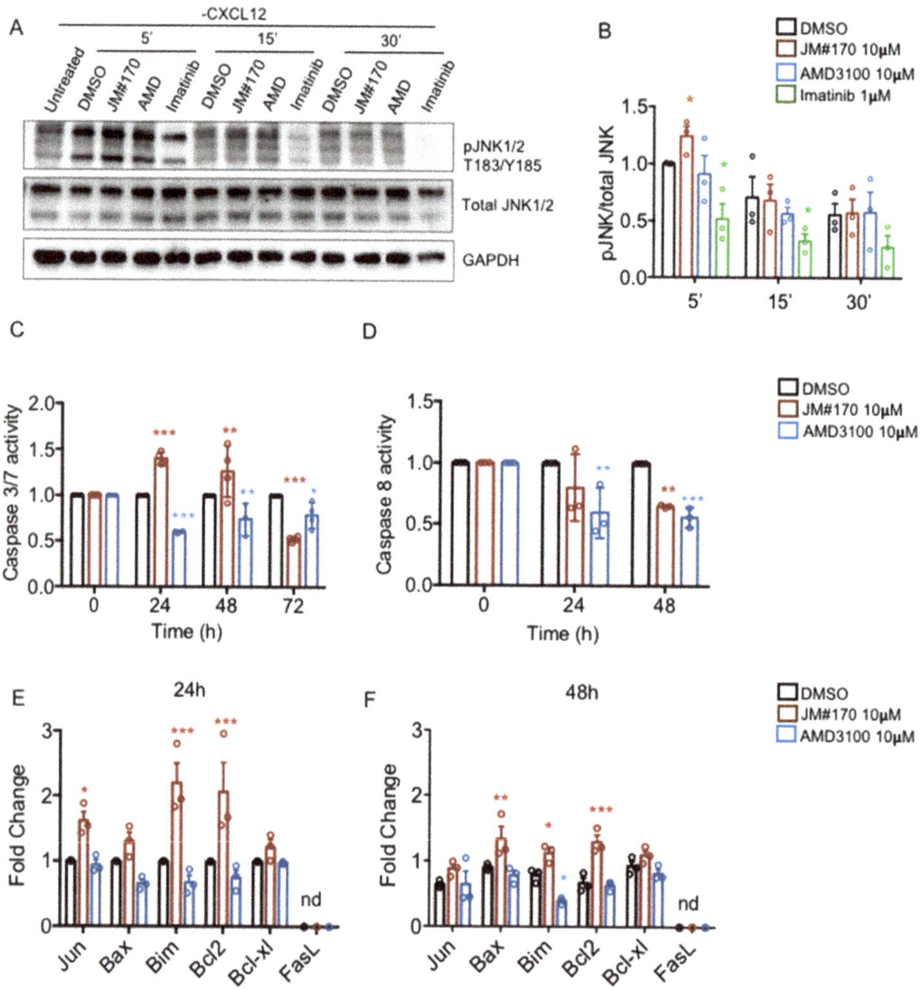

Figure 4. JM#170 induces intrinsic apoptosis in BCR–ABL1 cells. (**A**) Western blot analysis depicting the level of JNK1/2 phosphorylation in BCR–ABL1 cells treated with DMSO, 10 μM of JM#170 or AMD3100, and 1 μM Imatinib for the indicated time period in the absence of any CXCL12 stimulation. GAPDH was used as the loading control. Image representative of $n = 3$ independent experiments. (**B**) Quantification of JNK1/2 phosphorylation, as shown in (**A**). The band intensity of the phosphoprotein was normalized with respect to the total protein for each treatment and is represented as fold change with respect to 5 min DMSO (considering 5 min DMSO as 1). Bar represents mean ± SEM, $n = 3$. Each circle represents one individual experiment. Statistical analysis—two-way ANOVA with Dunnett's multiple comparison test. * $p < 0.05$. (**C**,**D**) Analysis of caspase 3/7 (**C**) and caspase 8 (**D**) activity in BCR–ABL1 cells treated with DMSO or 10 μM each of JM#170 and AMD3100 for the indicated time period. Values of each time point were normalized with respect to the corresponding DMSO. Bar represents mean ± SEM, $n = 3$. Statistical analysis—two-way ANOVA with Dunnett's multiple comparison test. * $p < 0.05$, ** $p < 0.01$, *** $p < 0.001$. (**E**,**F**) Real-time gene expression analysis depicting the relative expression of the pro/anti-apoptotic genes in BCR–ABL1 cells treated with DMSO, 10 μM JM#170 or AMD3100 for 24 (**E**) and 48 h (**F**). Bar represents mean ± SEM, $n = 3$. Statistical analysis—two-way ANOVA with Dunnett's multiple comparison test. * $p < 0.05$, ** $p < 0.01$, *** $p < 0.001$. nd: not detected.

2.5. Combined Imatinib and JM#170 Treatment Kills BCR–ABL1 Cells More Effectively

Since both JM#170 and Imatinib could effectively kill BCR–ABL1-transformed B cells, we checked whether combination of the two inhibitors had an additive effect. We treated the cells with lower doses of Imatinib (10 and 100 nM instead of 1 μM) in the presence or absence of 10 μM JM#170 and measured the cell growth via real-time live cell imaging in IncuCyte, as stated before. The results suggested that in comparison to the control DMSO, Imatinib alone at 10 nM did not have any effect on BCR–ABL1 cell growth (Figure 5A,B) while at 100 nM, a mild but significant growth inhibition was observed specifically after ~72 h (Figure 5A,C,D, Supplementary Table S1). The combination of 10nM Imatinib with 10 μM JM#170 induced a stronger inhibition of cell growth, but the effect was comparable to that of JM#170 alone (Figure 5A,B, dark red and olive green lines). Thus, the inhibition observed here could be attributed to JM#170 alone. However, when co-treated with 100 nM of Imatinib, a complete block of cell growth was observed, which was stronger than that achieved with JM#170 alone (Figure 5A,C,D, Supplementary Table S1). Therefore, in combination with 10 μM JM#170, a 10-fold lower dose of Imatinib can completely block BCR–ABL1-transformed cell growth.

2.6. JM#170 Is Lethal for BCR–ABL1$^+$ Human ALL Cell Line

So far, we tested the activity of CXCR4 inhibitors in transformed mouse B cells. To investigate whether JM#170 is also effective in killing human ALL cell lines, we first screened several ALL cell lines for surface CXCR4 expression. Compared to healthy human-blood-derived B cells, CXCR4 expression was found to be the highest in 697 cells and the lowest in SD1 cells (Supplementary Figure S4A). SupB15 and Tom1 expressed intermediate levels of CXCR4. Therefore, we selected SupB15 cells as the BCR–ABL1$^+$ ALL cell line and 697 as the BCR–ABL1$^-$ cell line for further analysis. When tested for CXCL12-induced calcium mobilization; both JM#170 and AMD3100 completely blocked the calcium flux in SupB15 (Figure 6A,C) and 697 (Figure 6B,D) cell lines at 1 μM. To further assess the CXCR4-specific effect of the inhibitors, we performed an anti-CXCR4 antibody competition assay, as described before. SupB15 cells were treated with increasing concentrations of JM#170, AMD3100, and Imatinib in the presence of a fixed concentration of anti-CXCR4 antibody 12G5. The result suggested that both JM#170 and AMD3100 significantly inhibited 12G5 binding to CXCR4 (Supplementary Figure S4B), with JM#170 being more potent than AMD3100. Imatinib, as expected, had no effect on 12G5 binding to CXCR4 (Supplementary Figure S4B). This clearly suggests that, similar to BCR–ABL1-transformed cells, JM#170 specifically targets CXCR4 in the human ALL cell line SupB15.

Next, we tested if treatment with JM#170 and AMD3100 at 10 μM and Imatinib at 1 μM concentrations, as used previously, had any effect on the viability of these ALL cell lines over time. As depicted in Figure 6E and Supplementary Figure S5C, in comparison to DMSO-treated cells, JM#170 significantly reduced SupB15 cell survival at 48 and 96 h after treatment. Imatinib exerted a stronger and more persistent killing effect over time, while AMD3100, as also observed for mouse cells, had no effect on SupB15 cell survival (Figure 6E). The 697 cells, on the other hand, were resistant to Imatinib treatment, most likely due to the lack of the BCR–ABL1 fusion protein (Figure 6F). Surprisingly, JM#170 also had no effect on the survival of these cells (Figure 6F). This indicates that the cytotoxic effect of JM#170 is dependent on the presence of the BCR–ABL1 protein. A similar observation was obtained from the growth monitoring of these cells using IncuCyte. We observed that 10 μM JM#170 and 1 μM Imatinib significantly reduced SupB15 cell growth when compared to the DMSO-treated cells (Supplementary Figure S5A,B, upper panel) but had no effect on the 697 cells (Supplementary Figure S5B lower panel). Notably, the inhibitory effect of JM#170, as observed in SupB15 cells, was lower than that observed in BCR–ABL1-transformed mouse primary pre-B cells.

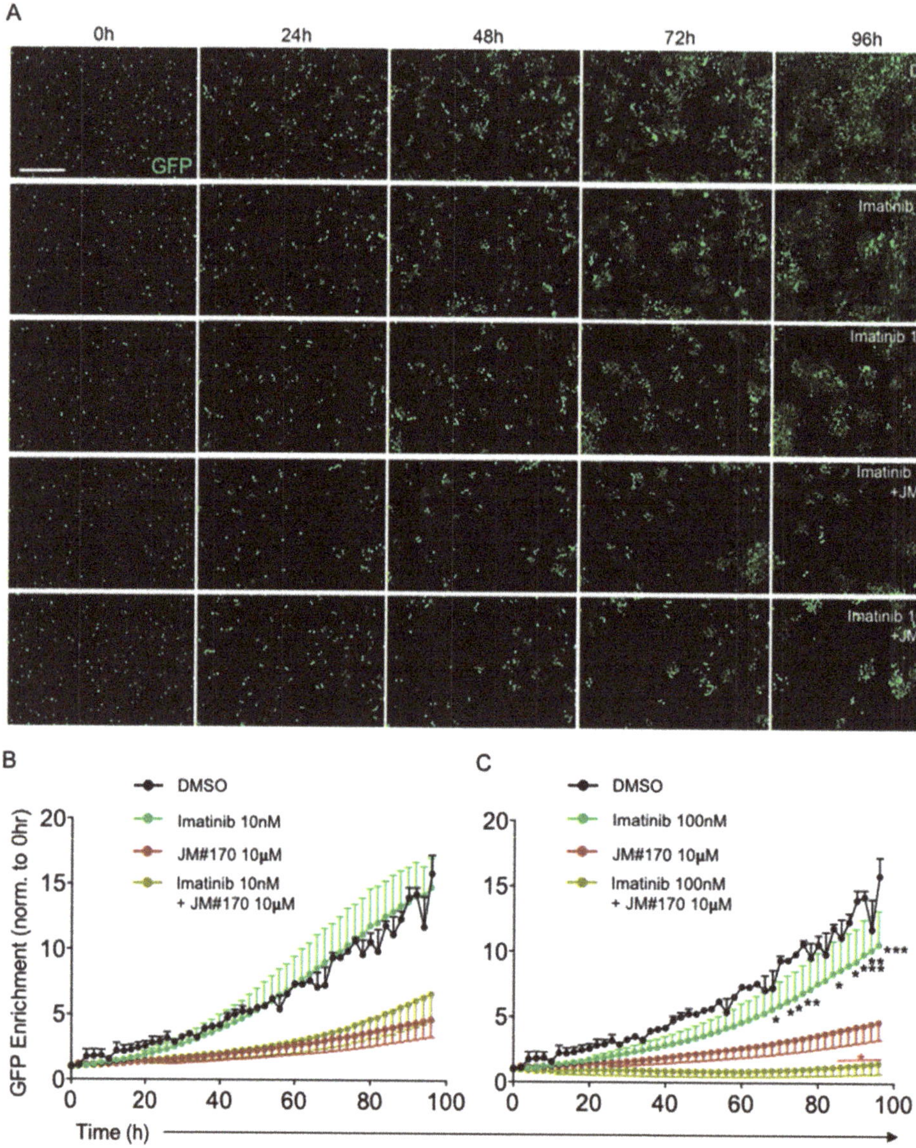

D

Time (h)	DMSO		JM#170 10µM		Imatinib 100nM		Imatinib 100nM + JM#170 10µM	
	Mean	SEM	Mean	SEM	Mean	SEM	Mean	SEM
0	1	0	1	0	1	0	1	0
24	2.925	0.357	1.443	0.252	1.892	0.32	0.911	0.4
48	5.257	0.069	2.185	0.557	3.421	0.936	0.843	0.404
72	9.396	0.088	3.222	0.938	6.244	2.005	0.979	0.485
96	15.849	1.413	4.679	1.336	10.605	2.625	1.517	0.82

Figure 5. JM#170 acts synergistically with Imatinib to strongly inhibit BCR–ABL1 cell survival. (**A**) Real-time imaging of BCR–ABL1 cells treated with DMSO, 10 or 100 nM Imatinib, and 10 or 100 nM Imatinib in combination with 10 µM JM#170 over 96 h. Images are representative of three independent experiments. Scale bar: 200 µm. (**B**) Quantification of GFP enrichment as a marker of

BCR–ABL1 cell growth in DMSO, 10 nM Imatinib, and 10 nM Imatinib in combination with 10 µM JM#170 treated cells over 96 h. The count of GFP+ cells for each time point for each treatment was normalized with respect to the corresponding count at 0 h. The 10 µM JM#170 plot (dark red) was taken from Figure 1B to facilitate comparison. (**C**) Similar quantification of GFP enrichment in DMSO, 100 nM Imatinib, and 100 nM Imatinib in combination with 10 µM JM#170. Graph represents mean ± SEM, $n = 3$. Statistical analysis—two-way ANOVA with Dunnett's multiple comparison test. Black *: comparison with respect to DMSO, dark red *: comparison with JM#170 alone. * $p < 0.05$, ** $p < 0.01$, *** $p < 0.001$. (**D**) Table representing the normalized GFP+ cell counts for the different treatment groups at the indicated time points.

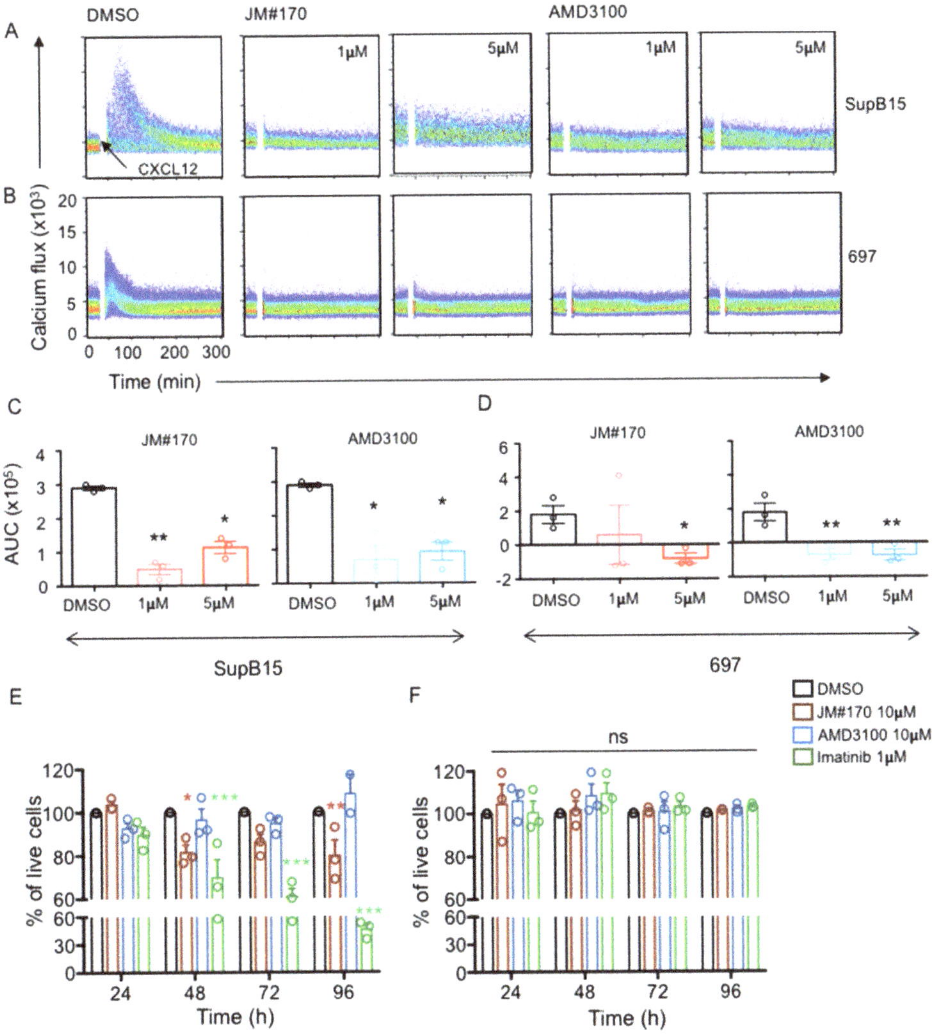

Figure 6. JM#170 efficiently blocks CXCR4 activation in BCR–ABL1-positive human ALL cell line and induces cell death. (**A**,**B**) Flow cytometric measurement of CXCL12-driven calcium flux in SupB15 (**A**) and 697 (**B**) cells treated with solvent (DMSO), 1 or 5 µM JM#170, and 1 or 5 µM AMD3100. The baseline was measured for 30 s, which was followed by the addition of 100 ng/mL

human CXCL12 (black arrow), and the signal was recorded for a total of 5 min. Images representative of three independent experiments. (**C**,**D**) Quantification of the above calcium flux analysis for SupB15 (**C**) and 697 (**D**) cells treated with DMSO (black), 1 μM (light red) and 10 μM (red) JM#170 and 1 μM (light blue) and 10 μM (blue) AMD3100. The area under the curve (AUC) for each measurement was calculated, and the AUC of the water control (solvent control of CXCL12) was subtracted from each measurement. The subtracted values are plotted as mean ± SEM, $n = 3$. Statistical analysis—one-way ANOVA with Dunnett's multiple comparison test. * $p < 0.05$, ** $p < 0.01$. (**E**,**F**) Flow cytometric analysis of cell survival of SupB15 (**E**) and 697 (**F**) cells treated with solvent DMSO, 10 μM JM#170 or AMD3100, or 1 μM Imatinib over the indicated time period. The live cell count for each treatment for each time point was normalized to the corresponding live cell count for DMSO and is represented as a percentage. Graph represents mean ± SEM, $n = 3$. Each circle represents one individual experiment. Statistical analysis—two-way ANOVA with Dunnett's multiple comparison test. * $p < 0.05$, ** $p < 0.01$, *** $p < 0.001$.

In addition to the ALL cell lines, we also assessed the efficacy of JM#170 on primary Ph^+ ALL cells. To this end, we used ALL blast cells isolated from the spleen of immunodeficient mice that were previously xenografted with Imatinib-resistant Ph^+ ALL primary cells. The xenograft cells ($hCD19^+$ $mCD45^-$) were cultured and treated with control DMSO, 10 μM JM#170, and 1 μM Imatinib; cellular growth was measured using real-time imaging using IncuCyte for a period of 6 days. Although the xenograft cells survived in culture, they did not proliferate, as observed from their growth curve in the control (Supplementary Figure S6A, black line). JM#170 clearly exhibited a significant growth inhibitory effect on these cells compared to DMSO, whereas no effect was seen for Imatinib treatment, as the primary samples were resistant to Imatinib (Supplementary Figure S6A,B).

Taken together, our data suggest that in addition to BCR–ABL1-transformed mouse B cells, JM#170 is effective in killing the $BCR\text{-}ABL^+$ human ALL cell line and primary Ph^+ ALL xenograft cells.

3. Discussion

The seven-transmembrane G-protein-coupled chemokine receptor CXCR4 plays an essential role in the homing and retention of tumor cells in the protective bone marrow niches, thereby preventing their culmination by therapeutic agents and increasing the risk of disease relapses [21]. The elevated expression of CXCR4 in hematological malignancies as well as in solid tumors is associated with poor prognosis. Consequently, targeting CXCR4 activation through antagonists leads to the egress of hiding cancer cells from bone marrow to the periphery, a process known as chemosensitization, which therefore possesses great therapeutic potential. Several small molecules, peptides, neutralizing antibodies, as well as antibody–drug conjugates are being tested for their efficacy in antagonizing CXCR4 function in different cancers. For instance, the small-molecule inhibitor AMD3100, the peptide-based inhibitors BL-8040 and LY2510924, and anti-CXCR4 monoclonal antibodies have been used in several clinical trials for patients with acute myeloid leukemia (AML) and ALL, both as monotherapies and in combination with chemotherapy (as reviewed in [22]). Although the trials have demonstrated that targeting the CXCR4 axis in vivo is feasible and safe, the clinical outcome in many cases does not prove to be beneficial compared with that of chemotherapy alone. This therefore warrants new improved CXCR4 antagonists.

Ph^+ B-ALL represents a group of ALL cases that expresses the oncogenic BCR–ABL1 fusion protein. Although the invention of Imatinib, a tyrosine kinase blocker of BCR–ABL1, greatly improved the outcome of the disease, resistance to Imatinib is a major problem that can lead to relapse. It is therefore crucial to identify other contributing pathways that can be additionally targeted in this disease. A previous study from our laboratory identified both CXCR4 and IL7R pathways as contributing to the pathology of BCR–ABL1 [10]. The complete deletion of CXCR4 was found to be sufficient to block BCR–ABL1 cell growth in vitro. Therefore, the aim of the current work was to study the effect of CXCR4 inhibition on BCR–ABL1-mediated transformation.

EPI-X4, a 16-amino-acid peptide derived from the proteolysis of serum albumin, is a naturally occurring CXCR4 antagonist that prevents CXCR4-tropic HIV-1 virus entry [13]. Using a molecular docking study to predict the EPI-X4 binding sites to CXCR4 and QSAR to identify modifications that might enhance the binding and functional efficacy of EPI-X4, several optimized EPI-X4 derivatives were generated [14]. Many of these derivatives effectively block the CXCL12-induced calcium mobilization in BCR–ABL1-transformed mouse B cells, showing much higher efficacy than parental EPI-X4, indicating that they could inhibit CXCR4 signaling in these cells [14,17].

In the current manuscript, we presented data that the inhibition of CXCR4 by a lipid-conjugated truncated version of EPI-X4, namely JM#170, induced rapid and strong cell death in BCR–ABL1-transformed malignant mouse cells, whereas it remained inactive against the WT B cells. Live cell imaging of BCR–ABL1 cells in the presence of different inhibitors clearly indicated that JM#170 potently blocked cellular growth within 24 h of treatment, while AMD3100 showed an effect at a much later time point (~60 h post treatment, Figure 1A–C). Notably, for cells treated with JM#170, a slight increase in GFP^+ cell accumulation was observed 72 and 96 h post treatment (Figure 1A). This could be explained by the relatively lower stability of peptide-based inhibitors in serum containing cell culture media. Although the optimized derivatives are significantly more stable in blood plasma than the mother peptide EPI-X4 [17], 72–96 h could still be long. The cells that remained resistant to JM#170 until ~48 h may have started proliferating after the degradation of the inhibitor, which in turn increased the GFP^+ cell density. Interestingly, neither JM#170 nor AMD3100 had any growth inhibitory effect on untransformed bone-marrow-derived B cells (Figure 2 and Supplementary Figure S3C). This may have arisen from the relatively high rate of cell proliferation observed in the transformed cells compared to the WT cells, which was clearly evident from the growth curve of the two cell types in live cell imaging (Figure 1B black line vs. Figure 2B black line). As the requirement for CXCR4 signaling for survival and proliferation of transformed cells is higher than that of normal cells, the effect of CXCR4 inhibition is also stronger on these cells than on normal cells. This selectivity is a very important aspect for JM#170 to be potentially used as an anticancer peptide drug.

Although both JM#170 and AMD3100 blocked BCR–ABL1 cell growth (Figure 1A–C), as well as CXCL12-induced AKT and ERK1/2 phosphorylation (Figure 3B,C), the end effect was different for the two inhibitors. While JM#170 effectively killed BCR–ABL1 cells, AMD3100 halted the proliferation, with no cell killing effect observed within the experimental timeline (Figure 1E–G). This clearly indicates that JM#170 has a different mechanism of action other than blocking ligand-induced CXCR4 activation in BCR–ABL1-transformed cells. Indeed, we observed that JM#170 spontaneously induced transient JNK1/2 phosphorylation (Figure 4A,B), leading to the enhanced expression of JNK-downstream genes such as *cJun*, *Bax*, and *Bim* (Figure 4E,F) and triggered the intrinsic apoptotic pathway in BCR–ABL1-expressing cells (Figure 4C,D). JNK, also known as stress-activated protein kinase (SAPK), is activated upon various kinds of cellular stress, including treatment with drugs or signaling pathway inhibitors; depending on the context and specific cell types, it can act as both a pro-survival as well as a pro-apoptotic signaling cascade [20]. In this case, treatment with the inhibitor JM#170 exerted cellular stress, thereby activating the JNK-mediated pro-apoptotic pathway.

The strong cytotoxic effect exerted by JM#170 on BCR–ABL1 cells prompted us to check if it could be used in combination with Imatinib, specifically with a lower dose of Imatinib. This would be particularly interesting in terms of reducing the side effects of Imatinib. Co-treatment of JM#170 at 10 μM with Imatinib at 100 nM (10-fold lower than usual) induced a complete block of BCR–ABL1 cell growth, which was even stronger than that achieved with JM#170 alone (Figure 5A,C,D). Another 10-fold reduction in Imatinib concentration (10 nM) did not impart any effect on BCR–ABL1 cell growth; the co-treatment yielded an effect similar in magnitude to that of JM#170 alone (Figure 5A,B). This suggests that the combinatorial treatment of JM#170 and Imatinib could be very effective against BCR–ABL1-induced transformation, which not only allows the lowering of Imatinib doses but might also be helpful for Imatinib-resistant cases.

In addition to its effect on BCR–ABL1-transformed mouse B cells, JM#170 was also active against human BCR–ABL1$^+$ ALL cell line SupB15. Although JM#170 blocked the CXCL12-induced calcium flux in both SupB15 and 697 cell lines (human BCR–ABL1$^-$ ALL cell line, Figure 6A–D), the killing effect was only observed in BCR–ABL1$^+$ SupB15 cells (Figure 6E, Supplementary Figure S5). This suggests that the presence of BCR–ABL1 is essential for the inhibitory action of JM#170. It is important to mention that the level of CXCR4 expression on the surface of 697 cells was very high compared to that on other cells, such as SupB15 or healthy human-blood-derived B cells (Supplementary Figure S4A). It is therefore possible that the maximum concentration of JM#170 used here (10 μM), though sufficient to block ligand-induced calcium mobilization, was not enough to impart an ultimate effect on the survival of these cells. Additionally, as pointed out before, the magnitude of the inhibitory effect observed in the SupB15 cell line was lower compared to that of BCR–ABL1-transformed mouse cells. This indicates the robust nature of the ALL cell lines: in addition to BCR–ABL1 transformation, there might be additional growth-promoting and death-evading mechanisms making these cell lines difficult to target. The mouse cells, on the other hand, with a single transformation event, could be highly susceptible, as observed in this study.

Our experiment with the xenografted primary Ph+ ALL cells also indicated an important aspect of the inhibitory effect of JM#170 (Supplementary Figure S6A). The relative growth inhibition of the xenografted cells by JM#170 was much milder compared to its effect on BCR–ABL1-transformed cells or the human ALL cell line. This, in our view, is due to the lack of proliferation ability of these cells under in vitro conditions. As revealed from their growth curve, the xenografted cells could survive in culture but never proliferated (Supplementary Figure S6A). Since CXCR4 is more involved in proliferating cells than in resting ones, the effect of JM#170 may be milder in resting cells, leading to subtle growth inhibition.

In conclusion, we provide evidence that JM#170, a lipid-modified EPI-X4-derived CXCR4 antagonist, is a potent inhibitor of BCR–ABL1-positive ALL cell growth in vitro. An interesting question would be why, among all the derivatives, JM#170 was found to be the most active. Among the derivatives tested in this study, JM#170 has the lowest molecular weight (Table 1). It could be possible that this size is optimum for fitting into the binding pocket of CXCR4, thereby preventing ligand-induced activation. In addition, such tight interaction might trigger non-classical signal pathway activation such as JNK as observed here. Further structural studies might shed light on this finding. As the next step for therapeutic application, the effect of JM#170 should be investigated using in vivo ALL models.

4. Materials and Method

4.1. Reagents and Optimized EPI-X4 Derivatives

Optimized EPI-X4 peptide derivatives (Table 1) were synthesized as described previously [17]. Briefly, the peptides were synthesized via standard Fmoc solid-phase peptide synthesis using a Liberty Blue microwave synthesizer (CEM Corporation, Matthews, NC, USA) and then purified using reversed-phase high-performance liquid chromatography (Waters, Milford, MA, USA), employing an acetonitrile/water gradient under acidic conditions on a Phenomenex C18 Luna column (particle size 5 μm, pore size 100 Å). Purified peptides were lyophilized on a freeze-dryer (Labconco, Kansas City, MI, USA), and the molecular mass was verified by liquid chromatography–mass spectrometry (LC-MS; Waters, Milford, MA, USA). The peptides were dissolved in dimethyl sulfoxide (DMSO, Sigma-Aldrich, Hamburg, Germany) at a stock concentration of 3 mM and further diluted in phosphate-buffered saline (PBS) /complete cell culture media before usage. AMD3100 octahydrochloride hydrate (#A5602) and Imatinib mesylate (#SML1027) were purchased from Sigma-Aldrich, Hamburg, Germany and dissolved in H_2O and DMSO respectively to create a 10 mM stock. Human and mouse CXCL12 were purchased from Peprotech, Hamburg, Germany (#300-28A, #250-20A) and dissolved at 100 µg/mL in H_2O.

4.2. Cell Culture

BCR–ABL1-transformed mouse pre-B cells were generated in-house, as described previously [10]. Briefly, wild-type (WT) mouse bone marrow B cells were cultured in Iscove's modified Dulbecco's media (Sigma- Aldrich, Hamburg, Germany) supplemented with 10% heat-inactivated fetal bovine serum (FBS, PAN Biotech, Aidenbach, Germany), 2 mM L-glutamine (Gibco, Dreieich, Germany), 100 units/mL of penicillin/streptomycin (Gibco), 50 µM beta-marcaptoethanol (Gibco), and 1 ng/mL of recombinant mouse interleukin 7 (IL7, Immunotools, Friesoythe, Germany) for 4–7 days at 37 °C in a 7.5% CO_2 incubator. The cells were then retrovirally transduced with a BCR–ABL1 construct cloned in pMIG vector containing an EGFP marker. Two days after transduction, cells were tested for GFP expression via FACS, and positive cells were selected via IL7 withdrawal from culture medium. BCR–ABL1 transduction transforms the cell, leading to uncontrolled growth and eventually enriching the culture. $Rag2^{-/-}$ $\lambda5^{-/-}$ $Spl65^{-/-}$ TKO mouse pro-B cells were cultured in similar IL7 containing Iscove's media at 37 °C in a 7.5% CO_2 incubator and transduced with either BCR–ABL1 construct (TKO-BCR–ABL1) or empty pMIG vector containing an EGFP marker (TKO-EV). Selection and enrichment of TKO-BCR–ABL1 cells were performed as stated before. Human ALL cell lines SupB15 (ACC 389), Tom1 (ACC 578), SD1 (ACC 366), and 697 (ACC 42) were purchased from DSMZ. SupB15 cells were maintained in McCoy's 5A (Biowest, Nuaillé, France) and the rest of the cells in RPMI media (Gibco), supplemented with 20% heat-inactivated FBS, 2 mM L-glutamine, and 100 units/mL of penicillin/streptomycin at 37 °C in a 5% CO_2 incubator.

4.3. Isolation of Ph+ ALL Cells Form Xenografted NSG Mice

Xenografting of immunodeficient NOD.Cg-Prkdcscid Il2rgtm1Wjl/SzJ (NSG) mice with an Imatinib-resistant ALL sample from a patient was described in [10]. Animals showing clinical symptoms of leukemia or with >75% leukemic blasts in blood were sacrificed, and total splenic cells were isolated and frozen for future use.

4.4. Real-Time Cell Growth Analysis by IncuCyte

A flat-bottom 96-well plate was coated with 0.01% poly-L ornithine (#P4957, Sigma-Aldrich, Hamburg, Germany) for 1 h at room temperature (RT). BCR–ABL1, SupB15, and 697 cells were counted as 0.5×10^5 cells/well, while TKO-BCR–ABL1 and TKO-EV cells as 1×10^5 cells/well, which were labeled with IncuCyte Cytotox Red dye (#4632, Sartorius, Ulm, Germany) as per the manufacturer's protocol. The cells were plated in 100 µL complete medium. The solvent control DMSO, peptide inhibitors, AMD3100 or Imatinib were diluted in complete medium at 2X concentration and mixed with the cells in a 1:1 ratio. Plate was prewarmed at 37 °C for 30 min prior to placing in the IncuCyte chamber. Scanning was conducted every two hours for total of 4 days. Images were acquired using a 20X objective in phase contrast and fluorescence mode at 4 images/well and analyzed using the cell-by-cell analysis module of IncuCyte software version 2020B (Essen Bioscience, Ann Arbor, MI, USA).

For Ph+ ALL cells isolated from the xenografted NSG mice, frozen cells were thawed and cultured in MEM-alpha (Gibco) media supplemented with 20% FBS and 100 units/mL of penicillin/streptomycin for 5–16 h in a 5% CO_2 incubator. Next, the cells were overlaid on 10 mL Ficoll-Paque™PLUS (#17144003, Cytiva, Freiburg, Germany) in 50 mL tubes and centrifuged at 400 g without break for 10 min at RT. The cells were collected from the interface of Ficoll and media and washed once with PBS. Viable cells were counted and plated into previously coated 48-well plates at 4.25×10^5 cells/well in 250 µL of media with or without the inhibitors. Scanning was conducted every two hours for total of 6 days in phase contrast mode and analyzed using the cell-by-cell analysis module of IncuCyte software version 2020B (Essen Bioscience).

4.5. Flow Cytometry

Cells treated with either solvent control DMSO or different concentrations of inhibitors for different time points were collected and washed with ice-cold PBS. Cells were then stained with efluor 450-labeled fixable viability dye (FVD, #65-0863-14, eBioscience, San Diego, CA, USA) at 1:1000 dilution at 4 °C or using 50 µg/mL propidium iodide (PI, #P3566, Thermo Fisher, Dreieich, Germany) solution at RT for 15 min in the dark. After washing, labeled cells were resuspended in 100 µL of PBS and acquired using LSR-Fortessa (BD Bioscience, Heidelberg, Germany). FACS data were analyzed with FlowJo software version 10.0.

To determine the expression of CXCR4 on the cell surfaces, 0.5×10^6 BCR–ABL1 and TKO-EV cells were collected, washed with FACS buffer (PBS containing 3% FBS), and stained with a 1:100 dilution of BV421-labeled anti-mouse CXCR4 antibody (#146511, Biolegend, San Deago, CA, USA). Human ALL cell lines were similarly collected and stained with a 1:100 dilution of Alexa flour 488-labeled antihuman CD19 (#53-0199-42, Invitrogen, Dreieich, Germany) and APC-Cy7-labeled anti-human CXCR4 (#306527, Biolegend) antibodies at 4 °C for 15 min in the dark. Cells were then washed with FACS buffer and analyzed using LSR-Fortessa (BD Bioscience).

Human peripheral blood mononuclear cells (PBMCs) were isolated using Ficoll-Paque™PLUS density gradient centrifugation as per the manufacturer's instructions. Mononuclear cells were collected from the interface of plasma and Ficoll–Paque media, then washed several times with PBS. Cells were then counted and either used directly for experimentation or frozen in 10% DMSO-containing media for future use.

4.6. Cell Proliferation Assay

BCR–ABL1 cells were collected at 0.5×10^5 cells/well of a 96-well plate and labeled with cell trace far red cell proliferation dye (#C34564, Invitrogen, Dreieich, Germany), according to the manufacturer's instructions. Labeled cells were plated in 100 µL of complete media and were mixed with equal volume of 2X DMSO or inhibitor-containing media. A small part of the labeled cells was measured in FACS to determine the fluorescence signal on day 0. After specific time periods (48 and 72 h), cells were collected, washed with FACS buffer, and analyzed using LSR-Fortessa (BD Bioscience).

4.7. Anti-CXCR4 Antibody Competition Assay

An anti-CXCR4 competition assay was conducted as previously described [14,17]. Briefly, 1×10^5 BCR–ABL1-transformed mouse B cells were incubated with serially diluted (10 µM to 1 nM) JM#170, AMD3100, and Imatinib in the presence of a fixed concentration of BV421-labeled antimouse CXCR4 antibody (clone L276F12, #146511, Biolegend) for 2 h at 4 °C. Afterward, the cells were washed to remove unbound inhibitors and antibody, and measured via FACS for the fluorescence signal of the bound antibody. The fluorescence signal corresponding to only antibody (no inhibitor) was considered to be 100% antibody binding. For SupB15 cells, a similar experiment was carried out using APC-Cy7-labeled anti-human CXCR4 antibody (clone 12G5, #306527, Biolegend).

4.8. Calcium Flux Analysis

Ca^{2+} signaling was analyzed as described previously [14]. Briefly, SupB15 and 697 cells were collected at 1×10^6 cells/treatment and loaded with calcium-sensitive dye Indo-1 AM (#I1223, Invitrogen) and 0.5 mg/mL of pluronic F-127 (#P3000MP, Invitrogen) in their respective media supplemented with 1% FBS at 37 °C for 45 min. Cells were then washed and treated with the inhibitors for 10 min at 37 °C. Baseline signal for calcium was measured for 30 s via flow cytometry, followed by stimulation with 100 ng/mL human CXCL12. The area under the curve (AUC) of each calcium flux plot was determined using FlowJo. The

AUC of the water control (solvent for CXCL12) was subtracted from each treatment to obtain the correct estimation of the calcium signal upon CXCL12 stimulation.

4.9. Western Blotting

BCR–ABL1 cells were collected as 5×10^6 cells/500 µL complete media and treated either with DMSO or different inhibitors in the absence and presence of 100 ng/mL mouse CXCL12 for 5, 15, and 30 min at 37 °C. Cells were then immediately transferred onto ice to stop the reaction and washed with ice-cold PBS. Cell extract was prepared by resuspending the cell pellet in 100 µL of radio-immunoprecipitation assay (RIPA) buffer supplemented with 1X protease inhibitor cocktail (#78429, Thermo Fisher), 1 mM sodium orthovanadate (Sigma-Aldrich), and 10 mM beta-glycerophosphate (Sigma-Aldrich). For each treatment, 15 µL of cell extract was mixed with 5 µL of 4X Laemmli buffer (reducing), boiled at 95 °C for 10 min, and run on 10% SDS-PAGE. Gels were wet-transferred to PVDF membranes (Millipore, Burlington, MA, USA) and stained with 0.1% ponceau-S solution to check for efficient blotting. The membranes were blocked with 3% BSA solution and incubated with primary antibodies at 4 °C overnight. The next day, primary antibodies were washed, and membranes were probed with horseradish peroxidase (HRP)-conjugated secondary antibodies at RT for 2 h. After washing, the blots were developed using Immobilon ECL Ultra Western HRP Substrate (#WBULS0500, Millipore), and images were acquired with a Fusion SL gel imaging system (Vilber Lourmat, Eberhardzell, Germany). The following primary antibodies from Cell Signaling were used: anti-Phospho-Akt (Ser473, #4060), anti-AKT (#9272), anti-Phospho-p44/42 MAPK (Thr202/Tyr204, #4370), anti-p44/42 MAPK (137F5, #4695), anti-Phospho-SAPK/JNK (Thr183/Tyr185) (81E11, #4668), anti-SAPK/JNK (#9252), and anti-GAPDH (14C10, #2118) antibody. Anti-rabbit IgG, HRP-linked (#7074, Cell Signaling technology, Danvers, MA, USA) was used as secondary antibody.

4.10. Caspase 3/7 and Caspase 8 Activation Assay

BCR–ABL1 cells were plated at 0.5×10^5 cells/well of a 96-well plate in 100 µL of complete media and treated with DMSO or various inhibitors. At specific time points (24, 48 and 72 h), activation of caspases was measured with a Caspase-Glo® 3/7 Assay (#G8090) and Caspase-Glo® 8 Assay (#G8200, Promega, Madison, WI, USA) following the manufacturer's instructions.

4.11. RNA Isolation and Real-Time Gene Expression Analysis

BCR–ABL1 cells were plated at 1×10^6 cells/well of a 12-well plate in 1 mL of complete media and treated with DMSO or various inhibitors. After specific time points (24 and 48 h), RNA was isolated from cells using a ReliaPrep Cell RNA miniprep kit (#Z6011, Promega). Fifty nanograms of total RNA was reverse-transcribed using a high-capacity RNA to cDNA kit (#4387406, Thermo Fisher), and gene expression was measured via Taqman assay using Taqman Gene expression master mix (#4369016, Thermo Fisher) following ghd manufacturer's protocol. The following Taqman probes were used: Jun (Mm07296811_s1), Bax (Mm00432051_m1), Bim (Mm00437796_m1), Bcl2 (Mm00477631_m1), Bcl-xl (00437783_m1), FasL (Mm00438864_m1), and beta actin (04394036_g1).

4.12. Statistical Analysis

Statistical analysis was performed using GraphPad Prism 6.0 software. Specific statistical tests are mentioned in the figure legends. Unless otherwise mentioned, all experiments were independently conducted at least three times.

Supplementary Materials: The following supporting information can be downloaded at: https://www.mdpi.com/article/10.3390/ijms25158306/s1.

Author Contributions: Conceptualization, M.D.; data curation, M.D.; formal analysis, J.P., A.L. and M.D.; funding acquisition, H.J.; investigation, J.P., A.L., O.E.A. and M.D.; methodology, A.R.-A. and L.S.; project administration, H.J.; resources, M.H. and J.M.; supervision, H.J. and M.D.; validation,

M.D.; writing—original draft, M.D.; writing—review and editing, A.R.-A., M.H., J.M., H.J. and M.D. All authors have read and agreed to the published version of the manuscript.

Funding: This study was supported by the German Research Foundation (DFG) through the CRC 1279 (Project ID 316249678) to L.S, J.M. and H.J. M.H. was funded by the "Bausteinprogramm", Projektnummer: L.SBN.0209, of Ulm University. M.H. also received funding from the Baden-Württemberg Foundation.

Institutional Review Board Statement: Not applicable.

Informed Consent Statement: Not applicable.

Data Availability Statement: All data supporting the findings of this study are available within the article and its supplementary information files.

Acknowledgments: We thank Corinna Setz for her help with the IncuCyte experiment and Merve Karacan and Nico Preising for the peptide synthesis. We also thank Marc Young and Oles Havryliuk for their excellent technical support.

Conflicts of Interest: M.H. and J.M. are co-inventors of pending and issued patents that claim to use EPI-X4 (ALB408-423) and its derivatives for the therapy of CXCR4-associated diseases.

References

1. Ribeiro, R.C.; Abromowitch, M.; Raimondi, S.C.; Murphy, S.B.; Behm, F.; Williams, D.L. Clinical and biologic hallmarks of the Philadelphia chromosome in childhood acute lymphoblastic leukemia. *Blood* **1987**, *70*, 948–953. [CrossRef] [PubMed]
2. Rowley, J.D. Letter: A new consistent chromosomal abnormality in chronic myelogenous leukaemia identified by quinacrine fluorescence and Giemsa staining. *Nature* **1973**, *243*, 290–293. [CrossRef] [PubMed]
3. Collins, S.J.; Groudine, M.T. Rearrangement and amplification of c-abl sequences in the human chronic myelogenous leukemia cell line K-562. *Proc. Natl. Acad. Sci. USA* **1983**, *80*, 4813–4817. [CrossRef] [PubMed]
4. Ottmann, O.G.; Pfeifer, H. Management of Philadelphia chromosome-positive acute lymphoblastic leukemia (Ph+ ALL). *Hematol. Am. Soc. Hematol. Educ. Program.* **2009**, 371–381. [CrossRef] [PubMed]
5. Cross, S.A.; Lyseng-Williamson, K.A. Imatinib: In relapsed or refractory Philadelphia chromosome-positive acute lymphoblastic leukaemia. *Drugs* **2007**, *67*, 2645–2654. [CrossRef] [PubMed]
6. Biondi, A.; Schrappe, M.; De Lorenzo, P.; Castor, A.; Lucchini, G.; Gandemer, V.; Pieters, R.; Stary, J.; Escherich, G.; Campbell, M.; et al. Imatinib after induction for treatment of children and adolescents with Philadelphia-chromosome-positive acute lymphoblastic leukaemia (EsPhALL): A randomised, open-label, intergroup study. *Lancet Oncol.* **2012**, *13*, 936–945. [CrossRef]
7. Silva, W.; Rego, E. How to Manage Philadelphia-Positive Acute Lymphoblastic Leukemia in Resource-Constrained Settings. *Cancers* **2023**, *15*, 5783. [CrossRef]
8. Jabbour, E.; Short, N.J.; Jain, N.; Huang, X.; Montalban-Bravo, G.; Banerjee, P.; Rezvani, K.; Jiang, X.; Kim, K.H.; Kanagal-Shamanna, R.; et al. Ponatinib and blinatumomab for Philadelphia chromosome-positive acute lymphoblastic leukaemia: A US, single-centre, single-arm, phase 2 trial. *Lancet Haematol.* **2023**, *10*, e24–e34. [CrossRef] [PubMed]
9. Schultz, K.R.; Carroll, A.; Heerema, N.A.; Bowman, W.P.; Aledo, A.; Slayton, W.B.; Sather, H.; Devidas, M.; Zheng, H.W.; Davies, S.M.; et al. Long-term follow-up of Imatinib in pediatric Philadelphia chromosome-positive acute lymphoblastic leukemia: Children's Oncology Group study AALL0031. *Leukemia* **2014**, *28*, 1467–1471. [CrossRef]
10. Abdelrasoul, H.; Vadakumchery, A.; Werner, M.; Lenk, L.; Khadour, A.; Young, M.; El Ayoubi, O.; Vogiatzi, F.; Kramer, M.; Schmid, V.; et al. Synergism between IL7R and CXCR4 drives BCR-ABL induced transformation in Philadelphia chromosome-positive acute lymphoblastic leukemia. *Nat. Commun.* **2020**, *11*, 3194. [CrossRef]
11. Hendrix, C.W.; Collier, A.C.; Lederman, M.M.; Schols, D.; Pollard, R.B.; Brown, S.; Jackson, J.B.; Coombs, R.W.; Glesby, M.J.; Flexner, C.W.; et al. Safety, pharmacokinetics, and antiviral activity of AMD3100, a selective CXCR4 receptor inhibitor, in HIV-1 infection. *J. Acquir. Immune Defic. Syndr.* **2004**, *37*, 1253–1262. [CrossRef] [PubMed]
12. Hoy, S.M. Motixafortide: First Approval. *Drugs* **2023**, *83*, 1635–1643. [CrossRef] [PubMed]
13. Zirafi, O.; Kim, K.A.; Standker, L.; Mohr, K.B.; Sauter, D.; Heigele, A.; Kluge, S.F.; Wiercinska, E.; Chudziak, D.; Richter, R.; et al. Discovery and characterization of an endogenous CXCR4 antagonist. *Cell Rep.* **2015**, *11*, 737–747. [CrossRef] [PubMed]
14. Harms, M.; Habib, M.M.W.; Nemska, S.; Nicolo, A.; Gilg, A.; Preising, N.; Sokkar, P.; Carmignani, S.; Raasholm, M.; Weidinger, G.; et al. An optimized derivative of an endogenous CXCR4 antagonist prevents atopic dermatitis and airway inflammation. *Acta Pharm. Sin. B* **2021**, *11*, 2694–2708. [CrossRef] [PubMed]
15. Harms, M.; Fabech Hansson, R.; Gilg, A.; Almeida-Hernandez, Y.; Loffler, J.; Rodriguez-Alfonso, A.; Habib, M.M.W.; Albers, D.; Ahmed, N.S.; Abadi, A.H.; et al. Development of N-Terminally Modified Variants of the CXCR4-Antagonistic Peptide EPI-X4 for Enhanced Plasma Stability. *J. Med. Chem.* **2023**, *66*, 15189–15204. [CrossRef] [PubMed]
16. Gaonkar, R.H.; Schmidt, Y.T.; Mansi, R.; Almeida-Hernandez, Y.; Sanchez-Garcia, E.; Harms, M.; Munch, J.; Fani, M. Development of a New Class of CXCR4-Targeting Radioligands Based on the Endogenous Antagonist EPI-X4 for Oncological Applications. *J. Med. Chem.* **2023**, *66*, 8484–8497. [CrossRef] [PubMed]

17. Harms, M.; Haase, A.; Rodriguez-Alfonso, A.; Löffler, J.; Almeida-Hernández, Y.; Ruiz-Blanco, Y.B.; Albers, D.; Gilg, A.; von Bank, F.; Zech, F.; et al. Fatty acid conjugated EPI-X4 derivatives with increased activity and in vivo stability. *J. Control. Release* **2024**.
18. Duhren-von Minden, M.; Ubelhart, R.; Schneider, D.; Wossning, T.; Bach, M.P.; Buchner, M.; Hofmann, D.; Surova, E.; Follo, M.; Kohler, F.; et al. Chronic lymphocytic leukaemia is driven by antigen-independent cell-autonomous signalling. *Nature* **2012**, *489*, 309–312. [CrossRef]
19. Iype, J.; Datta, M.; Khadour, A.; Ubelhart, R.; Nicolo, A.; Rollenske, T.; Duhren-von Minden, M.; Wardemann, H.; Maity, P.C.; Jumaa, H. Differences in Self-Recognition between Secreted Antibody and Membrane-Bound B Cell Antigen Receptor. *J. Immunol.* **2019**, *202*, 1417–1427. [CrossRef]
20. Dhanasekaran, D.N.; Reddy, E.P. JNK-signaling: A multiplexing hub in programmed cell death. *Genes Cancer* **2017**, *8*, 682–694. [CrossRef]
21. Peled, A.; Klein, S.; Beider, K.; Burger, J.A.; Abraham, M. Role of CXCL12 and CXCR4 in the pathogenesis of hematological malignancies. *Cytokine* **2018**, *109*, 11–16. [CrossRef] [PubMed]
22. Cancilla, D.; Rettig, M.P.; DiPersio, J.F. Targeting CXCR4 in AML and ALL. *Front. Oncol.* **2020**, *10*, 1672. [CrossRef] [PubMed]

International Journal of
Molecular Sciences

MDPI

Article

Metabolic Profiling as an Approach to Differentiate T-Cell Acute Lymphoblastic Leukemia Cell Lines Belonging to the Same Genetic Subgroup

Husam B. R. Alabed [1], Roberto Maria Pellegrino [1], Sandra Buratta [1,2], Anair Graciela Lema Fernandez [3], Roberta La Starza [3], Lorena Urbanelli [1,2], Cristina Mecucci [3], Carla Emiliani [1,2,*] and Paolo Gorello [1,2,*]

1 Department of Chemistry, Biology and Biotechnology, University of Perugia, 06100 Perugia, Italy; roberto.pellegrino@unipg.it (R.M.P.); sandra.buratta@unipg.it (S.B.); lorena.urbanelli@unipg.it (L.U.)
2 Centro di Eccellenza sui Materiali Innovativi Nanostrutturati (CEMIN), University of Perugia, Via del Giochetto, 06123 Perugia, Italy
3 Hematology and Bone Marrow Transplantation Unit, Laboratory of Molecular Medicine (CREO), Department of Medicine and Surgery, University of Perugia, 06132 Perugia, Italy; anairgraciela.lemafernandez@unipg.it (A.G.L.F.); cristina.mecucci@unipg.it (C.M.)
* Correspondence: carla.emiliani@unipg.it (C.E.); paolo.gorello@unipg.it (P.G.)

Abstract: T-cell acute lymphoblastic leukemia (T-ALL) is an aggressive tumor mainly affecting children and adolescents. It is driven by multiple genetic mutations that together define the leukemic phenotype. Interestingly, based on genetic alterations and/or deregulated expression, at least six genetic subgroups have been recognized. The TAL/LMO subgroup is one of the most represented genetic subgroups, characterizing 30–45% of pediatric T-ALL cases. The study of lipid and metabolic profiles is increasingly recognized as a valuable tool for comprehending the development and progression of tumors. In this study, metabolic and lipidomic analysis via LC/MS have been carried out on four T-ALL cell lines belonging to the TAL/LMO subgroup (Jurkat, Molt-4, Molt-16, and CCRF-CEM) to identify new potential metabolic biomarkers and to provide a subclassification of T-ALL cell lines belonging to the same subgroup. A total of 343 metabolites were annotated, including 126 polar metabolites and 217 lipid molecules. The statistical analysis, for both metabolic and lipid profiles, shows significant differences and similarities among the four cell lines. The Molt-4 cell line is the most distant cell line and CCRF-CEM shows a high activity in specific pathways when compared to the other cell lines, while Molt-16 and Jurkat show a similar metabolic profile. Additionally, this study highlighted the pathways that differ in each cell line and the possible enzymes involved using bioinformatic tools, capable of predicting the pathways involved by studying the differences in the metabolic profiles. This experiment offers an approach to differentiate T-ALL cell lines and could open the way to verify and confirm the obtained results directly in patients.

Keywords: untargeted metabolomics; lipidomics; T-ALL; lymphoblastic leukemia; TAL/LMO

1. Introduction

T-cell acute lymphoblastic leukemia (T-ALL) is a highly aggressive form of lymphoid tumor caused by the malignant transformation of T cells [1]. T-ALL represents approximately 15% of pediatric cases and 25% of adult cases among all lymphoblastic leukemia instances [2–4]. Patients show symptoms that are typically linked to anemia, thrombocytopenia, and neutropenia due to the infiltration of the bone marrow by tumor cells [5].

In recent years, the genetic basis of T-ALL has been largely explored [6–9]. Genomic studies have provided the genetic classification of T-ALL based on alterations/deregulated expression of transcription factors with pivotal roles in T-cell differentiation. In this context, at least six subgroups have been recognized. They are TAL/LMO, HOXA, TLX3, TLX1, NKX2-1/2-2, and BCL11B. In addition, abnormalities of other gene classes that control self-renewal capacity, cell cycle, proliferation, apoptosis, and/or differentiation cooperate in the leukemia phenotype [10,11].

While most efforts are directed toward the genetic characterization of tumors, it is becoming evident that the study of metabolic and lipid profiles provides additional insight into the pathogenesis and progression of tumors [12,13].

Metabolomics and lipidomics are emerging fields of biochemistry that study metabolic pathways and metabolic processes in a biological system [14–16]. Recently, liquid chromatography/mass spectrometry (LC/MS) has become the most used approach in laboratories to study metabolic and lipid profiles [17,18]. This analytical approach allows the generation of complex data matrices that can be studied and analyzed with several bioinformatics tools such as the MetaboAnalyst 5.0 web platform for statistical and pathway analysis [19], the OmicsNet web platform for biological networks [20], LipidOne for lipidomic data analysis [21], and Biopan for lipid metabolic pathways [22].

In the field of research, these methods offer priceless insights into biological pathways and processes, helping scientists better understand how diseases, genetic mutations, and the environment affect these pathways [23–25] and allowing them to find potential therapeutic targets or biomarkers [26–29]. In this context, it would be particularly interesting to deepen the metabolic and lipid studies of T-ALL to identify and highlight the significant differences between the different forms of leukemia. Such investigation could provide a deep understanding of these types of tumors, opening new research perspectives and potentially revealing important diagnostic and therapeutic information.

The TAL/LMO transcriptional complex subgroup constitutes a substantial proportion of T-ALL cases, comprising 30–45% of pediatric T-ALL cases and 10–15% of adult T-ALL cases [10]. In light of this, it would be interesting to investigate the metabolomic and lipidomic profiles of T-ALL tumor cells taken from multiple sources and belonging to this subgroup to study any metabolic similarity or differences inside the same subgroup. Four cell lines have been selected for this study: Jurkat, CCRF-CEM, MOLT-16, and MOLT-4. All of them belong to the TAL/LMO transcriptional complex subgroup and all represent in vitro models of acute lymphoblastic leukemia. By digging into the molecular phenotype of these cell lines, we aim to identify potential variations among them, possibly allowing for the classification and stratification of the different cell lines at the metabolic level, unraveling differences, or similarities, in the same genetic subgroup. This characterization could offer valuable insights for further subclassification of this type of leukemia, shedding light on statistically significant differences in metabolites and lipids, which can eventually be verified in clinical cases.

To achieve this aim, metabolomic and lipidomic analyses were conducted on the selected T-ALL cell lines. At the level of polar metabolites, statistical and pathway analyses were performed. Regarding the study of lipids, statistical analyses were conducted at three different levels: lipid classes, lipid molecular species, and lipid building blocks.

2. Results

2.1. Polar Metabolite Analysis

Untargeted metabolomics analysis allowed the annotation of 126 polar metabolites: complete information is listed in Table S1. The data were normalized via the median and Log transformation (base 10) and were scaled with Pareto scaling.

Unsupervised principal component analysis (PCA) on the polar metabolite matrix was performed (Figure 1).

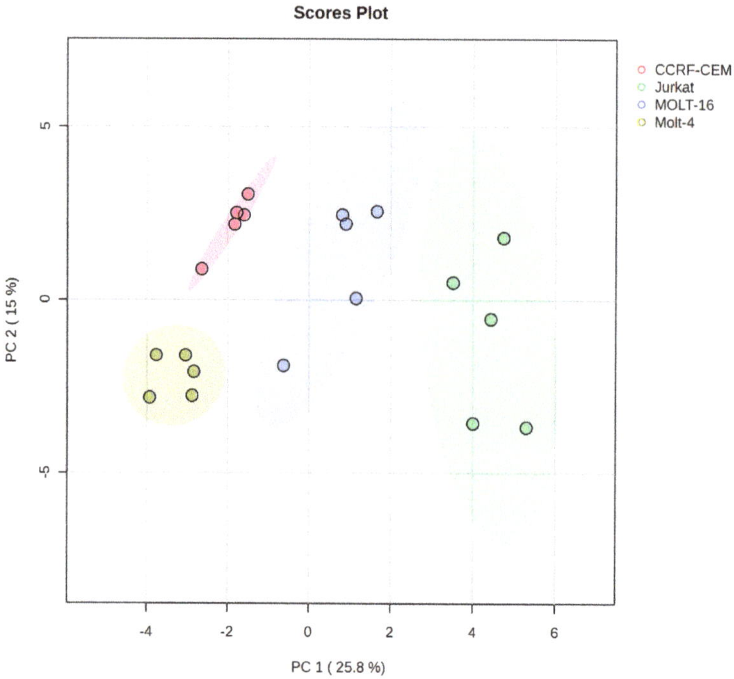

Figure 1. The figure shows the PCA scores plot; the ellipses enclose the scores inside a region with 95% confidence. The colors indicate the cell line type, and the symbols indicate the sample. The platform Metaboanalyst was used to generate these score plots.

The PCA score of polar metabolites demonstrates clear separation among the different cell lines. In fact, the first component (that explains 25.8% of variance) divides the Jurkat and Molt-16 cell lines from the CCRF-CEM and Molt-4 cell lines, while the second component (15%) was able to separate between the CCRF-CEM and Molt-4 cell lines. In fact, according to the classification proposed by Burger, Renate, et al., which classify the cells based on their immunophenotype, the CCRF-CEM cell line is considered pre-T, while Jurkat and Molt-16 lines are classified as mature T and Molt-4 as cortical T [30]. This classification could provide an explanation regarding the marked separation of the CCRF-CEM cell line from the other three lines. Similarly, the separation of the cortical cell line, Molt-4, and ultimately the separation at the first component level of the two mature T-type cell lines, Jurkat and Molt-16, from the other two can be explained. Moreover, the cell lines are from different genders and ages (Jurkat: 14-year-old male, CCRF-CEM: 3-year-old girl, Molt-4: 19-year-old man, and Molt-16: 5-year-old girl); however, it appears that the sex and age of the patients from whom these lines were derived do not influence or explain the clustering shown in the PCA analysis.

A one-way ANOVA test with a q-value (FDR) cut-off of 0.05 was performed to highlight the statistically significant metabolites. The ANOVA test revealed 57 significant metabolites (see Table S2), while the remaining metabolites did not show significant differences among the cell lines. Notably, several amino acids and their derivatives, dipeptides, and other metabolites vary among the different groups (Figure 2a), suggesting the presence of variations affecting cellular pathways. Most of these metabolites are involved in at least one metabolic pathway (See Table S3).

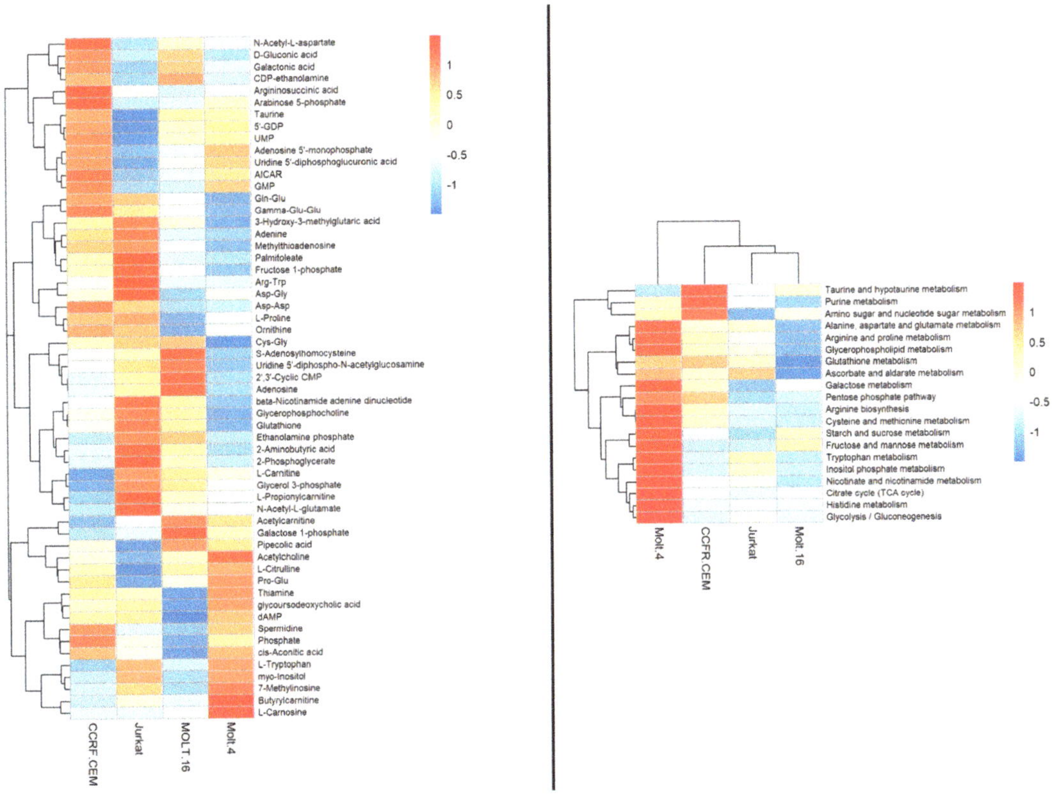

(a) (b)

Figure 2. The heatmaps: (**a**) Displays the correlation of the 57 statistically significant polar metabolites within each cell line. The colors indicate the expression level of each individual metabolite in each cell line based on their relative abundance. (**b**) Presents the results of pathway analysis conducted on each cell line sample, comparing them to medium bootstrap samples. The colors represent the significance based on the −log(*p*-value) of each pathway in each cell line. The analysis employed the Euclidean correlation index and the complete clustering method.

Pathway analysis was conducted on the entire polar metabolite matrix in order to highlight pathway variations in each cell line. The results were visualized using a heatmap to show the significance intensity of each pathway in each cell line (Figure 2b). Pathways with an impact of less than 0.1 were excluded.

As indicated in Figure 2b, different metabolic pathways exhibit statistical differences among specific cell lines. Notably, Molt-4 appears to be the most distinct cell line based on its metabolic profile. Several pathways, including tryptophan metabolism, show statistically significant differences in Molt-4 compared to the other cell lines. This is supported by the elevated abundance of tryptophan in Molt-4 cells when compared to the other lines (Figure 2a). Additionally, glutathione metabolism in Molt-4 varies significantly, attributed to the lower abundance of glutathione and Cys-Gly in Molt-4 compared to the other three cell lines. Arginine biosynthesis also appears to be decreased in Molt-4, potentially due to the lower abundance of N-(L-Arginino) succinate and ornithine. Inositol phosphate metabolism is another pathway exhibiting variations in Molt-4, likely linked to the higher abundance of myo-inositol in Molt-4 cells compared to the other lines.

The CCRF-CEM cell line emerges as the second most distinct based on its metabolic profile. Differences in multiple metabolic pathways, including purine metabolism, are evident, with CCRF-CEM exhibiting higher levels compared to other cell lines. This is supported by the elevated presence of metabolites like GDP, adenosine, AMP, GMP, and adenine, which also play roles in cellular signaling. Taurine and hypotaurine metabolism show a similar pattern, with CCRF-CEM displaying higher levels, possibly due to increased taurine abundance. Similar to Molt-4, CCRF-CEM also exhibits significant variation in glutathione metabolism, suggesting potential differences in oxidative stress response compared to Jurkat and Molt-16. Moreover, metabolites such as acetylcholine vary in different ways in these cell lines; in fact, Molt-4 demonstrates a high abundance of it; on the other hand, Molt-16 and CCRF-CEM demonstrate similar abundance, while Jurkat demonstrates a low abundance of this metabolite.

On the other hand, Molt-16 and Jurkat demonstrate similar metabolic profiles, with minor differences compared to the other two cell lines.

Finally, a cluster analysis was performed based on all polar metabolites detected with the Dendrogram function (see Figure 3).

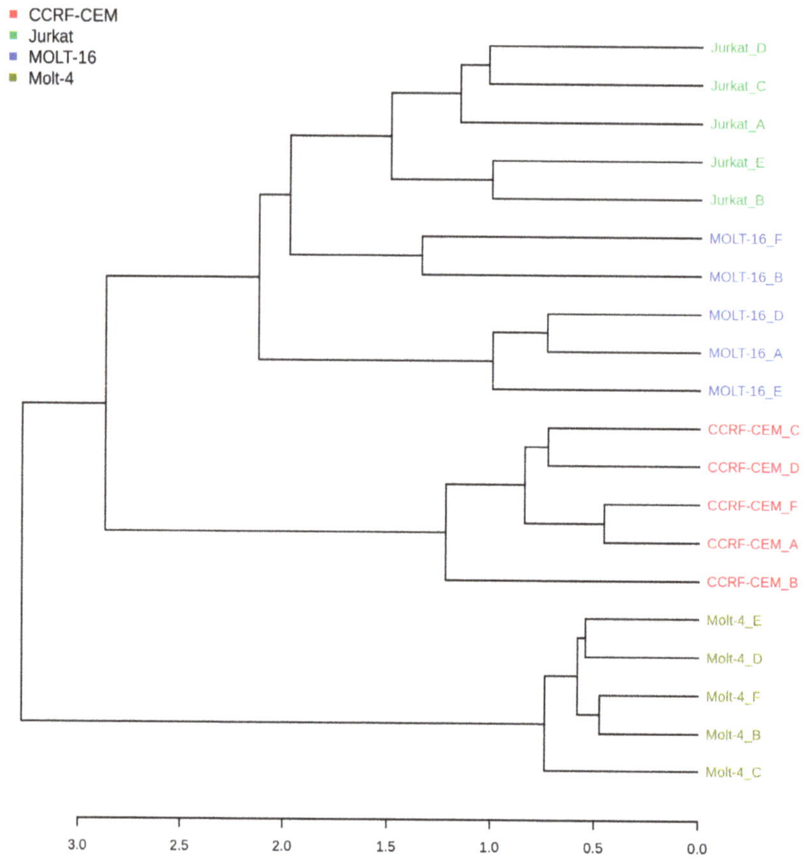

Figure 3. Hierarchical clustering dendrogram. The numbers below are the distances calculated with the Pearson algorithm. The tree was created by using the distance measure of the Pearson correlation and complete clustering algorithm.

Hierarchical cluster analysis revealed clear segregation of all the analyzed cell lines from the Molt-4 (Figure 3) cell line. In fact, this result could indicate that Molt-4 has an overall different metabolic profile when compared to the other three. The remaining cell lines can be separated into two sub-branches: one containing Molt-16 and Jurkat, which mostly demonstrate a similar metabolic profile, and the second one containing the CCRF-CEM cell line.

2.2. *Lipid Profile Analysis*

After lipidomic workflow, a data matrix was obtained containing qualitative and semi-quantitative information on 217 lipid molecular species divided into 19 classes (see Table S4). For a clearer and more detailed lipidomic analysis, qualitative and semiquantitative differences within lipid classes will be studied at first, then among molecular species, and finally among lipid building blocks.

2.2.1. Analysis at the Level of Lipid Classes

The results at the level of lipid classes are expressed as the average and standard error. The p-value of the comparison among these four cell lines was calculated using one-way ANOVA. The results are shown in Table 1. We also calculated the percentage of lipid classes among each cell line analyzed (see Figure 4).

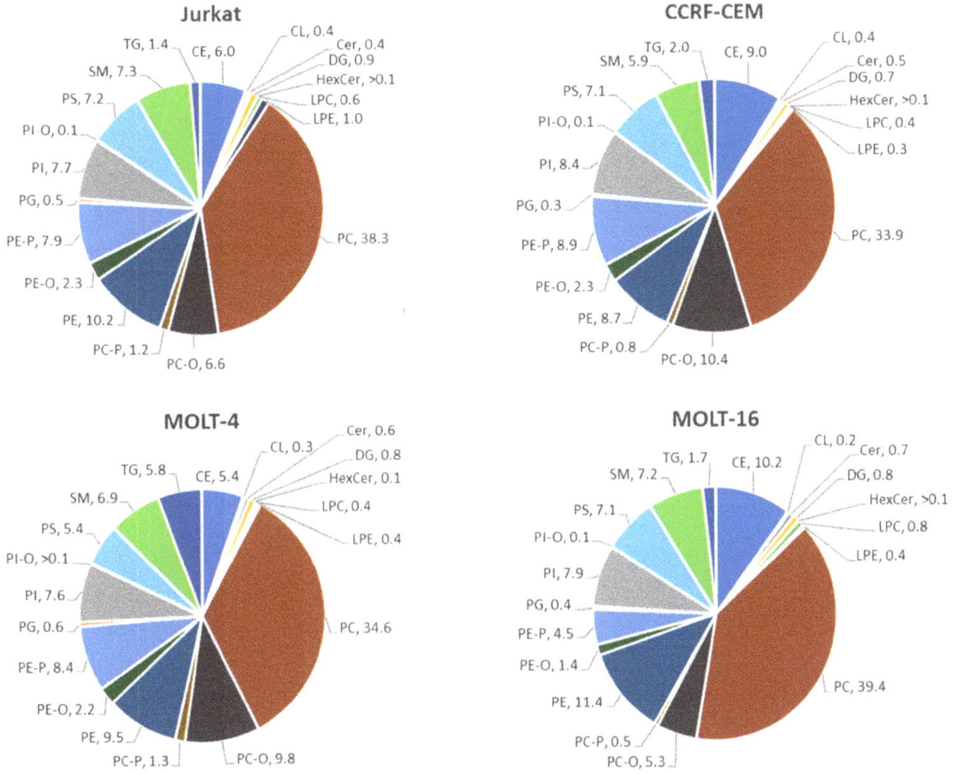

Figure 4. Pie chart: the figure shows the percentages of lipid classes referred to each cell line. Excel-Microsoft office 365 (version 2402) was used to create the charts after obtaining the percentages table by using an R script on the lipid data matrix. Every color represents one of the lipid classes.

Table 1. Comparison of the concentration of lipid classes of different T-cell lines; the number of replicates is 5. The average concentrations are reported in ug/10^6 cells. The number of annotated molecules is the number of single molecular species revealed.

Lipid Class Abbreviation	Explained Class Name	Number of Annotated Molecules	Average ± Exp Er (Jurkat)	Average ± Exp Er (CCRF-CEM)	Average ± Exp Er (MOLT-4)	Average ± Exp Er (MOLT-16)	p-Value
CE	Cholesteryl ester	6	0.54559 (±0.07061)	0.89815 (±0.06599)	0.69316 (±0.07075)	1.13462 (±0.12362)	0.001093
CL	Cardiolipin	9	0.03421 (±0.00316)	0.03732 (±0.00131)	0.04399 (±0.00265)	0.02556 (±0.00065)	0.000741
Cer	Ceramide	5	0.0371 (±0.00355)	0.04498 (±0.00264)	0.07195 (±0.01037)	0.08302 (±0.00841)	0.000205
DG	Diacylglycerol	9	0.08151 (±0.00735)	0.07011 (±0.00243)	0.10137 (±0.00789)	0.09266 (±0.00154)	0.006469
HexCer	Hexosylceramide	2	0.00399 (±0.00049)	0.00274 (±0.00011)	0.00754 (±0.00154)	0.00554 (±0.0003)	0.004946
LPC	Lysophophatidylcholine	3	0.05673 (±0.01429)	0.03656 (±0.00711)	0.04768 (±0.00934)	0.08803 (±0.02083)	0.094575
LPE	Lysophosphatidylethanolamine	1	0.09433 (±0.05043)	0.03227 (±0.00886)	0.0462 (±0.00317)	0.0435 (±0.01015)	0.37543
PC	Phosphatidylcholine	42	3.46958 (±0.21436)	3.36706 (±0.03942)	4.40161 (±0.06745)	4.39338 (±0.07721)	6.1×10^{-6}
PC-O	Alkyl Ether-linked phosphatidylcholine	10	0.59456 (±0.06462)	1.03528 (±0.03938)	1.25128 (±0.08139)	0.58819 (±0.05143)	1.01×10^{-6}
PC-P	Vinyl Ether-linked phosphatidylcholine	5	0.10567 (±0.01139)	0.08346 (±0.00222)	0.16357 (±0.00725)	0.05577 (±0.00151)	5.72×10^{-8}
PE	Phosphatidylethanolamine	20	0.92424 (±0.0747)	0.86159 (±0.03958)	1.20771 (±0.03715)	1.2668 (±0.02376)	2.27×10^{-5}
PE-O	Alkyl Ether-linked phosphatidylethanolamine	8	0.21023 (±0.02108)	0.23111 (±0.00425)	0.28497 (±0.0164)	0.15191 (±0.0111)	9.12×10^{-5}
PE-P	Vinyl Ether-linked phosphatidylethanolamine	18	0.71301 (±0.06548)	0.88215 (±0.02568)	1.06558 (±0.04709)	0.49967 (±0.02099)	7.29×10^{-7}
PG	Phosphatidylglycerol	2	0.04741 (±0.00487)	0.0251 (±0.00093)	0.07804 (±0.00477)	0.04413 (±0.00145)	1.42×10^{-7}
PI	Phosphatidylinositol	15	0.70036 (±0.08017)	0.83635 (±0.01766)	0.96282 (±0.04508)	0.87907 (±0.03204)	0.013254
PI-O	Ether-linked phosphatidylinositol	1	0.00489 (±0.00067)	0.00513 (±0.0003)	0.00523 (±0.00033)	0.00634 (±0.00061)	0.22212
PS	Phosphatidylserine	10	0.65673 (±0.05325)	0.70552 (±0.01925)	0.68516 (±0.01973)	0.79491 (±0.02234)	0.040757
SM	Sphingomyelin	9	0.65778 (±0.03399)	0.58726 (±0.01193)	0.87832(±0.04014)	0.80118 (±0.02078)	8.53×10^{-6}
TG	Triacylglycerol	42	0.12245 (±0.00637)	0.19821 (±0.0283)	0.73949 (±0.07466)	0.19183 (±0.02192)	3.39×10^{-8}
Total		217	9.06037 (±0.4956)	9.94036 (±0.15381)	12.73568 (±0.21066)	11.14609 (±0.13639)	7.45×10^{-7}

As indicated in Table 1, a significant difference appears in the total lipid content among the cell lines, especially between Jurkat and CCRF-CEM on the one hand and Molt-4 and Molt-16 on the other. Molt-4 exhibits the highest total lipid amount among the cell lines. Moreover, there are statistically significant differences in the amounts of specific lipid classes, including PC, PE, SM, TG, PC-O, PE-P, and others. In fact, both Molt-16 and Molt-4 demonstrate higher levels of PC and PE in comparison to the Jurkat and CCRF-CEM cell lines. Molt-4 also displays a remarkable quantity of TG compared to the other cell lines. Interestingly, Molt-16 presents a lower concentration of ether-linked lipids such as PE-P, PE-O, and PC-P when compared to the other cell lines.

In Figure 4, the percentage of each lipid class relative to the total lipids within each cell line is represented. The most represented lipid classes within all four cell lines are the phospholipids (PC, PE, PI, PG, PS, PE-O, PE-P, PC-O, PC-P, PI-O LPC, LPE, and SM) representing 90.9% in Jurkat, 87.4% in CCRF-CEM, 87.0% in Molt-4, and 86.2% in Molt-16. Notably, most lipids are distributed similarly among the cell lines and represent the majority of lipids inside them (PC, PE, PI, PG, PS, PE-O, PI-O, and SM). However, some lipid classes vary among the cell lines, as observed in Figure 4. Specifically, Molt-16 exhibits a relatively different distribution of certain lipid classes when compared to other cell lines, such as CE (10.2%), compared to Jurkat (6.0%) and Molt-4 (5.4%); PC-O (5.3%) compared to CCRF-CEM (10.4%), Jurkat (6.6%), and Molt-4 (9.8%); and PE-P (4.5%) compared to CCRF-CEM (8.9%), Jurkat (7.9%), and Molt-4 (8.4%). On the other hand, in Molt-4, the TG lipid class is uniquely distributed, representing 5.8% of total lipids and showing a higher percentage of this lipid class compared to Jurkat (1.4%), Molt-16 (1.7%), and CCRF-CEM (2.0%).

In this context, few studies on the lipid composition of T cells have been reported in the literature, which were mainly interested in T cells isolated from blood rather than immortalized cell lines or tumor models. A study from Alarcon-Barrera and colleagues on the lipid composition of CD4+ T cells [31] showed that the percentage of PC within these cells is 30% of lipids, while that of PE and SM is 20% and 30%, respectively. A subsequent study concerning differences in the lipid composition of the plasma membranes of T cells and B cells [32] showed that the percentages of PC within the cell membrane of T cells are about 65%, for PE the percentage is 8.6%, and for SM the percentage is 15.7%. Although these different results are due to noncomparable techniques, they provide indications about the most represented lipid classes within this cell type, which are precisely PC, PE, and SM. Our data confirmed this lipid composition on T-cell line models, and our matrix underlines the significant presence of other important lipid classes such as ether-linked PC, ether-linked PE, PI, and PS.

2.2.2. Analysis at the Level of Lipid Molecular Species

The one-way ANOVA test revealed 170 significant lipid species (Table S5); it also includes the Tukey's test.

The lipidomic data matrix was subjected to principal component analysis (PCA). The results are illustrated in Figure 5.

The principal component analysis in Figure 5a highlights a clear separation between the four cell lines, both in the first component (42% of explained variance), between Molt-16 and Jurkat on the one hand and Molt-4 and CCRF-CEM on the other, and in the second component (16.7% of explained variance), between Molt-4 and Jurkat on one side and Molt-16 and CCRF-CEM on the other. These results are very similar to the results of the PCA on the polar metabolites (Figure 1). Observing Figure 5b, it is possible to note the lipid molecular species that contribute the most to the separation and clustering; in fact, most of these molecules are PC, SM, PE, PI, and CE.

Heatmap visualization was applied on the lipidomic data matrix to study the quantitative differences among the single lipids inside the different cell lines. The results shown in Figure 6 highlight the main lipid molecular species with differences in expression.

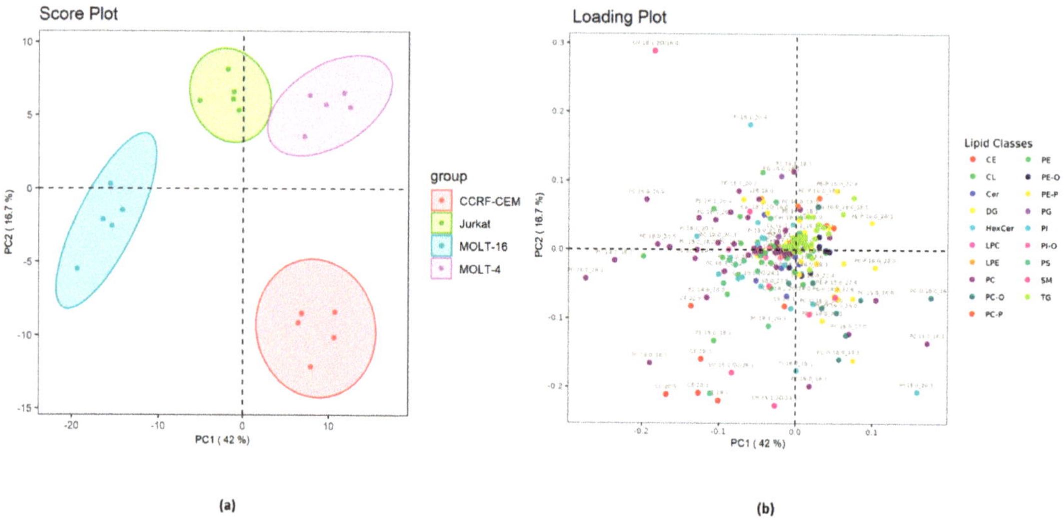

Figure 5. (**a**) PCA score plot of the lipid molecular species from the four cell lines. The ellipses enclose the scores inside a region with 95% confidence. (**b**) Loading plot of the lipid molecular species which contribute to the separation among the cell lines. Before the analysis, data matrix was normalized and pareto scaling was applied.

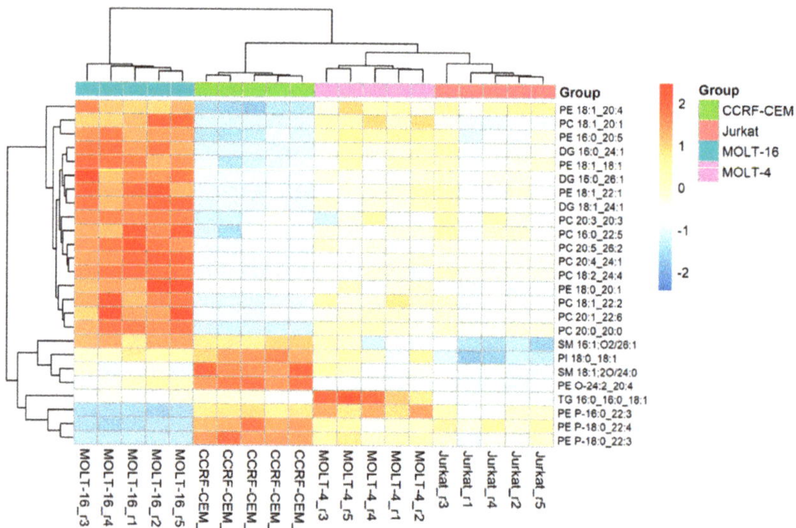

Figure 6. Heatmap: The figure shows the correlation of the 25 most significant lipid molecular species within each sample. The color shows the level of expression of each individual species in each sample based on their concentrations. The analysis was performed using the Pearson correlation index and the complete clustering method.

It is worth mentioning that some molecular species of the PE P lipid class, such as PE P-16:0_22:3, PE P-18:0_22:4, and PE P-18:0_22:3, are present in concentrations relatively high in the CCRF-CEM cell line compared to the other lines. On the contrary, relatively low concentrations of these three lipids are found in the Molt-16 line, while the other two cell lines show average concentrations compared to CCRF-CEM. On the other side, numerous molecular species belonging to the PE and PC lipid classes are present in relatively high concentrations in the Molt-16 line, whereas relatively low concentrations are found in the CCRF-CEM line and relatively medium concentrations in the Jurkat and Molt-4 lines. Furthermore, some molecular species, such as SM 16:1;O2/26:1, SM 18:1;O2/24:0, PI 18:0_18:1, and PE O-24:2_20:4, show relatively high concentrations in the CCRF-CEM line and relatively low concentrations in the other cell lines. These results at the two levels confirm that the lipidic profile of Molt-16 is highly different from the other cell lines, especially CCRF-CEM, while Jurkat and Molt-4 demonstrate a similar lipid profile.

2.2.3. Analysis of Lipid Building Blocks

Ultimately, we further analyzed the composition of the building blocks in the context of lipid molecular species. Specifically, we analyzed the lengths of the chains and the amount of unsaturation of the fatty acids that make up the various lipids. Figure 7 shows the differences in the concentrations of chains with different lengths (with different numbers of carbon atoms).

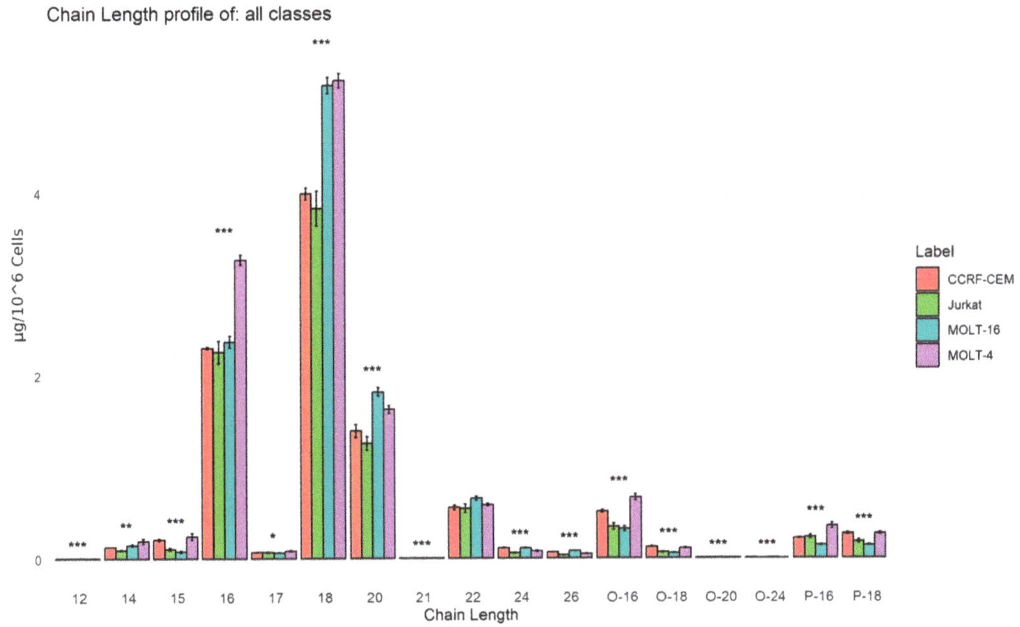

Figure 7. Bar graph: The figure shows the average concentrations (ug/10^6 of cells) of the chains with different lengths. Experimental error bar (n = 5) and ANOVA significance asterisks are represented (*** indicates p-value < 0.001, ** indicates p-value < 0.01, and * indicates p-value < 0.05). This graph was made with R program (R version 4.2.3 (2023-03-15 ucrt)).

The bar graph in Figure 7 shows that the most abundant chains are those composed of 16, 18, 20, and 22 carbon atoms. It is interesting to note that most of the chain lengths are statistically different: particularly, 18 and 20 carbon-atom chains are highly present in Molt-4 and Molt-16. Chains with 16 carbon atoms are predominantly present in Molt-4. Furthermore, a particular abundance of ether chains with 16 and 18 carbon atoms is observed, which are mostly present in the two cell lines Molt-4 and CCRF-CEM.

Regarding the unsaturation in the fatty acids of lipids, ratios of saturated fatty acids (SFA), monounsaturated fatty acids (MUFA), and polyunsaturated fatty acids (PUFA) were calculated based on the average amount (in μg/10^cells) of fatty acids with different types of saturation and unsaturation within the lipid species. Table 2 illustrates the results.

Table 2. Ratio of saturated fatty acids (SFA), monounsaturated fatty acids (MUFA), and polyunsaturated fatty acids (PUFA) using the average amount of chains with different types of saturations (n = 5) in μg/10^6 of cells.

Cell Line/Ratio	SFA/MUFA	SFA/PUFA
Jurkat	0.9393	1.7644
CCRF-CEM	0.9926	1.8439
Molt-4	0.9765	2.1925
Molt-16	0.8479	1.4532

As shown in Table 2, the SFA/MUFA ratio in all four cell lines is less than one, indicating a lower quantity of saturated fatty acids compared to monounsaturated fatty acids inside the cells. Conversely, the SFA/PUFA ratios are all higher than 1, signifying a greater presence of saturated fatty acids than polyunsaturated fatty acids inside the cells. However, differences in the ratios among the cell lines do not reach significance. Nevertheless, the lower ratios in the Molt-16 cell line could suggest a higher activity in pathways involving the desaturation of fatty acids compared to the other cell lines.

3. Discussion

Statistical analyses of the relative abundances of polar metabolites confirm the presence of significant differences in the metabolism of the four T-ALL analyzed cell lines. The results of principal component analysis (PCA) applied to polar metabolite and lipid matrices showed that differences in metabolic and lipid profiles are able to cluster cell lines according to their maturation status. Additionally, specific pathways emerge that vary among them, such as tryptophan metabolism, glutathione metabolism, arginine biosynthesis, purine metabolism, and others. The analysis showed a higher abundance of tryptophan in Molt-4 when compared to the other cell lines, suggesting a different metabolic behavior for this amino acid in Molt-4. The catabolism of this amino acid is generally correlated with peripheral immune tolerance [33]. Additionally, Molt-4 showed a low abundance of glutathione and other metabolites involved in its metabolism, indicating a different oxidative stress activity. Enzymes such as glutathione synthetase and glutamate cysteine ligase, which contribute to glutathione metabolism [34], may have a lower activity in Molt-4 when compared to the other cell lines. Studies have shown that this pathway is closely related to tumors; in fact, high levels of glutathione promote tumor progression and increased metastasis [35].

The pathway analysis has also demonstrated lower arginine biosynthesis in Molt-4 in comparison to the other cell lines. This result could also indicate a variation in the activity of enzymes involved in this pathway, such as ornithine transcarbamylase and argininosuccinate synthase 1. Arginine biosynthesis is one of the most important and sensitive pathways in cancer cells, regulating cell death [36]. The identified differences within these T-ALL cell lines highlight the possibility to further investigate their sensitivity to new personalized therapeutic approaches.

Our pathway analysis demonstrated higher abundance in specific metabolites related to purine metabolism in the CCRF-CEM cell line, suggesting its higher activity in CCR-CEM. Moreover, enzymes such as guanylate kinase 1, phosphodiesterase 10A, and adenosine kinase play key roles in purine metabolism and may be involved in the identified deregulation. Numerous studies have demonstrated the importance of this pathway in cancer biology; indeed, purine metabolism appears to be increased in tumors because purine nucleotide metabolism is crucial for cancer cell proliferation. Accordingly, this pathway is therefore one of the targets for cancer therapies including some types of leukemia [37–41].

These results, at the level of polar metabolites, highlight potential biomarkers and distinct behaviors for some cell line. For instance, purine metabolism is distinguishable

in CCRF-CEM, while the other cell lines exhibit similar characteristics. Moreover, Molt-4 exhibits a unique behavior in various metabolic pathways, particularly in arginine biosynthesis, the metabolism of glutathione, and tryptophan. The pathway analysis has also demonstrated a comparable metabolic profile in Jurkat and Molt-16.

The results of our hierarchical cluster analysis reveal a significant finding: the Molt-4 cell line exhibits the most distinct metabolic phenotype compared to the other three cell lines. It is noteworthy to highlight that the metabolic behavior of CCRF-CEM is also distinguishable, while Molt-16 and Jurkat show a similar metabolic profile.

Lipidomic analysis reveals a marked distinction among the four cell lines under study. The absolute amount of intracellular lipids manifests statistically significant differences, with the Molt-4 cell line having a higher amount overall than the other lines. In addition, significant variations are observed at the level of lipid classes. Lipid classes such as PC, PE, PS, PI, and SM manifest differences in at least one of the cell lines, suggesting a possible diversification in the lipid composition of both the cell membrane and the intracellular environment. Such changes in lipid classes may be attributable to changes in the activity of specific enzymes responsible for intracellular lipid synthesis, such as phosphotransferases, phospholipases, phosphatases, lipid kinases, and sphingosine kinases. It is relevant to note that numerous scientific studies have demonstrated activity variation with many of these enzymes in the context of cancer [42–45]. Interestingly, the percentages of lipid classes in each cell line confirm a uniform distribution of lipid classes across all the cell lines. Our results, based on semiquantitative lipid assessment, support the hypothesis that phospholipid transformation and synthesis pathways diverge among the four cell lines under study. This suggests the possibility of further classification of these tumors based on these lipid classes as biomarkers and even identifying specific pathways that could represent potential therapeutic targets.

Furthermore, specific molecular lipids with statistically significant variations were identified. The heatmap revealed that particular lipid species, such as PE P-16:0_22:3, PE P-18:0_22:4, PE P-18:0_22:3, SM 16:1;O2/26:1, SM 18:1;O2/24:0, PI 18:0_18:1, and PE O-24:2_20:4, show noticeable differences within at least one of the cell lines. These molecules could be the subject of further studies to identify potential biomarkers. In fact, at this level of analysis, the Molt-16 cell line demonstrates a unique lipidomic profile compared to the other cell lines, while Jurkat and Molt-4 share a similar lipid profile. CCRF-CEM also distinguishes itself from the others, albeit to a lesser extent than Molt-16.

Lipid building block analyses revealed significant variations in the levels of fatty acid chains within the lipids of the four cell lines. Specifically, Molt-4 and Molt-16 cells exhibit a relatively higher presence of long-chain fatty acids (with 16–18 carbon atoms) compared to the other two cell lines. Conversely, CCRF-CEM and Molt-16 cells show an increase in lipids with ether-linked chains when compared to Molt-4 and Jurkat lines. These differences suggest distinct activities of enzymes involved in the elongation of fatty acids, such as elongase. While the ratios of SFA/MUFA and SFA/PUFA, calculated to study differences in the unsaturation within the lipid chains, show minimal variations, Molt-16 demonstrates lower ratio values. These differences in lipid-building chains could be associated with higher activity in enzymes regulating these fatty acids, such as specific desaturases.

Studies in different types of tumors have shown an increase in the expression of specific elongases, including elongases 1, 5, and 6 [46]. These enzymes are responsible for elongation of long-chain fatty acids, which include chains of 16, 18, and 20 carbon atoms. Further study showed that elongase 5 plays a key role in lipid metabolism in T cells. This was confirmed by the observation of high expression of this enzyme in proliferating T cells and Jurkat cells compared with resting T cells [47]. The same study also documented increased expression of fatty acid desaturases 1 and 2, which are responsible for the desaturation of long-chain fatty acids.

Our results reveal distinct metabolic behaviors across the four cell lines grown and maintained at the same experimental conditions. Specific pathway shows enhanced activity in one cell line more than the others. This observation not only aids in further classification of these cell lines but also paves the way for in vivo studies to validate these pathways as potential biomarkers. Consequently, these findings could be considered as promising diagnostic biomarkers for T-ALL patients based on the metabolic phenotype. These biochemical features from our preliminary study could then be validated and confirmed in patients. They could then be used to monitor the tumor, track its severity or progression during treatment, and, within specific biological pathways, could also be used to identify new therapeutic targets, thus allowing the assignment of different therapeutic approaches to patients of the same genetic subgroup, based on this classification and stratification due to metabolic phenotype. This encourages a shift towards personalized therapy approaches grounded in metabolic classification to integrate the genetic approach. Moreover, this study could serve as a foundation for additional research exploring the metabolic behavior of T-ALL in other genetic subgroups, as well as those categorized as unclassified due to the absence of cytogenetic markers [10]. Notably, recent studies demonstrated the feasibility of stratifying patients with acute myeloid leukemia (AML) using a lipidomic approach, revealing different lipid profiles among patients with distinct cytogenetic alterations [48]. Nonetheless, it is still necessary to verify and validate these results on primary tumor cells or on samples taken directly from patients in order to translate these findings into potential clinical applications.

4. Materials and Methods

4.1. Chemicals and Reagents

LC/MS grade water (H_2O) (Merck KGaA, Darmstadt, Germany) (LiChrosolv), acetonitrile (ACN), methanol (MeOH), isopropanol (IPA), toluene (Tol) all (Carlo Erba, Milan, Italy), ammonium fluoride, ammonium acetate, methyl-t-butyl ether (MTBE), and chloroform ($CHCl_3$) were purchased from Sigma-Aldrich (Sigma-Aldrich GmbH, Hamburg, Germany). The internal standard (IS) for lipidomics analysis was EquiSPLASH Lipidomix (Avanti Polar, Alabaster, AL, USA): a mixture with known concentrations of the following lipids [100 μg/mL]: PC 15:0_18:1(d7); PE 15:0_18:1(d7); PS 15:0_18:1(d7); PG 15:0_18:1(d7); PI 15:0_18:1(d7); C15 Ceramide-d7; LPC 18:1(d7); LPE 18:1(d7); CE 18:1(d7); MG 18:1(d7); DG 15:0_18:1(d7); TG 15:0_18:1(d7)_15:0; SM 18:1;2O/18:1(d9); and cholesterol(d7). The cell culture reagents were from Euroclone S.p.A (Pero, Italy).

The Jurkat cell line (TIB-152) was purchased at American Type Culture Collection, Manassas, VA, U.S.A. CCRF-CEM (ACC 240), MOLT-4 (ACC 362), and MOLT-16 (ACC 29) cell lines were kindly provided by the laboratories of Prof. Giovanni Roti (University of Parma, Italy) and purchased at the DSMZ-German Collection of Microorganisms and Cell Cultures GmbH, Germany.

4.2. Samples and Sample Preparation

4.2.1. Cell Lines

This study was carried out on four T-acute lymphoblastic leukemia cell lines: Jurkat, CCRF-CEM, MOLT-16, and MOLT-4, all belonging to the TAL/LMO transcriptional complex [49,50], with a well-characterized immunophenotype [30]; see Table S6 for more details. The cell lines were cultured in RPMI 1640 medium with the addition of 10% heat-inactivated fetal bovine serum (FBS) and 1% penicillin/streptomycin (P/S). Cells were kept in the same experimental conditions: in T-75 flasks in a humidified atmosphere containing 5% CO_2 at a temperature of 37 °C. In order to obtain better results and minimize variations, cells from all four cell lines were seeded at the same concentration and, after 48 h, were harvested, counted, and collected into a pellet via centrifugation at 300× *g*, washed twice with phosphate-buffered saline (PBS), and stored at −80 °C until LC/MS analysis.

4.2.2. Preparation of Analytical Samples and Metabolites Extraction

For polar metabolite analyses, from each cell line, 5 experimental replicates were prepared in 5 different T-75 flasks. After incubation of the cells under physiological conditions for 48 h, 1 million cells were collected, pelleted, and washed twice with PBS.

The extraction of polar metabolites was performed following the biphasic method described by Cajka et al. [51], with some minor modifications. A total of 275 μL of MeOH was added to each cell pellet, followed by 30 s of vortexing. Subsequently, 1 mL of MTBE was added, and the sample was again vortexed and shaken for 20 min at 1500 rpm using a T-Shaker (Euroclone). After that, 275 μL of a 10% MeOH solution was added. The sample was centrifuged at 16,000× *g* for 10 min at 4 °C. After phase separation, the polar lower phase was transferred to a glass vial and evaporated with a gentle flow of nitrogen at 60 degrees. The dry residue was resuspended in 100 μL of ACN/H_2O 4:1 and then placed in the autosampler. The same procedures were followed on a pool of all cells and on an empty Eppendorf tube, which was subsequently used as a blank control.

For the lipidomic analysis, the sample pellet preparation procedure was identical to the previous one. With some modifications, lipid extraction was performed on the pellet following the lipid solubilization process described by Pellegrino et al. [52]. Initially, an extraction mixture was prepared consisting of 33 mL of MTBE, MeOH, and $CHCl_3$ at a ratio of 1:1:1 (MMC). The MMC consists of 1 mL of IS diluted 1:10 in MeOH, 10 mL of MeOH, 11 mL of MTBE, and 11 mL of $CHCl_3$. Subsequently, 1 mL of the MMC mixture was added to each sample pellet. After 30 s of vortexing, the samples were placed in a T-Shaker (Euroclone) and processed for 20 min at 1500 rpm at 20 °C. Afterward, the samples were centrifuged at 16,000× *g* for 10 min at 4 °C, and the supernatant was transferred to a glass vial. Following this, the supernatant was dried with a light stream of nitrogen. Dried residue was resuspended in 100 μL of MeOH/Tol 9:1 and placed in the autosampler. The same procedures were followed on a pool of all cells and on an Eppendorf containing only the solubilization solution (MMC), which was subsequently used as a blank control.

4.3. LC/MS Analysis

LC/MS analysis was conducted using an Agilent system consisting of an Agilent 1260 Infinity II liquid chromatograph consisted of a quaternary pump, a thermostatted column compartment, and an autosampler coupled to an Agilent 6530 Accurate-Mass Q-TOF (Quadrupole-Time-of-Flight) analyzer and an Agilent JetStream source.

4.3.1. Untargeted Polar Metabolomics

Untargeted polar metabolomics chromatographic separation was conducted by following the indications reported by Jian Li et al. [53]. For the immobile phase, a Waters XBridge BEH Amide (HILIC) column (150 mm, 2.1 mm, and 2.5 μm) at 25 °C with a flow rate of 0.35 mL/min was used. The mobile phase consisted of a mixture of water (A) and ACN (B), both with 0.2% formic acid. The gradient used was as follows: From 0 to 3 min, an isocratic gradient was maintained, with A at 10% and B at 90%. From 3 to 13 min, a linear gradient was used, with A at 52% and B at 48%. From 13 to 15 min, an isocratic gradient was maintained, with A at 52% and B at 48%. From 15 to 16 min, a linear gradient was used, with A at 10% and B at 90%. From 16 to 20 min, an isocratic gradient was maintained, with A at 10% and B at 90%. At 20 min, the run was stopped. Spectrometric data were acquired in the range of 40–1700 m/z in both negative and positive polarity. The Agilent JetStream source was used with the following settings: gas temperature (N_2) at 200 °C, drying gas flow at 10 L/min, nebulizer pressure at 50 psi, and sheath gas temperature at 300 °C with a flow of 12 L/min.

4.3.2. Untargeted Lipidomics

Lipid chromatographic separation was performed as previously described [25,54], employing the same column and conditions: a Supelco Ascentis Express 90A C18 column (100 mm × 2.1 mm, 2.0 μm) maintained at 50 °C with a flow rate of 0.25 mL/min. The mobile phase consisted of four eluents: water, ACN, MeOH, and IPA. All solvents were prepared with ammonium fluoride at a concentration of 0.2 mM. Additionally, IPA, MeOH, and water were prepared with ammonium acetate at a concentration of 10 mM.

In full scan mode, spectrometric data were collected in the range of 50–3200 m/z for both negative and positive polarity. The pool sample was analyzed five times using an iterative DDA acquisition mode to capture as many MS/MS spectra as possible. The Agilent JetStream source settings were consistent with those described in previous works [25,54].

4.4. Raw Data Processing

The raw data for metabolic and lipid analysis were processed using MS-DIAL software (version 4.9). This process included peak selection, alignment, and data annotation [55]. In the case of polar metabolites, the annotation was conducted using mass spectra (MS) and mass/tandem spectra (MS/MS) using the NIST2020 database. To conduct the statistical analysis of the polar metabolites, the relative abundances of the metabolites (in terms of areas under the peaks) were measured and normalized according to the number of cells. Subsequently, these data were compared and studied using the MetaboAnalyst platform [19]. The resulting matrix was imported into MetaboAnalyst, where a normalization of the samples was applied with the median. In addition, a logarithmic transformation of the data was performed, followed by pareto scaling. The MetaboAnalyst interface allowed the execution of various analyses, including principal component analysis (PCA), one-way ANOVA tests, and the creation of a hierarchical clustering dendrogram. In addition, the possibility was given to conduct pathway analyses to compare variations in biochemical pathways between different cell lines. These pathways and the enzymes involved are based on the Homo Sapiens KEGG databases.

For lipid annotation, following the guidelines dictated by the Lipid Standard Initiative (LSI), the annotation of lipid molecular species was performed at the molecular level using data acquired with mass spectrometry (MS) and tandem mass spectrometry (MS/MS) [56] using databases generated through the Lipid Spectrum Generator (LSG) tool [57]. Following the procedure outlined by Tsugawa H. et al. [55], lipid semiquantification was performed using the deuterated internal standard (EquiSPLASH Lipidomix) for each lipid class at levels 2 and 3 of the LSI recommendations (see Table S7). Semiquantification of the raw data was conducted using an R script developed within our laboratory. The semiquantification was based on the known concentrations of the standards added to the samples. At the end of this analytical step, a set of matrices was produced containing the expressive concentrations in μg/1 million cells of the lipid molecular species previously annotated and classified according to the different lipid classes. These matrices were subjected to median normalization and then pareto scaling was applied, helping to prepare the final matrix for subsequent analyses. Statistical analyses on the identified variations within the lipid profiles were performed using a one-way ANOVA test, PCA, and heatmap visualization. Specifically, the matrix of lipid concentrations was examined using LipidOne [21], supported with R scripts developed in-house to generate visualizations such as the PCA score graph, heatmap, and bar graphs.

5. Conclusions

In this study, metabolomics and lipidomics analyses of Jurkat, Molt-16, Molt-4, and CCRF-CEM cell lines allowed the annotation of 126 polar metabolites and 217 different lipid species.

The experimental data confirm the possibility to differentiate T-cell acute lymphoblastic leukemia cell lines belonging to the same genetic subgroup. Notably, when considering the overall metabolic profile, it becomes apparent that Molt-4 stands out as the most distinct among the cell lines. However, digging into the detailed pathway and lipidomic analysis allows for the differentiation and stratification of these cell lines based on specific pathways. For example, CCRF-CEM is distinguishable with its high-activity in purine metabolism, Molt-4 is distinguishable with its unique behavior regarding glutathione metabolism and acetylcholine, or the unique lipidomic profile of Molt-16. On the other hand, the results also show some similarities among the cell lines. The overall metabolic and lipidic profiles indicate a resemblance between Jurkat and Molt-16. Furthermore, these cell lines share similar behaviors in specific metabolic pathways, such as purine metabolism and glutathione metabolism.

Consequently, our study introduces the potential for an additional subclassification for T-ALL based on the metabolic and lipid phenotype. The identified differences among the four cell lines call for a more in-depth investigation utilizing cells directly sourced from patients with TAL/LMO rearrangements to validate these observed distinctions as metabolic biomarkers. Such biochemical features could be used to classify patients into multiple groups based on metabolomic profile. This could be useful at a clinical level for diagnosis, as well as for stratification of disease severity and risk. Furthermore, they could be used to monitor disease progression during specific treatments. Ultimately, this classification could be useful for the discovery of potential therapies, based on the altered metabolic pathways within patients in each metabolomic subclass.

Moreover, within the context of T-ALL, cases labeled as 'unclassified' due to the absence of cytogenetic markers could benefit from multiomics approaches, such as metabolomics and lipidomics. This could unveil underlying leukemogenic mechanisms, leading to the identification of new biomarkers specific to each tumor variant. Such insights could facilitate the identification of tailored therapeutic targets based on the metabolic behavior of each tumor variant.

In conclusion, this study demonstrates the potential of the metabolomic and lipidomic approach as valuable tools offering a comprehensive view of the cells and their progression. This opens the possibility of designing experiments to directly verify and confirm the obtained results in patients.

Supplementary Materials: The following supporting information can be downloaded at: https://www.mdpi.com/article/10.3390/ijms25073921/s1.

Author Contributions: Conceptualization, H.B.R.A., C.E., P.G. and R.M.P.; methodology, H.B.R.A.; software, R.M.P. and H.B.R.A.; validation, H.B.R.A. and R.M.P.; formal analysis, H.B.R.A.; investigation, H.B.R.A., R.M.P., A.G.L.F., S.B. and P.G.; resources, P.G., C.E., R.L.S. and C.M.; data curation, H.B.R.A. and R.M.P.; writing—original draft preparation, H.B.R.A.; writing—review and editing, R.M.P., H.B.R.A., S.B., P.G., L.U., C.E., R.L.S., A.G.L.F. and C.M.; visualization, H.B.R.A.; supervision, C.E.; project administration, C.E. and R.M.P.; funding acquisition, P.G., C.E. and C.M. All authors have read and agreed to the published version of the manuscript.

Funding: This research was supported by the European Union—NextGenerationEU under the Italian Ministry of University and Research (MUR) National Innovation Ecosystem grant ECS00000041—VITALITY.

Institutional Review Board Statement: Not applicable.

Informed Consent Statement: Not applicable.

Data Availability Statement: The datasets generated during and/or analyzed during the current study are available from the corresponding author on reasonable request.

Acknowledgments: We acknowledge the University of Perugia and MUR for support within the project Vitality.

Conflicts of Interest: The authors declare no conflicts of interest.

References

1. Van Vlierberghe, P.; Ferrando, A. The Molecular Basis of T Cell Acute Lymphoblastic Leukemia. *J. Clin. Investig.* **2012**, *122*, 3398–3406. [CrossRef] [PubMed]
2. Litzow, M.R.; Ferrando, A.A. How I Treat T-Cell Acute Lymphoblastic Leukemia in Adults. *Blood* **2015**, *126*, 833–841. [CrossRef] [PubMed]
3. Karrman, K.; Johansson, B. Pediatric T-cell Acute Lymphoblastic Leukemia. *Genes Chromos. Cancer* **2017**, *56*, 89–116. [CrossRef] [PubMed]
4. Chiaretti, S.; Foà, R. T-Cell Acute Lymphoblastic Leukemia. *Haematologica* **2009**, *94*, 160–162. [CrossRef] [PubMed]
5. Puckett, Y.; Chan, O. *Acute Lymphocytic Leukemia*; StatPearls Publishing: St. Petersburg, FL, USA, 2023.

6. Ferrando, A.A.; Look, A.T. Gene Expression Profiling in T-Cell Acute Lymphoblastic Leukemia. *Semin. Hematol.* **2003**, *40*, 274–280. [CrossRef] [PubMed]
7. La Starza, R.; Pierini, V.; Pierini, T.; Nofrini, V.; Matteucci, C.; Arniani, S.; Moretti, M.; Lema Fernandez, A.G.; Pellanera, F.; Di Giacomo, D.; et al. Design of a Comprehensive Fluorescence in Situ Hybridization Assay for Genetic Classification of T-Cell Acute Lymphoblastic Leukemia. *J. Mol. Diagn.* **2020**, *22*, 629–639. [CrossRef]
8. Atak, Z.K.; Gianfelici, V.; Hulselmans, G.; De Keersmaecker, K.; Devasia, A.G.; Geerdens, E.; Mentens, N.; Chiaretti, S.; Durinck, K.; Uyttebroeck, A.; et al. Comprehensive Analysis of Transcriptome Variation Uncovers Known and Novel Driver Events in T-Cell Acute Lymphoblastic Leukemia. *PLoS Genet.* **2013**, *9*, e1003997. [CrossRef]
9. Franciosa, G.; Smits, J.G.A.; Minuzzo, S.; Martinez-Val, A.; Indraccolo, S.; Olsen, J. V Proteomics of Resistance to Notch1 Inhibition in Acute Lymphoblastic Leukemia Reveals Targetable Kinase Signatures. *Nat. Commun.* **2021**, *12*, 2507. [CrossRef] [PubMed]
10. Bardelli, V.; Arniani, S.; Pierini, V.; Di Giacomo, D.; Pierini, T.; Gorello, P.; Mecucci, C.; La Starza, R. T-Cell Acute Lymphoblastic Leukemia: Biomarkers and Their Clinical Usefulness. *Genes* **2021**, *12*, 1118. [CrossRef] [PubMed]
11. Van Vlierberghe, P.; Pieters, R.; Beverloo, H.B.; Meijerink, J.P.P. Molecular-Genetic Insights in Paediatric T-Cell Acute Lymphoblastic Leukaemia. *Br. J. Haematol.* **2008**, *143*, 153–168. [CrossRef] [PubMed]
12. Lima, A.R.; Carvalho, M.; Aveiro, S.S.; Melo, T.; Domingues, M.R.; Macedo-Silva, C.; Coimbra, N.; Jerónimo, C.; Henrique, R.; Bastos, M.D.L.; et al. Comprehensive Metabolomics and Lipidomics Profiling of Prostate Cancer Tissue Reveals Metabolic Dysregulations Associated with Disease Development. *J. Proteome Res.* **2022**, *21*, 727–739. [CrossRef] [PubMed]
13. Armitage, E.G.; Southam, A.D. Monitoring Cancer Prognosis, Diagnosis and Treatment Efficacy Using Metabolomics and Lipidomics. *Metabolomics* **2016**, *12*, 146. [CrossRef]
14. Wang, R.; Li, B.; Lam, S.M.; Shui, G. Integration of Lipidomics and Metabolomics for In-Depth Understanding of Cellular Mechanism and Disease Progression. *J. Genet. Genom.* **2020**, *47*, 69–83. [CrossRef]
15. Wang, J.; Wang, C.; Han, X. Tutorial on Lipidomics. *Anal. Chim. Acta* **2019**, *1061*, 28–41. [CrossRef] [PubMed]
16. Hollywood, K.; Brison, D.R.; Goodacre, R. Metabolomics: Current Technologies and Future Trends. *Proteomics* **2006**, *6*, 4716–4723. [CrossRef] [PubMed]
17. Züllig, T.; Trötzmüller, M.; Köfeler, H.C. Lipidomics from Sample Preparation to Data Analysis: A Primer. *Anal. Bioanal. Chem.* **2020**, *412*, 2191–2209. [CrossRef] [PubMed]
18. Harrieder, E.-M.; Kretschmer, F.; Böcker, S.; Witting, M. Current State-of-the-Art of Separation Methods Used in LC-MS Based Metabolomics and Lipidomics. *J. Chromatogr. B Analyt. Technol. Biomed. Life Sci.* **2022**, *1188*, 123069. [CrossRef] [PubMed]
19. Pang, Z.; Chong, J.; Zhou, G.; de Lima Morais, D.A.; Chang, L.; Barrette, M.; Gauthier, C.; Jacques, P.-É.; Li, S.; Xia, J. MetaboAnalyst 5.0: Narrowing the Gap between Raw Spectra and Functional Insights. *Nucleic Acids Res.* **2021**, *49*, W388–W396. [CrossRef] [PubMed]
20. Zhou, G.; Pang, Z.; Lu, Y.; Ewald, J.; Xia, J. OmicsNet 2.0: A Web-Based Platform for Multi-Omics Integration and Network Visual Analytics. *Nucleic Acids Res.* **2022**, *50*, W527–W533. [CrossRef] [PubMed]
21. Pellegrino, R.M.; Giulietti, M.; Alabed, H.B.R.; Buratta, S.; Urbanelli, L.; Piva, F.; Emiliani, C. LipidOne: User-Friendly Lipidomic Data Analysis Tool for a Deeper Interpretation in a Systems Biology Scenario. *Bioinformatics* **2022**, *38*, 1767–1769. [CrossRef] [PubMed]
22. Gaud, C.; Sousa, B.C.; Nguyen, A.; Fedorova, M.; Ni, Z.; O'Donnell, V.B.; Wakelam, M.J.O.; Andrews, S.; Lopez-Clavijo, A.F. BioPAN: A Web-Based Tool to Explore Mammalian Lipidome Metabolic Pathways on LIPID MAPS. *F1000Research* **2021**, *10*, 4. [CrossRef]
23. Park, J.Y.; Lee, S.-H.; Shin, M.-J.; Hwang, G.-S. Alteration in Metabolic Signature and Lipid Metabolism in Patients with Angina Pectoris and Myocardial Infarction. *PLoS ONE* **2015**, *10*, e0135228. [CrossRef]
24. Kohno, S.; Keenan, A.L.; Ntambi, J.M.; Miyazaki, M. Lipidomic Insight into Cardiovascular Diseases. *Biochem. Biophys. Res. Commun.* **2018**, *504*, 590–595. [CrossRef]
25. Alabed, H.B.R.; Gorello, P.; Pellegrino, R.M.; Lancioni, H.; La Starza, R.; Taddei, A.A.; Urbanelli, L.; Buratta, S.; Fernandez, A.G.L.; Matteucci, C.; et al. Comparison between Sickle Cell Disease Patients and Healthy Donors: Untargeted Lipidomic Study of Erythrocytes. *Int. J. Mol. Sci.* **2023**, *24*, 2529. [CrossRef]
26. Wang, Y.-N.; Ma, S.-X.; Chen, Y.-Y.; Chen, L.; Liu, B.-L.; Liu, Q.-Q.; Zhao, Y.-Y. Chronic Kidney Disease: Biomarker Diagnosis to Therapeutic Targets. *Clin. Chim. Acta* **2019**, *499*, 54–63. [CrossRef]
27. Wood, P.L. Mass Spectrometry Strategies for Clinical Metabolomics and Lipidomics in Psychiatry, Neurology, and Neuro-Oncology. *Neuropsychopharmacology* **2014**, *39*, 24–33. [CrossRef]
28. Li, Y.; Liang, L.; Deng, X.; Zhong, L. Lipidomic and Metabolomic Profiling Reveals Novel Candidate Biomarkers in Active Systemic Lupus Erythematosus. *Int. J. Clin. Exp. Pathol.* **2019**, *12*, 857–866.
29. Farrokhi Yekta, R.; Rezaie Tavirani, M.; Arefi Oskouie, A.; Mohajeri-Tehrani, M.R.; Soroush, A.R. The Metabolomics and Lipidomics Window into Thyroid Cancer Research. *Biomarkers* **2016**, *22*, 595–603. [CrossRef]
30. Burger, R.; Hansen-Hagge, T.E.; Drexler, H.G.; Gramatzki, M. Heterogeneity of T-Acute Lymphoblastic Leukemia (T-ALL) Cell Lines: Suggestion for Classification by Immunophenotype and T-Cell Receptor Studies. *Leuk. Res.* **1999**, *23*, 19–27. [CrossRef]
31. Alarcon-Barrera, J.C.; von Hegedus, J.H.; Brouwers, H.; Steenvoorden, E.; Ioan-Facsinay, A.; Mayboroda, O.A.; Ondo-Mendez, A.; Giera, M. Lipid Metabolism of Leukocytes in the Unstimulated and Activated States. *Anal. Bioanal. Chem.* **2020**, *412*, 2353–2363. [CrossRef]

32. Kwon, H.-Y.; Kumar Das, R.; Jung, G.T.; Lee, H.-G.; Lee, S.H.; Berry, S.N.; Tan, J.K.S.; Park, S.; Yang, J.-S.; Park, S.; et al. Lipid-Oriented Live-Cell Distinction of B and T Lymphocytes. *J. Am. Chem. Soc.* **2021**, *143*, 5836–5844. [CrossRef]
33. van Baren, N.; Van den Eynde, B.J. Tryptophan-Degrading Enzymes in Tumoral Immune Resistance. *Front. Immunol.* **2015**, *6*, 34. [CrossRef]
34. Lu, S.C. Glutathione Synthesis. *Biochim. Biophys. Acta (BBA) Gen. Subj.* **2013**, *1830*, 3143–3153. [CrossRef]
35. Bansal, A.; Simon, M.C. Glutathione Metabolism in Cancer Progression and Treatment Resistance. *J. Cell Biol.* **2018**, *217*, 2291–2298. [CrossRef]
36. Cheng, C.-T.; Qi, Y.; Wang, Y.-C.; Chi, K.K.; Chung, Y.; Ouyang, C.; Chen, Y.-R.; Oh, M.E.; Sheng, X.; Tang, Y.; et al. Arginine Starvation Kills Tumor Cells through Aspartate Exhaustion and Mitochondrial Dysfunction. *Commun. Biol.* **2018**, *1*, 178. [CrossRef]
37. Yin, J.; Ren, W.; Huang, X.; Deng, J.; Li, T.; Yin, Y. Potential Mechanisms Connecting Purine Metabolism and Cancer Therapy. *Front. Immunol.* **2018**, *9*, 1697. [CrossRef]
38. Barfeld, S.J.; Fazli, L.; Persson, M.; Marjavaara, L.; Urbanucci, A.; Kaukoniemi, K.M.; Rennie, P.S.; Ceder, Y.; Chabes, A.; Visakorpi, T.; et al. Myc-Dependent Purine Biosynthesis Affects Nucleolar Stress and Therapy Response in Prostate Cancer. *Oncotarget* **2015**, *6*, 12587–12602. [CrossRef]
39. Goswami, M.T.; Chen, G.; Chakravarthi, B.V.S.K.; Pathi, S.S.; Anand, S.K.; Carskadon, S.L.; Giordano, T.J.; Chinnaiyan, A.M.; Thomas, D.G.; Palanisamy, N.; et al. Role and Regulation of Coordinately Expressed de Novo Purine Biosynthetic Enzymes PPAT and PAICS in Lung Cancer. *Oncotarget* **2015**, *6*, 23445–23461. [CrossRef]
40. Bahreyni, A.; Samani, S.S.; Rahmani, F.; Behnam-Rassouli, R.; Khazaei, M.; Ryzhikov, M.; Parizadeh, M.R.; Avan, A.; Hassanian, S.M. Role of Adenosine Signaling in the Pathogenesis of Breast Cancer. *J. Cell Physiol.* **2018**, *233*, 1836–1843. [CrossRef]
41. Yamauchi, T.; Miyawaki, K.; Semba, Y.; Takahashi, M.; Izumi, Y.; Nogami, J.; Nakao, F.; Sugio, T.; Sasaki, K.; Pinello, L.; et al. Targeting Leukemia-Specific Dependence on the de Novo Purine Synthesis Pathway. *Leukemia* **2022**, *36*, 383–393. [CrossRef]
42. Meana, C.; García-Rostán, G.; Peña, L.; Lordén, G.; Cubero, Á.; Orduña, A.; Győrffy, B.; Balsinde, J.; Balboa, M.A. The Phosphatidic Acid Phosphatase Lipin-1 Facilitates Inflammation-Driven Colon Carcinogenesis. *JCI Insight* **2018**, *3*, e97506. [CrossRef] [PubMed]
43. He, J.; Zhang, F.; Tay, L.W.R.; Boroda, S.; Nian, W.; Levental, K.R.; Levental, I.; Harris, T.E.; Chang, J.T.; Du, G. Lipin-1 Regulation of Phospholipid Synthesis Maintains Endoplasmic Reticulum Homeostasis and Is Critical for Triple-Negative Breast Cancer Cell Survival. *FASEB J.* **2017**, *31*, 2893–2904. [CrossRef] [PubMed]
44. Sanchez-Lopez, E.; Zimmerman, T.; Gomez del Pulgar, T.; Moyer, M.P.; Lacal Sanjuan, J.C.; Cebrian, A. Choline Kinase Inhibition Induces Exacerbated Endoplasmic Reticulum Stress and Triggers Apoptosis via CHOP in Cancer Cells. *Cell Death Dis.* **2013**, *4*, e933. [CrossRef] [PubMed]
45. Arora, G.K.; Palamiuc, L.; Emerling, B.M. Expanding Role of PI5P4Ks in Cancer: A Promising Druggable Target. *FEBS Lett.* **2022**, *596*, 3–16. [CrossRef]
46. Yamashita, Y.; Nishiumi, S.; Kono, S.; Takao, S.; Azuma, T.; Yoshida, M. Differences in Elongation of Very Long Chain Fatty Acids and Fatty Acid Metabolism between Triple-Negative and Hormone Receptor-Positive Breast Cancer. *BMC Cancer* **2017**, *17*, 589. [CrossRef]
47. Robichaud, P.-P.; Munganyiki, J.E.; Boilard, E.; Surette, M.E. Polyunsaturated Fatty Acid Elongation and Desaturation in Activated Human T-Cells: ELOVL5 Is the Key Elongase. *J. Lipid Res.* **2018**, *59*, 2383–2396. [CrossRef] [PubMed]
48. Stefanko, A.; Thiede, C.; Ehninger, G.; Simons, K.; Grzybek, M. Lipidomic Approach for Stratification of Acute Myeloid Leukemia Patients. *PLoS ONE* **2017**, *12*, e0168781. [CrossRef] [PubMed]
49. Sanda, T.; Lawton, L.N.; Barrasa, M.I.; Fan, Z.P.; Kohlhammer, H.; Gutierrez, A.; Ma, W.; Tatarek, J.; Ahn, Y.; Kelliher, M.A.; et al. Core Transcriptional Regulatory Circuit Controlled by the TAL1 Complex in Human T Cell Acute Lymphoblastic Leukemia. *Cancer Cell* **2012**, *22*, 209–221. [CrossRef] [PubMed]
50. Sharma, A.; Mistriel-Zerbib, S.; Najar, R.A.; Engal, E.; Bentata, M.; Taqatqa, N.; Dahan, S.; Cohen, K.; Jaffe-Herman, S.; Geminder, O.; et al. Isoforms of the TAL1 Transcription Factor Have Different Roles in Hematopoiesis and Cell Growth. *PLoS Biol.* **2023**, *21*, e3002175. [CrossRef] [PubMed]
51. Cajka, T.; Hricko, J.; Rudl Kulhava, L.; Paucova, M.; Novakova, M.; Kuda, O. Optimization of Mobile Phase Modifiers for Fast LC-MS-Based Untargeted Metabolomics and Lipidomics. *Int. J. Mol. Sci.* **2023**, *24*, 1987. [CrossRef] [PubMed]
52. Pellegrino, R.M.; Di Veroli, A.; Valeri, A.; Goracci, L.; Cruciani, G. LC/MS Lipid Profiling from Human Serum: A New Method for Global Lipid Extraction. *Anal. Bioanal. Chem.* **2014**, *406*, 7937–7948. [CrossRef] [PubMed]
53. Li, J.; Ma, J.; Li, Q.; Fan, S.; Fan, L.; Ma, H.; Zhang, Y.; Zheng, L. Determination of 35 Free Amino Acids in Tea Using Ultra-Performance Liquid Chromatography Coupled with Quadrupole Time-of-Flight Mass Spectrometry. *Front. Nutr.* **2021**, *8*, 767801. [CrossRef] [PubMed]
54. Alabed, H.B.R.; Del Grosso, A.; Bellani, V.; Urbanelli, L.; Carpi, S.; De Sarlo, M.; Bertocci, L.; Colagiorgio, L.; Buratta, S.; Scaccini, L.; et al. Untargeted Lipidomic Approach for Studying Different Nervous System Tissues of the Murine Model of Krabbe Disease. *Biomolecules* **2023**, *13*, 1562. [CrossRef] [PubMed]
55. Tsugawa, H.; Ikeda, K.; Takahashi, M.; Satoh, A.; Mori, Y.; Uchino, H.; Okahashi, N.; Yamada, Y.; Tada, I.; Bonini, P.; et al. A Lipidome Atlas in MS-DIAL 4. *Nat. Biotechnol.* **2020**, *38*, 1159–1163. [CrossRef] [PubMed]

56. Liebisch, G.; Fahy, E.; Aoki, J.; Dennis, E.A.; Durand, T.; Ejsing, C.S.; Fedorova, M.; Feussner, I.; Griffiths, W.J.; Köfeler, H.; et al. Update on LIPID MAPS Classification, Nomenclature, and Shorthand Notation for MS-Derived Lipid Structures. *J. Lipid Res.* **2020**, *61*, 1539–1555. [CrossRef] [PubMed]
57. Gertner, D.S.; Violi, J.P.; Bishop, D.P.; Padula, M.P. Lipid Spectrum Generator: A Simple Script for the Generation of Accurate In Silico Lipid Fragmentation Spectra. *Anal. Chem.* **2023**, *95*, 2909–2916. [CrossRef] [PubMed]

International Journal of
Molecular Sciences

MDPI

Review

Haploidentical HSCT in the Treatment of Pediatric Hematological Disorders

Anna Marszołek [1], Maria Leśniak [1], Anna Sekunda [1], Aleksander Siwek [1], Zuzanna Skiba [1], Monika Lejman [2,†] and Joanna Zawitkowska [3,*,†]

1 Student Scientific Society of Department of Pediatric Hematology, Oncology and Transplantology, Medical University of Lublin, 20-093 Lublin, Poland; anna.marszolek@gmail.com (A.M.); marialesniak68@gmail.com (M.L.); annasekunda00@gmail.com (A.S.); aleksiwek12@gmail.com (A.S.); zuzannaskiba01@o2.pl (Z.S.)

2 Independent Laboratory of Genetic Diagnostics, Medical University of Lublin, 20-093 Lublin, Poland; monika.lejman@umlub.pl

3 Department of Pediatric Hematology, Oncology and Transplantology, Medical University of Lublin, 20-093 Lublin, Poland

* Correspondence: joannazawitkowska@umlub.pl

† These authors contributed equally to this work.

Abstract: Allogeneic hematopoietic stem cell transplantation has become a treatment option for otherwise non-curative conditions, both malignant and benign, affecting children and adults. Nevertheless, the latest research has been focusing extensively on transplantation from related and unrelated haploidentical donors, suitable for patients requiring emergent hematopoietic stem cell transplantation (HSCT) in the absence of an HLA-matched donor. Haploidentical HSCT (haplo-HSCT) can be an effective treatment for non-malignant pediatric disorders, such as primary immunodeficiencies or hemoglobinopathies, by enabling a much quicker selection of the appropriate donor for virtually all patients, low incidence of graft-versus-host disease (GVHD), and transplant-related mortality (TRM). Moreover, the outcomes of haplo-HSCT among children with hematological malignancies have improved radically. The most demanding tasks for clinicians are minimizing T-cell-mediated alloreactivity as well as early GVHD prevention. As a result, several T-cell depletion approaches, such as ex vivo T-cell depletion (TCD), and T-cell replete approaches, such as a combination of anti-thymocyte globulin (ATG), post-transplantation cyclophosphamide (PTCy), cyclosporine/tacrolimus, mycophenolate mofetil, or methotrexate, have been taken up. As more research is needed to establish the most beneficial form of therapy, haplo-HSCT is currently considered an alternative donor strategy for pediatric and adult patients with complications like viral and bacterial infections, invasive fungal disease, and GVHD.

Keywords: haplo-HSCT; GVHD; pediatrics; pediatric hematology; leukemia; AML; transplantation

1. Introduction

Hematopoietic stem cell transplantation (HSCT) became a treatment option over 60 years ago, and due to immense progress in the medical field, it has been used to treat various diseases, including both malignant and non-malignant hematological conditions [1]. The procedure is based on the administration of hematopoietic stem cells from the donor to replace the recipient's malfunctioning hematopoietic system [2]. HSCT can be categorized depending on the relationship between the donor and recipient, as well as the source of the graft [3]. The great limitation in the general application of HSCT is the difficulty in finding a compatible donor in the context of the human leukocyte antigen (HLA) [4]. The concept of haploidentical HSCT (haplo-HSCT) was developed to serve as an alternative to allogenic HSCT (allo-HSCT), requiring an HLA-identical donor, whereas haplo-HSCT is conducted with at least a half-matched identical donor [5]. Histocompatibility genes are inherited as a group (haplotype) both from the mother and the father (Figure 1) [6,7].

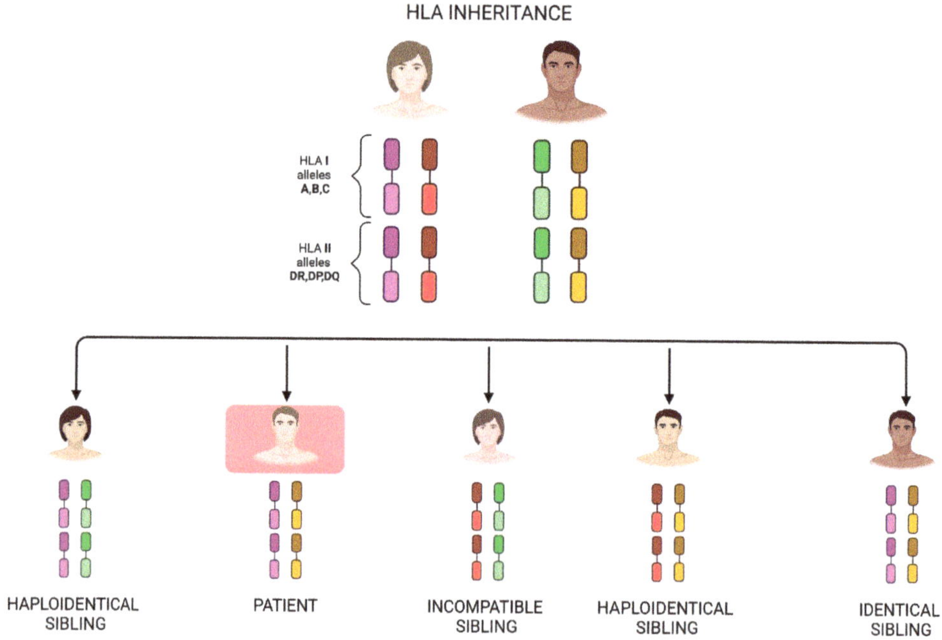

Figure 1. HLA gene inheritance. Image created with biorender.com (accessed on 2 April 2024). HLA genes are inherited according to classic Mendelian genetics, with HLA molecules being codominantly expressed. An HLA-haploidentical donor is a related donor who shares exactly 1 HLA haplotype and differs by a variable number of HLA genes on the unshared haplotype. Siblings have a 25% chance of being identical at the genotypic level of HLA molecules.

Minimal residual disease (MRD), defined as the lasting presence of leukemia cells after a chemotherapy/radiotherapy regimen, can be used to evaluate the risk of relapse and reaction to a therapy plan [8]. The assessment of the MRD status before transplantation is a crucial and significant prognostic factor in children and adolescents with hematological malignancies, as patients with negative MRD before haplo-HSCT tend to achieve substantially longer overall survival (OS) and event-free survival (EFS) [9].

The greatest advantage of haplo-HSCT is that it considerably widens the pool of potential donors, as over 95% of patients can find a donor among their parents, siblings, or children who share one HLA haplotype with the patient. Such donors are easily accessible, which is particularly beneficial for patients who are in an urgent need of HSCT [10]. Nevertheless, due to imperfectly matched HLA, haplo-HSCT is more prone to graft-versus-host disease (GVHD) and poorer graft function [5]. The negative response of the patient's immune system is prompted by alloreactive T-cells, either from the donor against the recipient's tissues or from the patient against the graft [11]. High tumor-related mortality (TMR) has primarily been associated with acute GVHD (aGVHD), whereas chronic GVHD (cGVHD) is said to be the leading cause of poor quality of life of children who have received haplo-HSCT [12].

2. GVHD Management

Although haplo-HSCT significantly increases the number of possible donors and offers a low toxicity rate and stable engraftment, it involves a greater risk of GVHD and treatment-related fatality. Children are affected by transplant-related toxicities at a very young age, which has life-long consequences, with cGVHD being one of the most serious complications [13]. Previously, it was believed that total T lymphocyte depletion from the graft was the only method of GVHD prophylaxis. Despite being successful, such an approach led to an increased rate of severe infections and patient mortality [14,15].

To provide higher rates of successful engraftment and better GVHD management, different strategies regarding alloreactive T-cells were developed, resulting in haplo-HSCT no longer being perceived as a last-resort treatment [16]. Presently, there are two main pathways of T-cell depletion (TCD), ex vivo and in vivo.

The ex vivo pathway involves $CD34^+$ cell selection with a subsequent infusion of a megadose of purified $CD34^+$ cells, $CD3/CD19^-$ negative selection, and T-cell receptor (TCR) α/β with CD19 depletion, as well as depletion of CD45RA naive T-cells [17–20]. In the past, $CD34^+$ cell selection was the most frequently used method. Even though it was associated with a lower risk of GVHD, it could delay the patient's immune reconstitution and slow down viral clearance [21]. The latest study results acknowledge haplo-HSCT with TCR$\alpha\beta$ and CD19 depletion as a choice for pediatric patients with non-malignant hematological and immunological conditions, due to satisfactory immune reconstitution [22]. This kind of graft manipulation results in stem cell transplants that are highly enriched in natural killer (NK) cells and TCRγ/δ^+ T-cells that are essential for viral protection [23–25]. Additionally, the depletion of B lymphocytes with anti-CD19 is performed to decrease the risk of Epstein–Barr virus (EBV) reactivation [26].

A recent study indicates that GVHD, particularly after TCRα/β and CD19 depletion haplo-HSCT, can be managed by the administration of multiple doses of zoledronic acid in the post-transplant course. The substance is said to enhance TCRγ/δ^+ lymphocyte action after depleted haplo-HSCT without life-threatening side effects, such as commonly observed asymptomatic hypocalcemia and flu-like symptoms after infusion. The research proved that three or more infusions of zoledronic acid were associated with a decreased frequency of aGVHD and cGVHD, as well as reduced transplant-related mortality (TRM), compared to one or two doses. As zoledronic acid is safe and provides a positive post-transplant response, it can be administered to children a few weeks after haplo-HSCT [27].

The in vivo pathway covers methods based on low-dose post-transplantation cyclophosphamide (PTCy) and anti-thymocyte globulin (ATG) treatment, as well as a combination of PTCy and ATG with cyclosporine (CsA) and mycophenolate mofetil (MMF) [18–20]. Recent research suggests that the PTCy-based method provides better leukemia-free survival (LFS) as well as GVHD-free survival [19]. The positive effect of haplo-HSCT with PTCy on GVHD risk has been proven in both adult and pediatric patients who qualified for a transplant [28]. Cyclophosphamide is also used in various non-malignant hematological disorders, not only in sickle cell disease (SCD), but also in thalassemia, primary immunodeficiencies (PIDs), severe aplastic anemia (SAA), and osteopetrosis [26,29]. The effect caused by PTCy is selective depletion of alloreactive donor T-cells that are responsible for GVHD and graft rejection, while preserving the non-alloreactive resting memory T-cells responsible for adaptive immunity and the blood stem cells necessary for successful engraftment. The crucial part of the process is the administration of cyclophosphamide during the appropriate time frame [25]. It is most often administered on the 3rd and 4th days after graft transplantation [30,31]. GVHD prophylaxis may also include tacrolimus and MMF administered during the 5th post-transplant day [30]. Furthermore, even though TCRα/β and CD19 depletion are also affiliated with successful GVHD prevention in children and adults, the application of PTCy enables haplo-HSCT without ex vivo TCD [13,32]. It has been observed that maternal- and collateral-related donor transplants lead to a greater prevalence of GVHD and reduced survival, in comparison to the direct family. Nonetheless, compared to other ATG-based or PTCy-based regimens, the low-dose PTCy/ATG regimen considerably constricted the cumulative incidence of aGVHD and did not worsen the relapse risk, thus making maternal/collateral donor transplants a safer option [33].

Another approach using basiliximab, a chimeric monoclonal antibody aiming at alpha chain of interleukin-2 receptors (CD25 antigen), has been proposed as a form of treatment of steroid-refractory (SR) aGVHD [34]. Basiliximab is used in both adult and pediatric patients after haplo-HSCT as a satisfactory second-line treatment. It has been demonstrated that the patient response rate to corticosteroids reaches only 50%, whereas SR aGVHD is responsible for a long-term mortality rate as high as 70%. As basiliximab mostly affects activated T lymphocytes without suppressing the resting T lymphocytes, it does not alter engraftment or the incidence of infectious complications. The effectiveness of SR aGVHD management differs depending on the distressed organ, with the best response to basiliximab being in skin involvement, followed by gut and liver involvement. Furthermore, no significant adverse effects were observed, thus enabling the usage of basiliximab as a recommended strategy [35].

3. Malignant Disorders

Despite the continuous development of new treatment options for pediatric acute lymphoblastic (ALL) and myeloid leukemia (AML), there is still a group of patients who are not eligible for aggressive induction chemotherapy, which results in a poor overall prognosis and a limited choice of therapies [36,37], and for whom HSCT remains a relevant and effective medical procedure [38,39]. Although allo-HSCT continues to be the first-line treatment, haplo-HSCT is gaining increased attention, due to its many advantages, such as a significant increase in the number of possible donors, low toxicity rate, wide availability for therapeutic procedures after transplantation, and a greater spectrum of immunologic reactions against tumor cells [40].

3.1. *Haplo-HSCT with Ex Vivo T-Cell Depletion*

The first approaches to performing bone marrow transplantation from related, not fully matched donors in patients with hematologic malignancies consisted of a conditioning regimen analogous to the one used with matched sibling donors; however, they did not yield satisfactory results, because of poor OS rates [41]. The implementation of transplantation TCD led to improved GVHD prevention in children with severe combined immunodeficiency (SCID) [21], but could not be used in patients with leukemia due to frequent graft failure, despite the benefits of improved GVHD prevention [42,43]. Eventually, a haplo-HSCT with the positive selection of $CD34^+$ peripheral stem cells preceded by myeloablative conditioning including myeloablative drugs, such as the alkylating agent thiotepa, total-body irradiation (TBI), busulfan-based conditioning regimens, and advanced engraftment in the treatment of adult and pediatric AML [44,45].

In recent years, the transplantation of T- and B-cell-depleted allografts from haploidentical family donors was assessed by Lang et al. in a prospective Phase II trial in pediatric patients with acute leukemias and myelodysplastic syndrome. A total of 46 patients received $CD3^+/CD19^+$-depleted peripheral allografts after a melphalan-based conditioning regimen. Twelve patients survived free of disease, with a median follow-up of 4.3 years; however, over 60% of patients died, with relapse being the most common cause of death. In terms of GVHD, a greater rate was observed in comparison with a historical cohort of patients who received $CD34$-selected grafts with similar numbers of stem cells (26% vs. 7% grades II–IV and 21% vs. 13% cGVHD) [46]. On the other hand, the incidence of GVHD was more favorable than in two similar pediatric trials regarding $CD3^+/CD20^+$-depleted allografts with serotherapy [47] and $CD3^+/CD19^+$-depleted allografts without serotherapy [48] (41% and 33% aGVHD II–IV and 22% and 13% cGVHD, respectively) [49].

Currently, novel studies aim to test a new graft manipulation involving $\alpha\beta^+$ T-cell removal, while retaining both NK and $\gamma\delta^+$ T-cells in the graft [35]. During a Phase I–II clinical trial (NCT01810120), Locatelli et al. noted that patients who underwent TCR $\alpha\beta$/CD19-depleted haplo-HSCT achieved survival outcomes comparable to patients who received an unmanipulated transplant from an HLA-compatible donor. In addition, this type of transplant was associated with a low incidence of aGVHD as well as cGVHD [50].

Seven years later, after a longer follow-up period and the use of the aforementioned transplant, the authors reanalyzed 213 pediatric patients diagnosed with ALL (n = 152) and AML (n = 61). The median age at the time of transplantation was 9.5 years. All patients were in morphologic complete remission (CR) at the time of transplantation. A total of 18 patients were positive for MRD before transplantation. All patients received fully conditioned myeloablation including a regimen based on TBI and/or cytostatic treatment. None of the patients received prophylactic pharmacotherapy for the prevention of GVHD, and aGVHD grades II–III occurred with a combined incidence of 14.7%. A total of 129 children developed viral infections due to cytomegalovirus (CMV), adenovirus (ADV), and human herpesvirus 6 (HHV-6). It is worth mentioning that the survival rates or relapse rates did not differ between patients who developed or did not develop the mentioned infections. The main reason for treatment failure was relapse. Children diagnosed with ALL who had low/negative MRD prior to HSCT, early-stage disease prior to transplantation, and received a TBI-based myeloablative conditioning regimen had a prolonged disease-free survival (DFS). In addition, it was noted that, compared to other regimens, the use of TBI, thiotepa, and fludarabine improved the DFS rate [51]. Another study regarding TCD graft modification compared outcomes of HLA-matched unrelated donor (MUD) transplantation and ex vivo $\alpha\beta^+$ T-cell-depleted haplo-HSCT among pediatric patients diagnosed with high-risk acute leukemias. The 5-year OS and relapse-free survival (RFS) rates in the group of haplo-HSCT patients were similar to those in the MUD group. After transplantation, 15 of the 53 patients died, including 5 who received haplo-HSCT. The most common cause of death was relapse. Furthermore, the incidence rates of grades II–IV aGVHD and cGVHD occurrence in MUD patients were higher than in haplo-HSCT patients, while GVHD prophylaxis differed between the groups [27]. As of right now, there is no evidence as to which platform, ex vivo T-cell depletion or PTCy, is better. A retrospective and multicenter study by Pérez-Martínez et al. intended to compare the viability of two cohort groups of haplo-HSCT platforms in children and young adults with high-risk hematological malignancies and PTCy and ex vivo TCD grafts. The second cohort of patients was divided into four groups, each of which received differently modified T-cells: highly purified $CD34^+$ cells (n = 13), combined depletion of $CD3^+$ donor T-cells and $CD19^+$ B-cells (n = 82), combined depletion of αβ T-cells and $CD19^+$ B-cells (n = 34), and highly purified $CD34^+$ cell transplantation with the addition of a product depleted of naive $CD45RA^+$ lymphocytes to the transplant. Only patients receiving haplo-HSCT in the form of repeated transplantation were given ATG as a preparative regimen. The other patients received total lymphoid irradiation (TLI), TBI, or high doses of methylprednisolone. The cumulative incidence rates of aGVHD grades I–II or grades III–IV were significantly lower in the case of children treated with TCD; however, the 2-year OS and DFS rates did not particularly differ between patient groups, as both major platforms for haplo-HSCT were proven to be effective. Based on the study, a young donor, negative MRD, and myeloid pathology are promising prognostic factors [52].

$\alpha\beta^+$ T-cell-depleted transplantation is expected to sustain anti-tumor and anti-infectious features, due to the ability of $CD3^+$ cells with TCR $\gamma\delta^+$ receptors to impose graft-versus-tumor activity [53–55]. Greater recovery of $\gamma\delta^+$ T-cells after transplantation has been connected with better EFS, fewer infectious complications, and longer DFS rates in both pediatric and adult populations [56,57]. Such findings correlate with the results of a study conducted by Dadi et al. to investigate the impact of increased $\gamma\delta^+$ T-cell content in the engraftment. Researchers analyzed the treatment outcomes in 38 children and adolescents diagnosed with acute leukemias who underwent haplo-HSCT with depletion of $\alpha\beta^+$ T-cells and $CD19^+$ B-cells. Six patients in this study received a reduced-intensity conditioning regimen that included fludarabine, thiotepa, melphalan, and ATG. However, because of frequent graft failure, the TBI regimen with additional drugs was implemented. The study demonstrated that a graft with a content of $\gamma\delta^+$ T-cells equal or higher than 9.5×10^6/kg was associated with notably higher EFS rates [58].

It is crucial to optimize treatment approaches for high-risk treatment failure patients to reduce the risk of relapse. Patients undergoing transplantation during an active stage of ALL have previously obtained highly unsatisfying results [46,59]. The reported survival rates after haplo-HSCT in relapsed or chemotherapy-resistant AML patients fluctuated between 9% and 44% [60,61]. Because ATG given at the time of the graft infusion may inactivate grafted NK and $\gamma\delta^{+}$ cells, replacing it with non-lymphodepleting targeted immunomodulation could protect the transplant. Promising results were achieved by Shelikhova et al., who analyzed 22 pediatric patients diagnosed with primary refractory (n = 10) or relapsed refractory (n = 12) AML in active disease status, who were administered haplo-HSCT with peripheral blood stem cells engineered by the depletion of $\alpha\beta^{+}$ T-cells and $CD19^{+}$ B-cells. Patients received fludarabine and cytarabine as a preparative regimen followed by treosulfan and thiotepa as a myeloablative conditioning regimen. Instead of ATG, patients were given tocilizumab, and an additional 10 children received abatacept. The infusion of donor lymphocytes containing a CD45RA-depleted fraction with or without a hypomethylating agent was used as prophylactic therapy post-transplantation. A total of 21 patients (95%) achieved CR. At the two-year follow-up, rates such as TRM, EFS, and OS were 9%, 49%, and 53%, respectively. The cumulative incidence rates of grades II–IV aGVHD and cGVHD were 18% and 23% [62].

Hematopoietic grafts infused with regulatory T-cells (Tregs) have been discovered to be protected from GVHD without decreasing conventional T-cell (Tcon) antileukemic activity in both murine and preclinical studies [63–65]. Pierini et al. researched outcomes of haplo-HSCT infused with donor Tcons under the protection of previously transferred donor Tregs as the exclusive GVHD prophylaxis. As expected, a significantly low relapse rate and a 75% cGVHD/relapse-free survival (CRFS) rate in adult AML patients were noted [66]. In this regard, Massei MS et al. aimed to test the efficacy of a newly developed haplo-HSCT variant with adoptive immunotherapy with thymic-derived $CD4^{+}$ $CD25^{+}$ $FoxP3^{+}$ Treg and Tcons in 20 children and adolescents diagnosed with high-risk ALL and AML. The conditioning regimen was based on TBI and chemotherapy. A total of 25% of the patients developed ≥grade II aGVHD, including one patient who developed grades III/IV and died 35 days after transplantation. A total of 75% of the patients included in the described analysis are alive and leukemia-free with a median follow-up time of 2.1 years. The feasibility of CRFS was 79% [67] (Table 1).

Table 1. Novel studies on haplo-HSCT with ex vivo T-cell depletion.

Number of Patients	Median Age	Transplant Type	Conditioning Regimen and GVHD Prophylaxis	Incidence of aGVHD	Incidence of cGVHD	Relapse NRM	OS Rate	Reference
80	9.7	haplo-HSCT with TCD	TBI + TT + Flu, TBI + TT + L-PAM, TT + Bu + Flu, Bu + Cy + L-PAM	I–II aGVHD 30%	5%	relapse 24% NRM 5%	Predicted 5-year OS 72%	[50]
213	9.5	haplo-HSCT with $\alpha\beta^+/CD19^+$ cell depletion	TBI + TT + Flu, TBI + TT + L-PAM, Bu + TT + Flu, Bu + Cy + L-PAM	II–III aGVHD 14.7%	8.1%	5-year NRM 5.2% 5-year CIR 22.7%	predicted 10-year OS 75.4%	[51]
53	No information	MUD (n = 32) haplo-HSCT with $\alpha\beta^+$ cell depletion (n = 21)	Bu + Cy ± r-ATG, Flu + TT + L-PAM + ATG + RTX	MUD: II–IV aGVHD 53.1% haplo-HSCT: II–IV GVHD 33.3%	MUD: 25% haplo-HSCT: 19%	Relapse MUD: 15.6% haplo-HSCT: 9.5% NRM MUD: 21.9% haplo-HSCT: 14.3%	MUD: 68.8% haplo-HSCT: 76.2%	[27]
192	8.6	haplo-HSCT with PTCy (n = 41) haplo-HSCT with TCD (n = 151)	Flu + TT + L-PAM + Bu + high-dose PT-Cy + MMF + TAC + mesna, Flu + TT + L-PAM + Bu + TLI or TBI or high-dose MP or ATG	PTCy: I–II aGVHD 52.6% III–IV aGVHD 28.2% TCD: I–II aGVHD 30.6% III–IV aGVHD 14.7%	2-year cGVHD PTCy: 47.7% TCD: 28.6%	predicted 2-year relapse PTCy: 26.8% TCD: 31.1%	2-year OS PTCy: 65.4% TCD: 52%	[52]
38	8.5	haplo-HSCT with $\alpha\beta^+/CD19^+$ cell depletion	Flu + TT + L-PAM + ATG + RTX, Flu + TT + Treo + ATG + RTX ± TBI	45%	7%	5-year NRM 36%	5-year OS 51%	[58]
22	9.6	PBSC haplo-HSCT with $\alpha\beta^+/CD19^+$ cell depletion	Flu + Ara-C + Treo + L-PAM + TT + RTX + bortezomib + tocilizumab + abatacept	II–IV aGVHD 18%	23%	2-year CIR 42%	2-year OS 53%	[62]
20	14.5	haplo-HSCT with adoptive immunotherapy with thymic-derived $CD4^+CD25^+FoxP3^+$ Tregs and Tcons	TBI + TT + Flu + Cy + RTX	≥II aGVHD 25%	5%	relapse 5% NRM 15%	No information	[67]

aGVHD—acute graft-versus-host disease, Ara-C—cytarabine, ATG—anti-thymocyte globulin, Bu—busulfan, cGVHD—chronic graft-versus-host disease, CIR—cumulative incidence of relapse/progression, Cy—cyclophosphamide, Flu—fludarabine, haplo-HSCT—haploidentical hematopoietic stem cell transplantation, L-PAM—melphalan, MMF—mycophenolate mofetil, MP—methylprednisolone, NRM—non-relapse mortality, OS—overall survival, PBSC—peripheral blood stem cells, PTCy—post-transplant cyclophosphamide, RTX—rituximab, TAC—tacrolimus, TBI—total body irradiation, Tcons—conventional T-cells, TLI—total lymphoid irradiation, Tregs—regulatory T-cells, Treo—treosulfan, TT—thiotepa.

3.2. Haplo-HSCT without Ex Vivo T-Cell Depletion

Due to the often-delayed reconstitution of the immune system, resulting in infectious complications and graft failure following TCD haplo-HSCT, current research is focusing extensively on developing new conditioning regimens and intensified GVHD prophylaxis combined with the T-cell replete approach (Table 2).

3.2.1. Granulocyte Colony-Stimulating Factor (G-CSF)/ATG-Based Protocol

Huang et al. proposed a novel strategy of GVHD prevention by incorporating G-CSF and ATG with unmanipulated allografts in a pilot cohort study known as the "Beijing Protocol" [68]. All patients achieved sustained, full donor-type engraftment. The authors noted 37.9% and 5.2% aGVHD rates (grades II–IV and III–IV) and a 61.9% cGVHD rate [69]. Studies have shown that a G-CSF (filgrastim) addition amplifies monocytic phenotype myeloid-derived suppressor cell (M-MDSC), promyelocytic-MDSC (P-MDSC), and granulocytic-MDSC (G-MDSC) expansion [70,71]. G-CSF is said to activate a subset of $CD34^+$ cells with monocyte functions [72]; moreover, it causes bone marrow regulatory B-cells (Bregs) to produce higher levels of interleukin 10 (IL-10) and transforming growth factor beta (TGF-β) [73]. Bregs influence T-cell tolerance by inhibiting T-cells of the Th1 phenotype in favor of the Th2 phenotype and heightening Treg levels [74]. All of the above-mentioned mechanisms of the G-CSF effects on the grafts were proven to lower the incidence of aGVHD and cGVHD [70–74]. Because the treatment approach has become successful, considerable progress has since been made to elongate patient survival [75–77]. Regarding AML, a study by Liu et al. declared a 73.3% 5-year OS rate in pediatric patients who underwent T-cell replete haplo-HSCT [75]. To focus more on a high-risk group of patients, a multicenter retrospective study was taken up to compare the outcomes between children who were exposed to unmanipulated haplo-HSCT with a G-CSF/ATG-based regimen or an identical sibling donor (ISD)-HSCT. Both transplant methods displayed comparable OS and DFS rates [78]. Bai et al. analyzed 200 pediatric patients diagnosed with high-risk AML who underwent their first unmanipulated haplo-HSCT. A total of 103 patients had a nondetectable MRD status prior to HSCT. The 4-year OS, EFS, and cumulative incidence of relapse (CIR) rates were 71,9%, 62,3%, and 32,4%, respectively. The above rates differed significantly between the two groups of patients, depending on the MRD status before transplantation. Patients who were MRD-negative achieved better OS, EFS, and CIR rates of 80.5%, 73.3%, and 23.8%, respectively, compared to MRD-positive children pre-transplant, for whom the aforementioned rates were 63.4%, 51.4%, and 41.0%, respectively [9].

BCR/ABL-positive ALL occurred in 3–5% of all pediatric ALL patients [79] and was associated with a poor overall outcome [80] before tyrosine kinase inhibitors (TKIs) came into play. Chen et al. performed haplo-HSCT in 50 Philadelphia chromosome-positive (Ph^+) ALL children. Patients received two myeloablative conditioning regimens, TBI or a combination of cytarabine, busulfan, and semustine (Me-CCNU), both combined with ATG. The 3-year incidence of relapse and non-relapse mortality rates were 22.7% and 16.4% [81].

Another study was conducted in order to compare the treatment outcomes between haplo-HSCT- and TKI-based chemotherapy for Ph^+ pediatric ALL patients. Mild grades I–II aGVHD and severe grades III–IV aGVHD occurred in 25 and 5 out of 68 patients undergoing haplo-HSCT, respectively. A total of 42 patients survived more than 100 days after transplantation. The CIR, EFS, and OS rates were 23.5%, 73.4%, and 80.3% in the transplantation group. The authors found no significant difference in the rates of the above-mentioned indicators between patients belonging to the standard risk group, regardless of whether they had a transplant or not. However, in patients with at least one adverse prognostic factor, the above rates were better in those who underwent transplantation, which showed that only in the high-risk group of patients did haplo-HSCT have a significant advantage in terms of prolonged survival [82].

Studies test the efficacy of the G-CSF/ATG regimen during haplo-HSCT in various diseases, many of which with a negative prognosis. Once more, Xue et al. compared

the results of unmanipulated haplo-HSCT with chemotherapy, this time among children with very high-risk (VHR) Philadelphia chromosome-negative (Ph^{-}) B-ALL. The 3-year estimated OS and EFS rates were better in children in the haplo-HSCT group than in the intensive chemotherapy group at 80.6% vs. 62.4% and 81.0% vs. 52.0%, respectively [83]. In another study, Bai et al. analyzed the outcomes of 38 patients with B-ALL with t(v;11q23) MLL-rearrangements. Similarly, the 4-year estimated OS and EFS rates were significantly greater in the haplo-HSCT cohort than in the intensive chemotherapy cohort [84].

A study by Hu GH et al. advocated the safety of combining chimeric antigen receptor T-cell (CAR-T) therapy with haplo-HSCT in patients suffering from relapsed B-ALL [85], which is said to have an extremely poor prognosis and be resistant to chemotherapy [86]. Earlier studies linked the MRD status with post-transplantation outcomes; therefore, relapsed B-ALL patients with lesser or undetectable MRD obtained significantly higher EFS and lower CIR rates [87]. In treatment based on the MRD status, the authors analyzed the effect of haplo-HSCT after CAR-T therapy or chemotherapy on the long-term survival and safety of pediatric patients with the first relapse of B-ALL. A total of 40 children were included in the analysis, 26 of whom received CAR-T-cells. At the time of the first remission, negative minimal residual disease was obtained by 21 patients in the CAR-T group and 10 patients in the chemotherapy group. The median MRD before haplo-HSCT in the group receiving chemotherapy (n = 14) was significantly higher than in the CAR-T group (n = 26). Post-haplo-HSCT complications in the form of infection, treatment-related mortality, aGVHD, and cGVHD were not significantly different between the two patient groups. A significant advantage was observed in the increase of 3-year leukemia-free survival (LFS) and 3-year OS in patients who received CAR-T therapy before haplo-HSCT, compared to patients receiving chemotherapy: (71.8% vs. 44.4%) and (84.6% vs. 40%), respectively. The results of the aforementioned study may suggest that the administration of CAR-T for positive pre-HSCT MRD has a beneficial effect on patient survival [88].

KMT2A is a frequently rearranged gene in leukemias, mostly in pediatric and infant AML [89,90]. In 21 patients diagnosed with AML with *t(v;11q23)/KMT2A*, rearrangement transplantation options were evaluated. A total of 17 of the 21 children underwent haplo-HSCT transplantation, while the others had a matched sibling donor. The Beijing protocol was used as myeloablative treatment, with no deaths related to myeloablation. Fully matched HSCT appeared to have a lower death rate, but the authors found no significant differences in the OS, EFS, or CIR rates between patient cohorts. The severity of aGVHD was higher in the group undergoing haplo-HSCT; however, only one haploidentical transplant patient died from aGVHD-related complications [91].

Rare acute leukemias occurring in children prior to 3 years of age are called infant leukemias [92]. While myeloid leukemias have similar outcomes in most children, the ones deriving from lymphoid progenitors have poorer disease progression and relapse-free survival, in comparison with ALL in older patients [93,94]. Allo-HSCT remains the first-line treatment for relapsed ALL [95]. To determine the safety of haplo-HSCT in such patient groups, the authors retrospectively analyzed a group of 97 infants and patients under 3 years of age diagnosed with acute leukemia. The most frequently identified gene fusion was *KMT2A* rearrangement found in 37 patients, of which 15 were infants. In children without the aforementioned gene fusion, the 3-year DFS and OS rates were significantly lower than in children with the identified *KMT2A* rearrangement at 63.8% vs. 78.4% and 66.9% vs. 86.1%, respectively. The median follow-up was 45 months. The 3-year OS and DFS rates in children diagnosed at <1 year of age and children diagnosed at ≥1 year were almost the same at 82.5% vs. 72.8% and 77.8% vs. 66.3%, respectively [96].

3.2.2. PTCy-Based Protocol

Cyclophosphamide (Cy) has been extensively studied for its immunosuppressive characteristics [97] in the context of bone marrow transplantation, and it is said to lower the chances of graft rejection, as well as GVHD, if given at an optimal time [98,99].

The first study to introduce the PTCy-based protocol was a clinical trial carried out by O'Donnell et al. regarding high-risk hematologic malignancy patients undergoing haplo-HSCT. Conditioning included fludarabine followed by TBI, PTCy that was given as GVHD prophylaxis at day 3 at a dose of 50 mg/kg with Mesna (80% of Cy dose in four divided doses over 8 h), mycophenolate mofetil, and tacrolimus. A total of 8 out of 13 patients obtained sustained engraftment [100]. Based on data from adult studies, haplo-HSCT with PTCy significantly reduces the risk of cGVHD and appears to be a better option than a MUD [101,102]. Sachdev et al. retrospectively examined the outcomes of 15 pediatric patients diagnosed with high-risk/relapsed ALL (n = 10) and AML (n = 5). A total of 3 patients received MUD transplantation, and 12 underwent haplo-HSCT. All patients accepted the transplant, except one who died before the procedure due to pneumonia. A total of 11 children achieved remission and were alive at a median follow-up time of 775 days. The cumulative incidences of aGVHD and cGVHD were 57.1% and 21.4%, respectively. The rates of relapse or mortality did not depend on the type of conditioning regimen used. The OS and EFS rates were 80% and 73.3% [103]. In another study, comparing haplo-HSCT and chemotherapy in children diagnosed with intermediate risk (IR) AML, the patients in the chemotherapy group had a higher CIR and worse EFS, but roughly equivalent OS. The results of the study indicated that haplo-HSCT is a beneficial therapeutic option for children with IR-AML in first complete remission (CR1), particularly for those patients who have MRD $\geq 10^{-3}$ after induction therapy [104]. Another study compared the treatment outcomes in 80 pediatric patients diagnosed with high-risk acute leukemia who, after myeloablative conditioning based on busulfan, received a transplant with PTCy from either not fully matched-related or MUD. The grades II–IV and grades III–IV aGVHD rates in the MUD group were higher than in the haploidentical related donor (HRD) group, i.e., 48.9% vs. 34.3% and 8.9% vs. 2.9%, respectively. The CIR of overall cGVHD and moderate to severe cGVHD was almost the same in both groups. Because of the similar outcomes and survival rates in both groups, PTCy haplo-HSCT should be given to patients requiring bone marrow transplantation who do not have an HLA-matched related or unrelated donor [28]. Tannumsaeung et al. aimed to determine the results of haplo-HSCT with PTCy preceded by either TBI- or thiotepa-based conditioning regimens. The percentage of graft-related complications and infections was comparable in both groups of patients [105].

3.3. Other Studies on Haplo-HSCT in Hematologic Malignancies

Apart from the above-mentioned trials or retrospective analyses, the available literature discussing haplo-HSCT in pediatric patients with hematologic malignancies contains a couple of single-institution reports (Table 3).

Table 2. Novel studies on haplo-HSCT without ex vivo T-cell depletion.

Number of Patients	Median Age	Transplant Type	Conditioning Regimen and GVHD Prophylaxis	Incidence of aGVHD	Incidence of cGVHD	Relapse NRM	OS Rate	Reference
179	ISD-HSCT 11 haplo-HSCT 12	ISD-HSCT (n = 23) haplo-HSCT (n = 156)	Ara-C + Bu + Cy + Me-CCNU + G-CSF + ATG + CSA + MMF + short-term MTX	ISD-HSCT II–IV aGVHD 13% haplo-HSCT II–IV aGVHD 34.8%	ISD-HSCT 14.1% haplo-HSCT 34.9%	Relapse ISD-HSCT 39.1% haplo-HSCT 16.4% NRM ISD-HSCT 0% haplo-HSCT 10.6%	3-year OS ISD-HSCT 73% haplo-HSCT 74.6%	[78]
200	10	haplo-HSCT	Ara-C + Bu + Cy + Me-CCNU + ATG + CSA + MMF + short-term MTX + G-CSF	II–IV aGVHD 41.1% III–IV aGVHD 9.5%	56.1%	Relapse 31% NRM 5%	4-year OS 80.5%	[9]
68	10	HSCT: haplo-HSCT (n = 37) MSD (n = 3) UCB (n = 4) chemotherapy and TKi (n = 24)	Ara-C + Bu + Cy + Me-CCNU + CSA + MMF + hydroxyurea (MSD) + ATG (UCB, haplo-HSCT) + G-CSF (MUD, haplo-HSCT) + short-term MTX (MSD, haplo-HSCT) + MP (UCB)	I–II aGVHD 56.8% III–IV aGVHD 11.4%	40.9%	Relapse no transplant: 45.8% transplant: 13.5%	3-year OS 80.3%	[82]
104	7	haplo-HSCT (n = 42) chemotherapy (n = 62)	Ara-C + Bu + Cy + Me-CCNU + ATG + G-CSF + CSA + MMF + short-term MTX	II–IV aGVHD 54.8% III–IV aGVHD 11.7%	55.8%	Relapse haplo-HSCT: 11.9% chemotherapy: 51.6% NRM haplo-HSCT: 9.5% chemotherapy: 0%	predicted 3-year OS haplo-HSCT: 80.6% chemotherapy: 62.4%	[83]
38	4	haplo-HSCT (n = 18) MUDT (n = 1) Chemotherapy (n = 18)	Ara-C + Bu + Cy + Me-CCNU + ATG + CSA + MMF + short-term MTX	II–IV aGVHD 37%	53.8%	predicted 4-year CIR 39.1%	predicted 4-year OS 69.8%	[84]
40	CAR-T-cell therapy before haplo-HSCT 9.5 chemotherapy before haplo-HSCT 9.0	CAR-T-cell therapy before haplo-HSCT (n = 26) chemotherapy before haplo-HSCT (n = 14)	TBI or Ara-C + Bu + Cy + ATG + Me-CCNU + G-CSF + CSA + MMF + short-term MTX	CAR-T-cells: II–IV aGVHD 26% chemotherapy: II–IV aGVHD 23%	CAR-T-cells: 53% chemotherapy: 50%	Relapse CAR-T-cells: 26.9% chemotherapy: 50% NRM CAR-T-cells: 3.8% chemotherapy: 7.14%	3-year OS CAR-T-cells: 84.6% chemotherapy: 40%	[88]
21	4.4	haplo-HSCT (n = 17) MSDT (n = 4)	Ara-C + Bu + Cy + Me-CCNU + ATG, CSA + MMF + short-term MTX (n = 17) Ara-C + Bu + Cy + CSA + short-term MTX (n = 4)	haplo-HSCT II–IV aGVHD 76.4%	No information	Relapse 14.3% NRM 9.5%	100%	[91]

Table 2. *Cont.*

Number of Patients	Median Age	Transplant Type	Conditioning Regimen and GVHD Prophylaxis	Incidence of aGVHD	Incidence of cGVHD	Relapse NRM	OS Rate	Reference
97	Patients diagnosed <1 year: 1.4 Patients diagnosed ≥1 year: 2.2	haplo-HSCT	Ara-C + Bu + Cy + Me-CCNU + ATG + CSA + MMF + short-term MTX	II–IV aGVHD 45.3% III–IV aGVHD 8.8%	36%	NRM 3.1% 3-year CIR 26.9%	3-year OS 74.2%	[96]
15	8.5	MUD (n = 3) haplo-HSCT (n = 12)	TBI + Cy, Flu + Bu, Flu + Bu + L-PAM, TT + Flu + Cy + TBI, Flu + Cy + TBI, PTCy + CSA/TAC + MMF, MTX + CSA + ATG + G-SCF,	57.1%	21.4%	NRM 26.7%	80%	[103]
80	haplo-HSCT: 10 chemotherapy: 8	haplo-HSCT (n = 33) chemotherapy (n = 47)	Ara-C + Bu + Cy + Me-CCNU + ATG	II–IV aGVHD 44.6% III–IV aGVHD 6%	60.6%	3-year CIR 25.4%	3-year OS 85.4%	[104]
80	haplo-HSCT with PTCy 7 MUD 8.9	haplo-HSCT with PTCy (n = 35) MUD (n = 45)	Bu + Flu ± etoposide + ATG + TAC + MMF, Bu + Flu + Cy + PTCy + TAC + MTX	MUD: II–IV aGVHD 48.9% III–IV aGVHD 8.9% haplo-HSCT with PTCy: II–IV aGVHD 34.3% III–IV aGVHD 2.9%	MUD: 18.3% haplo-HSCT with PTCy: 11.4%	Relapse MUD: 28% haplo-HSCT with PTCy: 25.6% NRM MUD: 2,2% haplo-HSCT with PTCy: 0%	3-year OS MUD: 83.7% haplo-HSCT with PTCy: 88.6%	[28]
43	TBI regimen 8.7 TT regimen 8.8	haplo-HSCT with PTCy	TBI + Cy + Flu + L-PAM, TT + Flu + Bu, PTCy + MMF + calcineurin inhibitor or sirolimus + G-CSF	aGVHD TBI regimen: 56.5% TT regimen: 45%	TBI regimen: 21.7% TT regimen: 10%	NRM TBI regimen 17.4% TT regimen 20%	3-year OS 62.4%	[105]

aGVHD—acute graft-versus-host disease, Ara-C—cytarabine, ATG—anti-thymocyte globulin, Bu—busulfan, CAR-T—chimeric antigen receptor T-cells, cGVHD—chronic graft-versus-host disease, CIR—cumulative incidence of relapse/progression, CSA—cyclosporin A, Cy—cyclophosphamide, Flu—fludarabine, G-CSF—granulocyte colony-stimulating factor, haplo-HSCT—haploidentical hematopoietic stem cell transplantation, ISD-HSCT—identical sibling donor hematopoietic stem cell transplantation, L-PAM—melphalan, Me-CCNU—methyl chloride hexamethylene urea nitrate (semustine), MMF—mycophenolate mofetil, MP—methylprednisolone, MUD—matched unrelated donor, MSDT—matched sibling donor transplant, MTX—methotrexate, NRM—non-relapse mortality, OS—overall survival, PTCy—post-transplant cyclophosphamide, TAC—tacrolimus, TBI—total body irradiation, TKi—tyrosine kinase inhibitor, TT—thiotepa, UCB—unrelated cord blood.

Table 3. Small cohort studies reporting haplo-HSCT results in the treatment of hematologic malignancies in children.

Condition/Disease	Study Group	Graft Characteristics	Transplant Type	Conditioning Regimen and GVHD Prophylaxis	Survival Rate	References
MDS: RCC, refractory anemia with excess of blasts	8 patients, 7 F, 1 M median age: 6.4 years	MNCs, $\times 10^8$/kg—19.8 The median $CD34^+$ cells, 10^6/kg—11.8	haplo-HSCT with PTCy	Cy at +3 and +4 days after transplantation, low-dose TAC, MMF	OS = 100% DFS = 100%	[106]
MDS: RCC, advanced MDS, MDR-AML	27 patients, 15 F, 12 M median age: 10 years	The median MNCs, $\times 10^8$/kg—8.6 The median $CD34^+$ cells, 10^6/kg—2.9	haplo-HSCT	Ara-C + Bu + Cy + Me-CCNU + ATG + CSA + MMF + short-term MTX	estimated 3-year rate probabilities for 10 patients diagnosed with RCC OS = 90% DFS = 90%, for 17 patients with advanced MDS/MDR-AML OS = 77.7% DFS = 77.7%	[107]
HLH	Case report First patient: 8 months/male Second patient: 10 years/male	The dose of $CD34^+$ cells, 10^6/kg First patient: 24.33 Second patient: 11.96	haplo-HSCT with PTCy	Cy at +3 and +4 days after transplantation + MMF, First patient: CSA + Flu + Treo + alemtuzumab Second patient: TAC + RTX + ATG + Flu + Cy + TBI	disease-free period of 912 and 239 days for the First and Second patients	[108]
HLH	12 patients 7 F, 5 M median age: 4.5 years	No information	haplo-HSCT with $\alpha\beta^+/CD19^+$ cell depletion (n = 2) and PTCy (n = 10)	Cy at +3 and +4 days after transplantation + Flu + Treo + ATG + TT ($\alpha\beta^+/CD19^+$ cell depletion group) + TBI (PTCy group)	OS = 66.7%	[109]

Ara-C—cytarabine, ATG—anti-thymocyte globulin, CSA—cyclosporine A, Cy—cyclophosphamide, F—female, Flu—fludarabine, HLH—hemophagocytic lymphohistiocytosis, M—male, MDR-AML—myelodysplasia-related acute myeloid leukemia, MDS—myelodysplatic syndrome, Me-CCNU—methyl chloride hexamethylene urea nitrate (semustine), MMF—mycophenolate mofetil, MNCs—median mononuclear cells, MTX—methotrexate, PTCy—post-transplant cyclophosphamide, RCC—refractory cytopenia of childhood, RTX—rituximab, TAC—tacrolimus, TBI—total body irradiation, Treo—treosulfan, TT—thiotepa.

4. Non-Malignant Disorders

Haplo-HSCT may be an effective treatment option not only for malignancies. Its wider application in pediatric non-malignant disorders has been thoroughly described in the literature. Haplo-HSCT usage ranges from primary immunodeficiencies (PIDs) to all kinds of anemias.

4.1. Primary Immunodeficiencies

PIDs comprise a large, heterogeneous group of diseases affecting all components of the immune system that may be caused by changes in over 300 genes [110,111]. One treatment option for the patients is hematopoietic stem cell transplantation [112]. The best option is a graft from a healthy HLA-genoidentical matched sibling donor. However, such transplants are possible in no more than 25% of the cases. Furthermore, less than 70% of the remaining patients will have a suitable matched unrelated donor, and chances are even slimmer for patients belonging to certain ethnic groups [113]. To avoid the delay due to a prolonged search for a matching donor, an HSCT from an HLA-haploidentical family donor (HIFD) can be performed, despite the fact that such a procedure is associated with a higher risk of GVHD and graft failure, which may lead to increased mortality rates [114–116]. The available literature discussing haploidentical HSCT in pediatric patients with PID consists of single-institution reports and multicenter retrospective analyses [117–122] (Table 4).

In the reviewed studies, researchers analyzed the impact of HSCT on patients with PIDs, ranging from trials where children were diagnosed with 12 different types of PIDs [117] to ones including only SCID patients [120]. The survival rates of patients after PID treatment with HSCT from an HLA-haploidentical donor ranged from 84% to 62.7%. There were numerous factors that contributed to the causes of death among patients, i.e., CMV infection, progressive respiratory failure, GVHD, or thrombotic microangiopathy. Regarding infectious complications after transplantation, one study reported a 63.6% incidence rate of post-HSCT CMV viremia [118], while another reported a 58.8% cumulative incidence rate of CMV and ADV infections [117]. At the same time, the incidence rate of significant GVHD in almost all the studies remained low. The rates of GVHD ranged from 54% to 27.2%; however, most of the studies revealed rates of GVHD lower than 40%. On top of that, most patients who developed a GVHD experienced it at a mild I or II grade. The time needed for immune reconstitution was also satisfactory [117–122]. One study reported that 75% (six out of eight) of survivors had a whole-blood chimerism greater than 95% [118], and in another trial, at the last follow-up, 76.1% of patients had a full donor chimerism [117]. However, in the case of an adenosine deaminase (ADA) deficiency, a type of PID, the results of haploidentical HSCT treatment were inconclusive. One study presented the OS rate of 68.4% (13/19 patients) [120], whereas the trial conducted by Hassan et al. suggested that haplo-HSCT is not an effective form of treatment in this PID type. The results of 106 patients showed that the HSCT OS rates from matched sibling and family donors were 86% and 81%, respectively. This proved to be a better result in comparison with patients receiving HSCT from haploidentical donors, many of who presented graft failure, with an OS rate of 43%. Having said that, long-term immune recovery showed that, regardless of the transplant type, the overall T-cell numbers were similar. Moreover, humoral immunity and donor B-cell engraftment were achieved in nearly all the survivors [123]. Those data stand in contrast to the satisfactory results of haploidentical HSCT in other types of immunodeficiencies. An explanation can include the fact that in the trial conducted on mice, the microenvironment of ADA-deficient bone marrow showed a reduced capacity to support in vitro or in vivo hematopoiesis. Therefore, patients with an ADA deficiency may fail to support engraftment of the transplanted HSCT [124].

In conclusion, a $CD3^{+}TCR\alpha\beta^{+}/CD19^{+}$-depleted HSCT from an HLA-haploidentical donor is an effective form of treatment for children with PIDs, especially when finding a matched sibling donor is not possible.

Table 4. Data summary regarding overall survival, graft modification, number of patients with GVHD prophylaxis, type of conditioning, cell dose, incidence and type of GVHD, and mean time of B- and T-cell recovery in different trials. Ranked by increasing survival rates.

Trial Name	Number of Patients Receiving Haplo-HSCT	Type of Graft Modification	Number of Patients with GVHD Prophylaxis	Type of Conditioning (Number of Patients Receiving at Least One of Listed Drug)	Cell Dose (Mean; Rage Dose)	Overall Survival Rate (%) (Number of Patients)	Incidence of GVHD (%) (Number of Patients)	Most Common Grade of GVHD (%)	Mean Time of T-Cell Recovery (days)	Mean Time of B-Cell Recovery (days)
Shah et al. [117]	25	TCRαβ$^+$/CD19$^+$	22	Treo, Flu, TT, ATG, Alemtuzumab 23	CD3: 3.3 (0.075–9.5) × 10^4/kg CD34: 17.8(4.7–50.9) × 10^6/kg	84 21/25	47.8 11/23	II	129	85
Brettig et al. [118]	11	TCRαβ$^+$/CD19$^+$	No information	Treo, Flu, TT 11	CD3: 1.5 (0.3–2) × 10^4/kg CD34: 14.1 (3.7–20.8) × 10^6/kg	81.8 8/11	27.2 3/11	II	132	93
Buckley et al. [119]	77	No information	0	0	No information	78 60/77	36.3 28/77	I or II	90–120	No information
Buckley et al. [120]	149	No information	0	0	No information	73 109/149	30.2 45/149	I or II	90–120	No information
Neven et at. [121]	22	No information	22	Flu, Bu, Cy, RTX, Alemtuzumab 22	CD3: 10.7 (2.6–30.2) × 10^7/kg CD34: 13.8 (2.6–47.7) × 10^6/kg	72.7 16/22	54 12/22	II	157	204
Holzer et al. [122]	19	CD34 selection; TCRαβ/CD19 depletion; TCRαβ depletion (+in vivo CD20-depletion); CD3/CD19 depletion	9	No information	No information	62.7 12/19	21 (acute) 15 (chronic)	I or II	30–365	No information

ATG—anti-thymocyte globulin, Bu—busulfan, Cy—cyclophosphamide, Flu—fludarabine, RTX—rituximab, Treo—treosulfan, TT—thiotepa.

4.2. Sickle Cell Disease

The course of SCD is highly variable. However, the one feature that unites the diverse nature of this disease is a shortened life expectancy and significant morbidity. Patients with SCD may experience hemolytic anemia, severe pain, vaso-occlusive crises, stroke, avascular necrosis, pulmonary hypertension, infections, renal failure, and thrombosis. Despite many genetic attempts, HSCT remains the only curative method [125]. The best outcomes are observed after HLA-matched sibling transplantation. However, approximately 70% of patients with SCD do not have an HLA-matched sibling. Alternative donor options include matched unrelated donor, unrelated umbilical cord blood transplantation, and mismatched related transplantation [14,126].

According to studies, haplo-HSCT exhibits high efficiency among pediatric patients. In the clinical trial carried out by J. Foell et al., 15 out of the 20 studied patients with high-risk SCD received a CD3/CD19-depleted graft and the rest received a TCRαβ/CD19-depleted graft. All patients experienced primary engraftments with stable grafts. The median time to reach leukocyte recovery was 16 days, and neutrophile recovery occurred after 19 days, and thrombocyte recovery occurred 10 days after the transplant. When it comes to lymphocytes, the median time of $CD3^+$ T-cell recovery was 173 days post-transplantation; it was 277 days for $CD4^+$ T-cells and 213 days for $CD8^+$ T-cells. B lymphocytes were restored around the 80th day after transplantation. According to these data, leucocytes, neutrophils, and thrombocytes recover rapidly, while T-cell recovery appears delayed. In this study group, the OS, EFS, and DFS were 90%. Total respiratory morbidity (TRM) was observed in 10% of the patients [127]. In another study conducted with a 9-year follow-up, haplo-HSCT did not bring satisfactory outcomes. The trial enrolled 22 patients with symptomatic SCD, 8 out of whom were recipients of a parental haploidentical donor graft. The median age of the patients was 9.0 ($\pm$5.0) years. All patients achieved donor engraftment with a 100% donor chimerism, with a median time to full engraftment amounting to 12.5 days. A total of 50% of the patients, however, developed evidence of graft rejection on approximately the 30th day post-transplant and required an additional stem cell infusion. After the infusion, 25% of the patients recovered with a sustained 100% donor chimerism, whereas the other patients progressed to graft failure with recurrence of disease. Donor engraftment was eventually sustained in 62% of the patients, and graft failure occurred in 38% of the subjects. A follow-up visit after 9 years post-transplantation indicated that 75% of the patients were alive, with 37.5% eventually experiencing sustained engraftment and remaining disease-free. However, SCD recurrence took place in another 37.5% of the studied population. The OS rate amounted to 75% [128].

Pawlowska et al. reported a complete engraftment with a 99.9% to 100% donor chimerism after T-cell replete haploidentical stem cell infusion. All patients maintained stable engraftment at the last follow-up (11 months). Additionally, neutrophil engraftment occurred between the 14th and 26th days post-transplant. Half of the patients presented high levels of donor-specific anti-HLA antibodies, which required the implementation of an antibody management protocol. This enabled neutrophil engraftment on days 16 and 26, respectively [30]. Similar results were reached by another research group [129]. Their follow-up was carried out 11, 14, and 30 months after HSCT transplant. The survival rate amounted to 100%, and all of the patients exhibited a complete donor chimerism. What is important, they did not have any more symptoms of SCD. Neutrophil engraftment was noted on days 12, 17, and 20. However, both of the studies above consisted of a low number of patients; therefore, the reliability of the results cannot be fully confirmed.

Despite the introduction of prophylaxis, GVHD still remains a critical issue. Nonetheless, it does not occur as often as previously and with significantly lower intensity. In a study of three patients, mild skin GVHD was observed in one patient. None of those patients experienced cGVHD, nor central nervous system toxicity. Surprisingly, two patients experienced an asymptomatic CMV reactivation [129]. In a study of four patients, one developed aGVHD grade I, while three of the patients experienced mild skin GVHD and responded well to immunosuppression therapy. Moreover, in three of the patients,

HHV-6 was detected, but resolved spontaneously without any treatment [30]. In the far-reaching study of eight patients, among which five underwent a successful engraftment, four experienced aGVHD. Two of those patients developed grade I, while the other two developed grade II aGVHD. Subsequently, three of those four patients developed cGVHD and two of them died from complications. In the study comparing T-haplo-HSCT and matched sibling donor grafts, 35% of the patients in the T-haplo-HSCT group experienced aGVHD. However, in all cases, GVHD resolved after a few days of low-dose prednisolone applications. None of the patients developed aGVHD grades III–IV. Nonetheless, four developed a steroid-sensitive cGVHD with cutaneous, oral, ocular, and fascial involvement responding to primary treatment. Apart from GVHD, haplo-HSCT complications included CMV, BK virus (BKV), EBV, HHV6 and ADV reactivation, BKV-associated nephritis, rotavirus diarrhea, CMV pneumonitis, and macrophage activation syndrome with a late graft failure [127].

These data indicate that cyclophosphamide, tacrolimus, and MMF usage is effective and extremely beneficial for patients with SCD as prophylaxis. Although it does not always guarantee 100% efficiency, such a treatment contributes to the development of less severe GVHD.

4.3. Severe Aplastic Anemia

Severe aplastic anemia (SAA) is a state of bone marrow failure resulting from its hypoplasia or aplasia. As a consequence, the bone marrow does not produce enough erythrocytes, leucocytes, and/or thrombocytes. Recently, SAA outcomes have significantly improved because of HSCT introduction and immunosuppressive treatments. HLA-matched sibling donor HSCT is a primary treatment option for pediatric SAA patients. However, due to the frequent lack of such donors, haplo-HSCT is most commonly performed instead [130]. Based on the little data available, this treatment seems to be very successful. In the multicenter trial conducted among 35 patients, all of them reached full engraftment with the median time for myeloid recovery amounting to 14 days and for platelet recovery to 18 days [131]. Another study proved a 98% success rate; however, 6% of the patients had a secondary graft rejection after more than 20 days post-transplant [130].

While haplo-HSCT usage decreases the severity of SAA symptoms, it also increases the risk of GVHD or post-transplant hemophagocytic syndrome (PTHPS), despite cyclophosphamide prophylaxis [131–133]. In both studies, the GVHD rate amounted to more than 50% of the cases. It included not only aGVHD grades I to IV, but also chronic GVHD involving the skin, liver, and gastrointestinal tract [130,131]. Nonetheless, previous research proved that the introduction of an immunosuppressive drug, inhibitor of mammalian target of rapamycin (mTOR), such as sirolimus on the 8th day before the transplant, significantly reduces this complication among adult patients [132,133]. Regarding pediatric patients, a co-stimulation blockade with cytotoxic T lymphocyte antigen-4 (CTLA4) IgA is a promising method of reducing GVHD and PTHPS occurrence. This approach has been described, inter alia, by Jaiswal et al. In their trial, two groups were compared. The first group received an extended T-cell co-stimulation blockade (COSBL) with abatacept, sirolimus, and post-transplantation cyclophosphamide, while the other—the control group—only received post-transplant cyclophosphamide. Both groups included 10 patients with SAA. The patients treated within the COSBL protocol had much better outcomes than those in the control group in terms of GVHD occurrence. The incidences of aGVHD were 10.5% and 50%, respectively. Moreover, approximately 12.5% of the patients in the COSBL group experienced cGVHD, while in the control group, it was 56% of the patients [132]. Those results confirm the previous thesis. Haplo-HSCT in combination with therapy involving COSBL, abatacept, sirolimus, and cyclophosphamide significantly decreases the GVHD incidence in pediatric patients with SAA.

Apart from GVHD, many patients experienced different complications of haplo-HSCT, such as bacterial, fungal, and viral (CMV and EBV) infections [131,133]. Wang et al.

additionally described a reversible posterior leukoencephalopathy syndrome that occurred in two patients in that study and ended with their death [131].

When it comes to the OS rate of haplo-HSCT used in SAA, the values fluctuated from 70% to approximately 86% [130–132].

4.4. Fanconi Anemia

Fanconi anemia (FA) is a rare, inherited condition characterized by congenital malformations, progressive marrow failure, and a predisposition to solid tumors, as well as acute myelogenous leukemia. Patients with FA are excellent candidates for haplo-HSCT because, without such a treatment, the prognosis is extremely poor [134,135]. The study of Ayas et al. enrolled 19 pediatric patients with FA. All of the patients experienced neutrophil engraftment at the median time of 14 days. On the other hand, platelet recovery occurred in 18 patients at the median time of 20.5 days. The overall incidence of aGVHD amounted to 42%, while extensive cGVHD occurred in only one patient. The follow-up examination was performed at the median time of 38 months, and the OS rate was set at 89% [134]. Another study included 24 pediatric patients who underwent haplo-HSCT for FA. Full engraftment was achieved in 22 patients (92%), with the median time for neutrophil and platelet recovery of 12 and 10 days, respectively. Eventual primary graft failure occurred in two patients. Four patients (16%) developed aGVHD grades I and II. Additionally, of the 22 patients at risk, only 1 developed mild, skin-only cGVHD (4.5%). On the follow-up after a median time of 5 years, all patients were alive; thus, the OS rate was 100%. Eleven patients (45.8%) developed post-HSCT viral reactivations or infections [136].

On the basis of this trial, a connection was made among older age, high transfusion burden, previous androgen exposure, development of clonal evolution, and lower survival rates. Moreover, children with FA undergoing haplo-HSCT are associated with a higher risk of developing severe aGVHD, due to the underlying DNA repair defect and deregulation of the apoptotic process [136].

5. Future Directions

Although haplo-HSCT became a point of interest over 20 years ago, to this day, there are several aspects that require further investigation, particularly in pediatric patients [137]. A lot of research focuses on the comparison of transplant results among MUD, HLA mismatched unrelated donor (MMUD), and HRD to determine the best choice for a patient lacking a family HLA-matched donor. For pediatric patients with acute leukemia, the 5-year OS rates between T-replete haplo-HSCT and transplant from MUD and MMUD appeared comparable. The relapse incidence (RI) and NRM also showed similar results [138]. Another study revealed that the results of haplo-HSCT with PTCy and the MAC regimen and the MUD HSCT with the ATG regimen were similar. Haplo-HSCT is recognized as an advantageous option for pediatric patients with high-risk leukemia, lacking a related or an unrelated HLA-identical donor. Moreover, a comparison between PTCy-based haplo-HSCT with MAC and non-MAC regimens exhibited similar toxicity [28]. CGVHD was observed more often in patients undergoing an MUD transplant rather than after haplo-HSCT. Pediatric patients with hematological malignancies can be successfully treated with haplo-HSCT, as the aGVHD and cGVHD incidence rates and OS rates are satisfactory [139].

Research on post-transplant immune recovery is still developing, as it is crucial to decrease the prevalence of infectious complications and relapse risks. Innate immunity, especially including NK cells, that exert both anti-leukemic and anti-viral effects, is responsible for such recovery. Despite that, TCD methods for haplo-HSCT cause around a 2-month delay for NK cells to be produced from donor hematopoietic stem cells. The study was conducted to determine if lower doses of anti-T lymphocyte globulin (ALTG) would affect the NK cell count after transplantation. It was revealed that the number of NK cells was indeed substantially elevated, which led to the conclusion that a higher concentration of ALTG might cause a lengthened immune readjustment. Nevertheless, because ALTG has a favorable effect on GVHD and graft rejection, it would be optimal to incorporate high pre-transplant ALTG doses with low post-transplant ALTG doses [140].

Another aspect worth further investigating is haplo-HSCT followed by donor lymphocyte infusion (DLI), which presents a distinct graft-versus-leukemia (GVL) effect. Data gathered from adult patients showed that ATG-based haplo-HSCT with subsequent prophylactic DLI reduced the risk of relapse, in addition to raising long-term survival among high-risk acute leukemia patients without enhancing the toxicity of the therapy [141]. Pediatric data are rather limited; however, a few studies were conducted and the results were analogous to those for the adult patients. Prophylactic DLI provided successful and safe outcomes in children with both malignant and non-malignant hematological diseases [142,143].

Moreover, haplo-HSCT is recognized as an independent risk factor for CMV infection. Statistically, the frequency of infections is higher after haplo-HSCT than after HLA-matched HSCT, which contributes to the extended mortality rate among pediatric patients [144]. Furthermore, the usage of PTCy is also associated with a greater rate of CMV infection, which suggested the need for an active prophylaxis regimen. As CMV-active anti-viral drugs, like valganciclovir or ganciclovir, present severe side effects, adding to the toxicity of the treatment, a new drug was developed. CMV DNA terminase inhibitor, letermovir, was introduced as prophylactic medication for HSCT recipients, including PTCy-based haplo-HSCT. The research showed that letermovir decreased the occurrence of CMV-related complications, as well as the necessity to use CMV-specific treatment, without altering the TRM or OS [145,146]. Data regarding the use of letermovir in pediatric patients are insufficient. However, recent studies confirm that it can be profitably and safely administered to children as a preventative measure against CMV reactivations [147,148].

6. Conclusions

Due to many its advantages, haplo-HSCT is becoming an increasingly popular form of transplantation in the absence of quick access to fully compatible donors. Although further research in the form of multicenter studies is needed to assemble larger, homogenous research groups with standardized peri-transplant treatment regimens to identify optimal GVHD prophylaxis and conditioning strategies, haplo-HSCT has proven to be an effective form of bone marrow transplantation in hematologic malignancies, both in active and refractory diseases with the OS and RFS rates similar to the MUD grafts. Moreover, it has been applied successfully in various non-malignant hematological disorders, such as SCD, PIDs, and SAA. Current research is focusing on post-transplant immune recovery to reduce the risk of infectious complications and relapses.

Author Contributions: M.L. (Monika Lejman) and J.Z. were responsible for the conception and design of the study; A.M., M.L. (Maria Leśniak), A.S. (Anna Sekunda), A.S. (Aleksander Siwek), and Z.S. were responsible for the acquisition of the literature for the manuscript. A.M., M.L. (Maria Leśniak), A.S. (Anna Sekunda), A.S. (Aleksander Siwek), and Z.S. wrote the original draft of the manuscript; M.L. (Maria Leśniak) was responsible for preparing figures; A.M., A.S. (Aleksander Siwek), and Z.S. were responsible for preparing tables. M.L. (Monika Lejman) and J.Z. reviewed and edited the manuscript. M.L. (Monika Lejman) and J.Z. supervised the paper. All authors have read and agreed to the published version of the manuscript.

Funding: This research received no external funding.

Institutional Review Board Statement: Not applicable.

Informed Consent Statement: Not applicable.

Data Availability Statement: Not applicable.

Conflicts of Interest: The authors declare no conflicts of interest.

References

1. Balassa, K.; Danby, R.; Rocha, V. Haematopoietic Stem Cell Transplants: Principles and Indications. *Br. J. Hosp. Med.* **2019**, *80*, 33–39. [CrossRef] [PubMed]
2. Sureda, A.; Bader, P.; Cesaro, S.; Dreger, P.; Duarte, R.F.; Dufour, C.; Falkenburg, J.H.F.; Farge-Bancel, D.; Gennery, A.; Kröger, N.; et al. Indications for Allo- and Auto-SCT for Haematological Diseases, Solid Tumours and Immune Disorders: Current Practice in Europe, 2015. *Bone Marrow Transplant.* **2015**, *50*, 1037–1056. [CrossRef] [PubMed]
3. Bazinet, A.; Popradi, G. A General Practitioner's Guide to Hematopoietic Stem-Cell Transplantation. *Curr. Oncol.* **2019**, *26*, 187–191. [CrossRef] [PubMed]
4. Hourigan, C.S. Haplo, We Have a Problem. *Blood* **2017**, *130*, 1180. [CrossRef] [PubMed]
5. Gao, Y.-Y.; Chen, X.-J.; Luo, R.-M. Research Advances on Haploidentical Hematopoietic Stem Cell Transplantation in the Treatment of Severe Aplastic Anemia in Children. *Zhongguo Dang Dai Er Ke Za Zhi* **2021**, *23*, 854–859. [CrossRef] [PubMed]
6. Cruz-Tapias, P.; Castiblanco, J.; Anaya, J.-M. Major Histocompatibility Complex: Antigen Processing and Presentation. In *Autoimmunity: From Bench to Bedside [Internet]*; El Rosario University Press: Bogota, Colombia, 2013.
7. Choo, S.Y. The HLA System: Genetics, Immunology, Clinical Testing, and Clinical Implications. *Yonsei Med. J.* **2007**, *48*, 11–23. [CrossRef]
8. Kruse, A.; Abdel-Azim, N.; Kim, H.N.; Ruan, Y.; Phan, V.; Ogana, H.; Wang, W.; Lee, R.; Gang, E.J.; Khazal, S.; et al. Minimal Residual Disease Detection in Acute Lymphoblastic Leukemia. *Int. J. Mol. Sci.* **2020**, *21*, 1054. [CrossRef]
9. Bai, L.; Zhang, Z.-X.; Hu, G.-H.; Cheng, Y.-F.; Suo, P.; Wang, Y.; Yan, C.-H.; Sun, Y.-Q.; Chen, Y.-H.; Chen, H.; et al. Long-Term Follow-up of Haploidentical Haematopoietic Stem Cell Transplantation in Paediatric Patients with High-Risk Acute Myeloid Leukaemia: Report from a Single Centre. *Br. J. Haematol.* **2024**, *204*, 585–594. [CrossRef] [PubMed]
10. Zachary, A.A.; Leffell, M.S. Desensitization for Solid Organ and Hematopoietic Stem Cell Transplantation. *Immunol. Rev.* **2014**, *258*, 183–207. [CrossRef]
11. Mancusi, A.; Kanakry, C.G.; Pierini, A. Editorial: The Immunobiology of HLA-Haploidentical Hematopoietic Cell Transplantation. *Front. Immunol.* **2020**, *11*, 1031. [CrossRef]
12. Choi, E.S.; Im, H.J.; Kim, H.; Koh, K.N.; Jang, S.; Park, C.-J.; Seo, J.J.; Park, H.R. Depletion of Aβ+ T Cells for a Haploidentical Hematopoietic Stem Cell Transplantation in Children. *J. Clin. Apher.* **2018**, *33*, 521–528. [CrossRef] [PubMed]
13. Shah, R.M. Contemporary Haploidentical Stem Cell Transplant Strategies in Children with Hematological Malignancies. *Bone Marrow Transplant.* **2021**, *56*, 1518–1534. [CrossRef] [PubMed]
14. Joseph, J.J.; Abraham, A.A.; Fitzhugh, C.D. When There Is No Match, the Game Is Not over: Alternative Donor Options for Hematopoietic Stem Cell Transplantation in Sickle Cell Disease. *Semin. Hematol.* **2018**, *55*, 94–101. [CrossRef] [PubMed]
15. Handgretinger, R. New Approaches to Graft Engineering for Haploidentical Bone Marrow Transplantation. *Semin. Oncol.* **2012**, *39*, 664–673. [CrossRef] [PubMed]
16. Bertaina, A.; Pitisci, A.; Sinibaldi, M.; Algeri, M. T Cell-Depleted and T Cell-Replete HLA-Haploidentical Stem Cell Transplantation for Non-Malignant Disorders. *Curr. Hematol. Malig. Rep.* **2017**, *12*, 68–78. [CrossRef] [PubMed]
17. Locatelli, F.; Vinti, L.; Palumbo, G.; Rossi, F.; Bertaina, A.; Mastronuzzi, A.; Bernardo, M.E.; Rutella, S.; Dellabona, P.; Giorgiani, G.; et al. Strategies to Optimize the Outcome of Children given T-Cell Depleted HLA-Haploidentical Hematopoietic Stem Cell Transplantation. *Best Pract. Res. Clin. Haematol.* **2011**, *24*, 339–349. [CrossRef] [PubMed]
18. Foell, J.; Kleinschmidt, K.; Jakob, M.; Troeger, A.; Corbacioglu, S. Alternative Donor: Aß/CD19 T-Cell-Depleted Haploidentical Hematopoietic Stem Cell Transplantation for Sickle Cell Disease. *Hematol. Oncol. Stem. Cell Ther.* **2020**, *13*, 98–105. [CrossRef] [PubMed]
19. Al Malki, M.M.; Jones, R.; Ma, Q.; Lee, D.; Reisner, Y.; Miller, J.S.; Lang, P.; Hongeng, S.; Hari, P.; Strober, S.; et al. Proceedings From the Fourth Haploidentical Stem Cell Transplantation Symposium (HAPLO2016), San Diego, California, December 1, 2016. *Biol. Blood Marrow Transplant.* **2018**, *24*, 895–908. [CrossRef] [PubMed]
20. Ciceri, F.; Bacigalupo, A.; Lankester, A.; Bertaina, A. Haploidentical HSCT. In *The EBMT Handbook: Hematopoietic Stem Cell Transplantation and Cellular Therapies*; Carreras, E., Dufour, C., Mohty, M., Kröger, N., Eds.; Springer: Cham, Switzerland, 2019; ISBN 978-3-030-02277-8.
21. Reisner, Y.; Kapoor, N.; Kirkpatrick, D.; Pollack, M.S.; Cunningham-Rundles, S.; Dupont, B.; Hodes, M.Z.; Good, R.A.; O'Reilly, R.J. Transplantation for Severe Combined Immunodeficiency with HLA-A,B,D,DR Incompatible Parental Marrow Cells Fractionated by Soybean Agglutinin and Sheep Red Blood Cells. *Blood* **1983**, *61*, 341–348. [CrossRef]
22. Giardino, S.; Bagnasco, F.; Falco, M.; Miano, M.; Pierri, F.; Risso, M.; Terranova, P.; Di Martino, D.; Massaccesi, E.; Ricci, M.; et al. Haploidentical Stem Cell Transplantation After TCR-Aβ+ and CD19+ Cells Depletion In Children With Congenital Non-Malignant Disease. *Transplant. Cell Ther.* **2022**, *28*, 394.e1–394.e9. [CrossRef]
23. Schumm, M.; Lang, P.; Bethge, W.; Faul, C.; Feuchtinger, T.; Pfeiffer, M.; Vogel, W.; Huppert, V.; Handgretinger, R. Depletion of T-Cell Receptor Alpha/Beta and CD19 Positive Cells from Apheresis Products with the CliniMACS Device. *Cytotherapy* **2013**, *15*, 1253–1258. [CrossRef] [PubMed]
24. Bertaina, A.; Merli, P.; Rutella, S.; Pagliara, D.; Bernardo, M.E.; Masetti, R.; Pende, D.; Falco, M.; Handgretinger, R.; Moretta, F.; et al. HLA-Haploidentical Stem Cell Transplantation after Removal of Aβ+ T and B Cells in Children with Nonmalignant Disorders. *Blood* **2014**, *124*, 822–826. [CrossRef]

25. Klein, O.R.; Chen, A.R.; Gamper, C.; Loeb, D.; Zambidis, E.; Llosa, N.; Huo, J.; Dezern, A.E.; Steppan, D.; Robey, N.; et al. Alternative-Donor Hematopoietic Stem Cell Transplantation with Post-Transplantation Cyclophosphamide for Nonmalignant Disorders. *Biol. Blood Marrow Transplant.* **2016**, *22*, 895–901. [CrossRef] [PubMed]
26. Oevermann, L.; Schulte, J.H.; Hundsdörfer, P.; Hakimeh, D.; Kogel, F.; Lang, P.; Corbacioglu, S.; Eggert, A.; Sodani, P. HLA-Haploidentical Hematopoietic Stem Cell Transplantation in Pediatric Patients with Hemoglobinopathies: Current Practice and New Approaches. *Bone Marrow Transplant.* **2019**, *54*, 743–748. [CrossRef]
27. Merli, P.; Algeri, M.; Galaverna, F.; Milano, G.M.; Bertaina, V.; Biagini, S.; Girolami, E.; Palumbo, G.; Sinibaldi, M.; Becilli, M.; et al. Immune Modulation Properties of Zoledronic Acid on TcRγδ T-Lymphocytes After TcRαβ/CD19-Depleted Haploidentical Stem Cell Transplantation: An Analysis on 46 Pediatric Patients Affected by Acute Leukemia. *Front. Immunol.* **2020**, *11*, 699. [CrossRef]
28. Hong, K.T.; Park, H.J.; Kim, B.K.; An, H.Y.; Choi, J.Y.; Kang, H.J. Post-Transplantation Cyclophosphamide-Based Haploidentical versus Matched Unrelated Donor Peripheral Blood Hematopoietic Stem Cell Transplantation Using Myeloablative Targeted Busulfan-Based Conditioning for Pediatric Acute Leukemia. *Transplant. Cell Ther.* **2022**, *28*, 195.e1–195.e7. [CrossRef]
29. Triozzi, P.L.; Laszlo, J. Optimum Management of Nausea and Vomiting in Cancer Chemotherapy. *Drugs* **1987**, *34*, 136–149. [CrossRef] [PubMed]
30. Pawlowska, A.B.; Cheng, J.C.; Karras, N.A.; Sun, W.; Wang, L.D.; Bell, A.D.; Gutierrez, L.; Rosenthal, J. HLA Haploidentical Stem Cell Transplant with Pretransplant Immunosuppression for Patients with Sickle Cell Disease. *Biol. Blood Marrow Transplant.* **2018**, *24*, 185–189. [CrossRef]
31. Brissot, E.; Labopin, M.; Labussière, H.; Fossard, G.; Chevallier, P.; Guillaume, T.; Yakoub-Agha, I.; Srour, M.; Bulabois, C.-E.; Huynh, A.; et al. Post-Transplant Cyclophosphamide versus Anti-Thymocyte Globulin after Reduced Intensity Peripheral Blood Allogeneic Cell Transplantation in Recipients of Matched Sibling or 10/10 HLA Matched Unrelated Donors: Final Analysis of a Randomized, Open-Label, Multicenter, Phase 2 Trial. *Blood Cancer J.* **2024**, *14*, 31. [CrossRef]
32. Trujillo, Á.M.; Karduss, A.J.; Suarez, G.; Pérez, R.; Ruiz, G.; Cardona, A.; Ramírez, M.; Betancur, J. Haploidentical Hematopoietic Stem Cell Transplantation with Post-Transplantation Cyclophosphamide in Children with High-Risk Leukemia Using a Reduced-Intensity Conditioning Regimen and Peripheral Blood as the Stem Cell Source. *Transplant. Cell Ther.* **2021**, *27*, 427.e1–427.e7. [CrossRef]
33. Li, T.; He, Q.; Yang, J.; Cai, Y.; Huang, C.; Xu, X.; Qiu, H.; Niu, J.; Zhou, K.; Zhang, Y.; et al. Low-Dose Anti-Thymocyte Globulin Plus Low-Dose Posttransplant Cyclophosphamide as an Effective Regimen for Prophylaxis of Graft Versus Host Disease After Haploidentical Peripheral Blood Stem Cell Transplantation With Maternal/Collateral Related Donors. *Cell Transplant.* **2022**, *31*, 9636897221139103. [CrossRef] [PubMed]
34. Huang, Z.; Yan, H.; Teng, Y.; Shi, W.; Xia, L. Lower Dose of ATG Combined with Basiliximab for Haploidentical Hematopoietic Stem Cell Transplantation Is Associated with Effective Control of GVHD and Less CMV Viremia. *Front. Immunol.* **2022**, *13*, 1017850. [CrossRef] [PubMed]
35. Tang, F.-F.; Cheng, Y.-F.; Xu, L.-P.; Zhang, X.-H.; Yan, C.-H.; Han, W.; Chen, Y.-H.; Huang, X.-J.; Wang, Y. Basiliximab as Treatment for Steroid-Refractory Acute Graft-versus-Host Disease in Pediatric Patients after Haploidentical Hematopoietic Stem Cell Transplantation. *Biol. Blood Marrow Transplant.* **2020**, *26*, 351–357. [CrossRef] [PubMed]
36. Hunger, S.P.; Raetz, E.A. How I Treat Relapsed Acute Lymphoblastic Leukemia in the Pediatric Population. *Blood* **2020**, *136*, 1803–1812. [CrossRef] [PubMed]
37. Zarnegar-Lumley, S.; Caldwell, K.J.; Rubnitz, J.E. Relapsed Acute Myeloid Leukemia in Children and Adolescents: Current Treatment Options and Future Strategies. *Leukemia* **2022**, *36*, 1951–1960. [CrossRef] [PubMed]
38. Fagioli, F.; Quarello, P.; Zecca, M.; Lanino, E.; Rognoni, C.; Balduzzi, A.; Messina, C.; Favre, C.; Foà, R.; Ripaldi, M.; et al. Hematopoietic Stem Cell Transplantation for Children with High-Risk Acute Lymphoblastic Leukemia in First Complete Remission: A Report from the AIEOP Registry. *Haematologica* **2013**, *98*, 1273–1281. [CrossRef] [PubMed]
39. Peters, C.; Schrappe, M.; von Stackelberg, A.; Schrauder, A.; Bader, P.; Ebell, W.; Lang, P.; Sykora, K.-W.; Schrum, J.; Kremens, B.; et al. Stem-Cell Transplantation in Children with Acute Lymphoblastic Leukemia: A Prospective International Multicenter Trial Comparing Sibling Donors with Matched Unrelated Donors-The ALL-SCT-BFM-2003 Trial. *J. Clin. Oncol.* **2015**, *33*, 1265–1274. [CrossRef] [PubMed]
40. Lang, P.; Handgretinger, R. Haploidentical SCT in Children: An Update and Future Perspectives. *Bone Marrow Transplant.* **2008**, *42* (Suppl. 2), S54–S59. [CrossRef] [PubMed]
41. Powles, R.L.; Morgenstern, G.R.; Kay, H.E.; McElwain, T.J.; Clink, H.M.; Dady, P.J.; Barrett, A.; Jameson, B.; Depledge, M.H.; Watson, J.G.; et al. Mismatched Family Donors for Bone-Marrow Transplantation as Treatment for Acute Leukaemia. *Lancet* **1983**, *1*, 612–615. [CrossRef]
42. Kernan, N.A.; Flomenberg, N.; Dupont, B.; O'Reilly, R.J. Graft Rejection in Recipients of T-Cell-Depleted HLA-Nonidentical Marrow Transplants for Leukemia. Identification of Host-Derived Antidonor Allocytotoxic T Lymphocytes. *Transplantation* **1987**, *43*, 842–847. [CrossRef]
43. Soiffer, R.J.; Mauch, P.; Tarbell, N.J.; Anderson, K.C.; Freedman, A.S.; Rabinowe, S.N.; Takvorian, T.; Murrey, C.I.; Coral, F.; Bosserman, L. Total Lymphoid Irradiation to Prevent Graft Rejection in Recipients of HLA Non-Identical T Cell-Depleted Allogeneic Marrow. *Bone Marrow Transplant.* **1991**, *7*, 23–33. [PubMed]

44. Aversa, F.; Tabilio, A.; Velardi, A.; Cunningham, I.; Terenzi, A.; Falzetti, F.; Ruggeri, L.; Barbabietola, G.; Aristei, C.; Latini, P.; et al. Treatment of High-Risk Acute Leukemia with T-Cell-Depleted Stem Cells from Related Donors with One Fully Mismatched HLA Haplotype. *N. Engl. J. Med.* **1998**, *339*, 1186–1193. [CrossRef] [PubMed]
45. Pasquini, M.C.; Devine, S.; Mendizabal, A.; Baden, L.R.; Wingard, J.R.; Lazarus, H.M.; Appelbaum, F.R.; Keever-Taylor, C.A.; Horowitz, M.M.; Carter, S.; et al. Comparative Outcomes of Donor Graft CD34+ Selection and Immune Suppressive Therapy as Graft-versus-Host Disease Prophylaxis for Patients with Acute Myeloid Leukemia in Complete Remission Undergoing HLA-Matched Sibling Allogeneic Hematopoietic Cell Transplantation. *J. Clin. Oncol.* **2012**, *30*, 3194–3201. [CrossRef] [PubMed]
46. Lang, P.; Greil, J.; Bader, P.; Handgretinger, R.; Klingebiel, T.; Schumm, M.; Schlegel, P.-G.; Feuchtinger, T.; Pfeiffer, M.; Scheel-Walter, H.; et al. Long-Term Outcome after Haploidentical Stem Cell Transplantation in Children. *Blood Cells Mol. Dis.* **2004**, *33*, 281–287. [CrossRef] [PubMed]
47. Chen, X.; Hale, G.A.; Barfield, R.; Benaim, E.; Leung, W.H.; Knowles, J.; Horwitz, E.M.; Woodard, P.; Kasow, K.; Yusuf, U.; et al. Rapid Immune Reconstitution after a Reduced-Intensity Conditioning Regimen and a CD3-Depleted Haploidentical Stem Cell Graft for Paediatric Refractory Haematological Malignancies. *Br. J. Haematol.* **2006**, *135*, 524–532. [CrossRef] [PubMed]
48. Pérez-Martínez, A.; González-Vicent, M.; Valentín, J.; Aleo, E.; Lassaletta, A.; Sevilla, J.; Vicario, J.L.; Ramírez, M.; Díaz, M.A. Early Evaluation of Immune Reconstitution Following Allogeneic CD3/CD19-Depleted Grafts from Alternative Donors in Childhood Acute Leukemia. *Bone Marrow Transplant.* **2012**, *47*, 1419–1427. [CrossRef] [PubMed]
49. Lang, P.; Teltschik, H.-M.; Feuchtinger, T.; Müller, I.; Pfeiffer, M.; Schumm, M.; Ebinger, M.; Schwarze, C.P.; Gruhn, B.; Schrauder, A.; et al. Transplantation of CD3/CD19 Depleted Allografts from Haploidentical Family Donors in Paediatric Leukaemia. *Br. J. Haematol.* **2014**, *165*, 688–698. [CrossRef] [PubMed]
50. Locatelli, F.; Merli, P.; Pagliara, D.; Li Pira, G.; Falco, M.; Pende, D.; Rondelli, R.; Lucarelli, B.; Brescia, L.P.; Masetti, R.; et al. Outcome of Children with Acute Leukemia given HLA-Haploidentical HSCT after Aβ T-Cell and B-Cell Depletion. *Blood* **2017**, *130*, 677–685. [CrossRef] [PubMed]
51. Merli, P.; Algeri, M.; Galaverna, F.; Bertaina, V.; Lucarelli, B.; Boccieri, E.; Becilli, M.; Quagliarella, F.; Rosignoli, C.; Biagini, S.; et al. TCRαβ/CD19 Cell-Depleted HLA-Haploidentical Transplantation to Treat Pediatric Acute Leukemia: Updated Final Analysis. *Blood* **2024**, *143*, 279–289. [CrossRef]
52. Pérez-Martínez, A.; Ferreras, C.; Pascual, A.; Gonzalez-Vicent, M.; Alonso, L.; Badell, I.; Fernández Navarro, J.M.; Regueiro, A.; Plaza, M.; Pérez Hurtado, J.M.; et al. Haploidentical Transplantation in High-Risk Pediatric Leukemia: A Retrospective Comparative Analysis on Behalf of the Spanish Working Group for Bone Marrow Transplantation in Children (GETMON) and the Spanish Grupo for Hematopoietic Transplantation (GETH). *Am. J. Hematol.* **2020**, *95*, 28–37. [CrossRef]
53. Otto, M.; Barfield, R.C.; Iyengar, R.; Gatewood, J.; Müller, I.; Holladay, M.S.; Houston, J.; Leung, W.; Handgretinger, R. Human Gammadelta T Cells from G-CSF-Mobilized Donors Retain Strong Tumoricidal Activity and Produce Immunomodulatory Cytokines after Clinical-Scale Isolation. *J. Immunother.* **2005**, *28*, 73–78. [CrossRef] [PubMed]
54. Gertner-Dardenne, J.; Castellano, R.; Mamessier, E.; Garbit, S.; Kochbati, E.; Etienne, A.; Charbonnier, A.; Collette, Y.; Vey, N.; Olive, D. Human Vγ9Vδ2 T Cells Specifically Recognize and Kill Acute Myeloid Leukemic Blasts. *J. Immunol.* **2012**, *188*, 4701–4708. [CrossRef]
55. Saitoh, A.; Narita, M.; Watanabe, N.; Tochiki, N.; Satoh, N.; Takizawa, J.; Furukawa, T.; Toba, K.; Aizawa, Y.; Shinada, S.; et al. Anti-Tumor Cytotoxicity of Gammadelta T Cells Expanded from Peripheral Blood Cells of Patients with Myeloma and Lymphoma. *Med. Oncol.* **2008**, *25*, 137–147. [CrossRef] [PubMed]
56. Godder, K.T.; Henslee-Downey, P.J.; Mehta, J.; Park, B.S.; Chiang, K.-Y.; Abhyankar, S.; Lamb, L.S. Long Term Disease-Free Survival in Acute Leukemia Patients Recovering with Increased Gammadelta T Cells after Partially Mismatched Related Donor Bone Marrow Transplantation. *Bone Marrow Transplant.* **2007**, *39*, 751–757. [CrossRef] [PubMed]
57. Perko, R.; Kang, G.; Sunkara, A.; Leung, W.; Thomas, P.G.; Dallas, M.H. Gamma Delta T Cell Reconstitution Is Associated with Fewer Infections and Improved Event-Free Survival after Hematopoietic Stem Cell Transplantation for Pediatric Leukemia. *Biol. Blood Marrow Transplant.* **2015**, *21*, 130–136. [CrossRef] [PubMed]
58. Dadi, G.; Jacoby, E.; Adam, E.; Hutt, D.; Varda-Bloom, N.; Bielorai, B.; Toren, A. Aβ+ /CD19+ -Depleted Haploidentical Stem Cell Transplantation for Children with Acute Leukemia: Is There a Protective Effect of Increased Γδ+ T-Cell Content in the Graft? *Pediatr. Transplant.* **2023**, *27*, e14531. [CrossRef] [PubMed]
59. Klingebiel, T.; Cornish, J.; Labopin, M.; Locatelli, F.; Darbyshire, P.; Handgretinger, R.; Balduzzi, A.; Owoc-Lempach, J.; Fagioli, F.; Or, R.; et al. Results and Factors Influencing Outcome after Fully Haploidentical Hematopoietic Stem Cell Transplantation in Children with Very High-Risk Acute Lymphoblastic Leukemia: Impact of Center Size: An Analysis on Behalf of the Acute Leukemia and Pediatric Disease Working Parties of the European Blood and Marrow Transplant Group. *Blood* **2010**, *115*, 3437–3446. [CrossRef] [PubMed]
60. Bunin, N.J.; Davies, S.M.; Aplenc, R.; Camitta, B.M.; DeSante, K.B.; Goyal, R.K.; Kapoor, N.; Kernan, N.A.; Rosenthal, J.; Smith, F.O.; et al. Unrelated Donor Bone Marrow Transplantation for Children with Acute Myeloid Leukemia beyond First Remission or Refractory to Chemotherapy. *J. Clin. Oncol.* **2008**, *26*, 4326–4332. [CrossRef] [PubMed]
61. O'Hare, P.; Lucchini, G.; Cummins, M.; Veys, P.; Potter, M.; Lawson, S.; Vora, A.; Wynn, R.; Peniket, A.; Kirkland, K.; et al. Allogeneic Stem Cell Transplantation for Refractory Acute Myeloid Leukemia in Pediatric Patients: The UK Experience. *Bone Marrow Transplant.* **2017**, *52*, 825–831. [CrossRef]

62. Shelikhova, L.; Ilushina, M.; Shekhovtsova, Z.; Shasheleva, D.; Khismatullina, R.; Kurnikova, E.; Pershin, D.; Balashov, D.; Radygina, S.; Trakhtman, P.; et al. Aβ T Cell-Depleted Haploidentical Hematopoietic Stem Cell Transplantation without Antithymocyte Globulin in Children with Chemorefractory Acute Myelogenous Leukemia. *Biol. Blood Marrow Transplant.* **2019**, *25*, e179–e182. [CrossRef]
63. Edinger, M.; Hoffmann, P.; Ermann, J.; Drago, K.; Fathman, C.G.; Strober, S.; Negrin, R.S. CD4+CD25+ Regulatory T Cells Preserve Graft-versus-Tumor Activity While Inhibiting Graft-versus-Host Disease after Bone Marrow Transplantation. *Nat. Med.* **2003**, *9*, 1144–1150. [CrossRef] [PubMed]
64. Di Ianni, M.; Falzetti, F.; Carotti, A.; Terenzi, A.; Castellino, F.; Bonifacio, E.; Del Papa, B.; Zei, T.; Ostini, R.I.; Cecchini, D.; et al. Tregs Prevent GVHD and Promote Immune Reconstitution in HLA-Haploidentical Transplantation. *Blood* **2011**, *117*, 3921–3928. [CrossRef] [PubMed]
65. Martelli, M.F.; Di Ianni, M.; Ruggeri, L.; Falzetti, F.; Carotti, A.; Terenzi, A.; Pierini, A.; Massei, M.S.; Amico, L.; Urbani, E.; et al. HLA-Haploidentical Transplantation with Regulatory and Conventional T-Cell Adoptive Immunotherapy Prevents Acute Leukemia Relapse. *Blood* **2014**, *124*, 638–644. [CrossRef] [PubMed]
66. Pierini, A.; Ruggeri, L.; Carotti, A.; Falzetti, F.; Saldi, S.; Terenzi, A.; Zucchetti, C.; Ingrosso, G.; Zei, T.; Iacucci Ostini, R.; et al. Haploidentical Age-Adapted Myeloablative Transplant and Regulatory and Effector T Cells for Acute Myeloid Leukemia. *Blood Adv.* **2021**, *5*, 1199–1208. [CrossRef] [PubMed]
67. Massei, M.S.; Capolsini, I.; Mastrodicasa, E.; Perruccio, K.; Arcioni, F.; Cerri, C.; Gurdo, G.; Sciabolacci, S.; Falzetti, F.; Zei, T.; et al. HLA-Haploidentical Hematopoietic Stem Cells Transplantation with Regulatory and Conventional T-Cell Adoptive Immunotherapy in Pediatric Patients with Very High-Risk Acute Leukemia. *Bone Marrow Transplant.* **2023**, *58*, 526–533. [CrossRef]
68. Xu, Z.-L.; Huang, X.-J. Haploidentical Transplants with a G-CSF/ATG-Based Protocol: Experience from China. *Blood Rev.* **2023**, *62*, 101035. [CrossRef]
69. Huang, X.J.; Han, W.; Xu, L.P.; Chen, H.; Liu, D.H.; Chen, Y.H.; Jiang, Q.; Lu, J.; Liu, K.Y.; Ren, H.Y.; et al. A novel approach to HLA-mismatched transplantation. *Beijing Da Xue Xue Bao Yi Xue Ban = J. Peking Univ. Health Sci.* **2004**, *36*, 229–233.
70. Vendramin, A.; Gimondi, S.; Bermema, A.; Longoni, P.; Rizzitano, S.; Corradini, P.; Carniti, C. Graft Monocytic Myeloid-Derived Suppressor Cell Content Predicts the Risk of Acute Graft-versus-Host Disease after Allogeneic Transplantation of Granulocyte Colony-Stimulating Factor-Mobilized Peripheral Blood Stem Cells. *Biol. Blood Marrow Transplant.* **2014**, *20*, 2049–2055. [CrossRef]
71. Lv, M.; Zhao, X.-S.; Hu, Y.; Chang, Y.-J.; Zhao, X.-Y.; Kong, Y.; Zhang, X.-H.; Xu, L.-P.; Liu, K.-Y.; Huang, X.-J. Monocytic and Promyelocytic Myeloid-Derived Suppressor Cells May Contribute to G-CSF-Induced Immune Tolerance in Haplo-Identical Allogeneic Hematopoietic Stem Cell Transplantation. *Am. J. Hematol.* **2015**, *90*, E9–E16. [CrossRef]
72. D'Aveni, M.; Rossignol, J.; Coman, T.; Sivakumaran, S.; Henderson, S.; Manzo, T.; Santos e Sousa, P.; Bruneau, J.; Fouquet, G.; Zavala, F.; et al. G-CSF Mobilizes CD34+ Regulatory Monocytes That Inhibit Graft-versus-Host Disease. *Sci. Transl. Med.* **2015**, *7*, 281ra42. [CrossRef]
73. Chang, Y.-J.; Zhao, X.-S.; Lv, M.; Zhao, X.-Y.; Han, T.-T.; Wang, H.-T.; Huang, X.-J. CD19+CD24highCD38high B Cells Exhibit Higher Ability in TGF-β and IL-10 Secretion and Suppressing of CD4+ T Cell Proliferation but Are Quantitatively Decreased in G-BM of Healthy Donors (P2146). *J. Immunol.* **2013**, *190*, 69.11. [CrossRef]
74. Hu, Y.; He, G.-L.; Zhao, X.-Y.; Zhao, X.-S.; Wang, Y.; Xu, L.-P.; Zhang, X.-H.; Yu, X.-Z.; Liu, K.-Y.; Chang, Y.-J.; et al. Regulatory B Cells Promote Graft-versus-Host Disease Prevention and Maintain Graft-versus-Leukemia Activity Following Allogeneic Bone Marrow Transplantation. *OncoImmunology* **2017**, *6*, e1284721. [CrossRef] [PubMed]
75. Liu, Q.-F.; Fan, Z.-P.; Wu, M.-Q.; Sun, J.; Wu, X.-L.; Xu, D.; Jiang, Q.-L.; Zhang, Y.; Huang, F.; Wei, Y.-Q.; et al. Allo-HSCT for Acute Leukemia of Ambiguous Lineage in Adults: The Comparison between Standard Conditioning and Intensified Conditioning Regimens. *Ann. Hematol.* **2013**, *92*, 679–687. [CrossRef] [PubMed]
76. Lv, M.; Chang, Y.; Huang, X. Update of the "Beijing Protocol" Haplo-Identical Hematopoietic Stem Cell Transplantation. *Bone Marrow Transplant.* **2019**, *54*, 703–707. [CrossRef] [PubMed]
77. Sun, Y.Q.; Xu, L.P.; Zhang, X.H.; Liu, D.H.; Chen, H.; Wang, Y.; Yan, C.H.; Wang, J.Z.; Wang, F.R.; Zhang, Y.Y.; et al. A Retrospective Comparison of BU-Fludarabine and BU–CY Regimens in Elderly Patients or in Patients with Comorbidities Who Received Unmanipulated Haploidentical Hematopoietic SCT. *Bone Marrow Transplant.* **2015**, *50*, 601–603. [CrossRef] [PubMed]
78. Zheng, F.-M.; Zhang, X.; Li, C.-F.; Cheng, Y.-F.; Gao, L.; He, Y.-L.; Wang, Y.; Huang, X.-J. Haploidentical- versus Identical-sibling Transplant for High-risk Pediatric AML: A Multi-center Study. *Cancer Commun.* **2020**, *40*, 93–104. [CrossRef] [PubMed]
79. Schlieben, S.; Borkhardt, A.; Reinisch, I.; Ritterbach, J.; Janssen, J.W.; Ratei, R.; Schrappe, M.; Repp, R.; Zimmermann, M.; Kabisch, H.; et al. Incidence and Clinical Outcome of Children with BCR/ABL-Positive Acute Lymphoblastic Leukemia (ALL). A Prospective RT-PCR Study Based on 673 Patients Enrolled in the German Pediatric Multicenter Therapy Trials ALL-BFM-90 and CoALL-05-92. *Leukemia* **1996**, *10*, 957–963. [PubMed]
80. Aricò, M.; Valsecchi, M.G.; Camitta, B.; Schrappe, M.; Chessells, J.; Baruchel, A.; Gaynon, P.; Silverman, L.; Janka-Schaub, G.; Kamps, W.; et al. Outcome of Treatment in Children with Philadelphia Chromosome–Positive Acute Lymphoblastic Leukemia. *N. Engl. J. Med.* **2000**, *342*, 998–1006. [CrossRef] [PubMed]
81. Chen, H.; Liu, K.; Xu, L.; Chen, Y.; Zhang, X.; Wang, Y.; Qin, Y.; Liu, Y.; Lai, Y.; Huang, X. Haploidentical Hematopoietic Stem Cell Transplantation for Pediatric Philadelphia Chromosome-Positive Acute Lymphoblastic Leukemia in the Imatinib Era. *Leuk. Res.* **2017**, *59*, 136–141. [CrossRef]

82. Xue, Y.-J.; Cheng, Y.-F.; Lu, A.-D.; Wang, Y.; Zuo, Y.-X.; Yan, C.-H.; Wu, J.; Sun, Y.-Q.; Suo, P.; Chen, Y.-H.; et al. Allogeneic Hematopoietic Stem Cell Transplantation, Especially Haploidentical, May Improve Long-Term Survival for High-Risk Pediatric Patients with Philadelphia Chromosome-Positive Acute Lymphoblastic Leukemia in the Tyrosine Kinase Inhibitor Era. *Biol. Blood Marrow Transplant.* **2019**, *25*, 1611–1620. [CrossRef]
83. Xue, Y.-J.; Suo, P.; Huang, X.-J.; Lu, A.-D.; Wang, Y.; Zuo, Y.-X.; Yan, C.-H.; Wu, J.; Kong, J.; Zhang, X.-H.; et al. Superior Survival of Unmanipulated Haploidentical Haematopoietic Stem Cell Transplantation Compared with Intensive Chemotherapy as Post-Remission Treatment for Children with Very High-Risk Philadelphia Chromosome Negative B-Cell Acute Lymphoblastic Leukaemia in First Complete Remission. *Br. J. Haematol.* **2020**, *188*, 757–767. [CrossRef] [PubMed]
84. Bai, L.; Cheng, Y.-F.; Lu, A.-D.; Suo, P.; Wang, Y.; Zuo, Y.-X.; Yan, C.-H.; Wu, J.; Jia, Y.-P.; Sun, Y.-Q.; et al. Prognosis of Haploidentical Hematopoietic Stem Cell Transplantation in Non-Infant Children with t(v;11q23)/MLL-Rearranged B-Cell Acute Lymphoblastic Leukemia. *Leuk. Res.* **2020**, *91*, 106333. [CrossRef] [PubMed]
85. Hu, G.-H.; Zhao, X.-Y.; Zuo, Y.-X.; Chang, Y.-J.; Suo, P.; Wu, J.; Jia, Y.-P.; Lu, A.-D.; Li, Y.-C.; Wang, Y.; et al. Unmanipulated Haploidentical Hematopoietic Stem Cell Transplantation Is an Excellent Option for Children and Young Adult Relapsed/Refractory Philadelphia Chromosome-Negative B-Cell Acute Lymphoblastic Leukemia after CAR-T-Cell Therapy. *Leukemia* **2021**, *35*, 3092–3100. [CrossRef] [PubMed]
86. Gaynon, P.S.; Angiolillo, A.L.; Carroll, W.L.; Nachman, J.B.; Trigg, M.E.; Sather, H.N.; Hunger, S.P.; Devidas, M. Children's Oncology Group Long-Term Results of the Children's Cancer Group Studies for Childhood Acute Lymphoblastic Leukemia 1983–2002: A Children's Oncology Group Report. *Leukemia* **2010**, *24*, 285–297. [CrossRef] [PubMed]
87. Bader, P.; Kreyenberg, H.; Henze, G.H.R.; Eckert, C.; Reising, M.; Willasch, A.; Barth, A.; Borkhardt, A.; Peters, C.; Handgretinger, R.; et al. Prognostic Value of Minimal Residual Disease Quantification before Allogeneic Stem-Cell Transplantation in Relapsed Childhood Acute Lymphoblastic Leukemia: The ALL-REZ BFM Study Group. *J. Clin. Oncol.* **2009**, *27*, 377–384. [CrossRef] [PubMed]
88. Hu, G.; Cheng, Y.; Zuo, Y.; Chang, Y.; Suo, P.; Jia, Y.; Lu, A.; Wang, Y.; Jiao, S.; Zhang, L.; et al. Comparisons of Long-Term Survival and Safety of Haploidentical Hematopoietic Stem Cell Transplantation After CAR-T Cell Therapy or Chemotherapy in Pediatric Patients With First Relapse of B-Cell Acute Lymphoblastic Leukemia Based on MRD-Guided Treatment. *Front. Immunol.* **2022**, *13*, 915590. [CrossRef] [PubMed]
89. Winters, A.C.; Bernt, K.M. MLL-Rearranged Leukemias—An Update on Science and Clinical Approaches. *Front. Pediatr.* **2017**, *5*, 4. [CrossRef] [PubMed]
90. Creutzig, U.; Zimmermann, M.; Reinhardt, D.; Rasche, M.; von Neuhoff, C.; Alpermann, T.; Dworzak, M.; Perglerová, K.; Zemanova, Z.; Tchinda, J.; et al. Changes in Cytogenetics and Molecular Genetics in Acute Myeloid Leukemia from Childhood to Adult Age Groups. *Cancer* **2016**, *122*, 3821–3830. [CrossRef] [PubMed]
91. Yang, W.; Qin, M.; Jia, C.; Yang, J.; Chen, W.; Luo, Y.; Jing, Y.; Wang, B. Pediatric Acute Myeloid Leukemia Patients with KMT2A Rearrangements: A Single-Center Retrospective Study. *Hematology* **2022**, *27*, 583–589. [CrossRef]
92. Bolouri, H.; Farrar, J.E.; Triche, T.; Ries, R.E.; Lim, E.L.; Alonzo, T.A.; Ma, Y.; Moore, R.; Mungall, A.J.; Marra, M.A.; et al. The Molecular Landscape of Pediatric Acute Myeloid Leukemia Reveals Recurrent Structural Alterations and Age-Specific Mutational Interactions. *Nat. Med.* **2018**, *24*, 103–112. [CrossRef]
93. Pieters, R.; Schrappe, M.; De Lorenzo, P.; Hann, I.; De Rossi, G.; Felice, M.; Hovi, L.; LeBlanc, T.; Szczepanski, T.; Ferster, A.; et al. A Treatment Protocol for Infants Younger than 1 Year with Acute Lymphoblastic Leukaemia (Interfant-99): An Observational Study and a Multicentre Randomised Trial. *Lancet* **2007**, *370*, 240–250. [CrossRef]
94. Creutzig, U.; Zimmermann, M.; Bourquin, J.-P.; Dworzak, M.N.; Kremens, B.; Lehrnbecher, T.; Von Neuhoff, C.; Sander, A.; Von Stackelberg, A.; Schmid, I.; et al. Favorable Outcome in Infants with AML after Intensive First- and Second-Line Treatment: An AML-BFM Study Group Report. *Leukemia* **2012**, *26*, 654–661. [CrossRef] [PubMed]
95. Peters, C.; Dalle, J.-H.; Locatelli, F.; Poetschger, U.; Sedlacek, P.; Buechner, J.; Shaw, P.J.; Staciuk, R.; Ifversen, M.; Pichler, H.; et al. Total Body Irradiation or Chemotherapy Conditioning in Childhood ALL: A Multinational, Randomized, Noninferiority Phase III Study. *JCO* **2021**, *39*, 295–307. [CrossRef] [PubMed]
96. Hu, G.-H.; Zhang, X.-H.; Wang, Y.; Xu, L.-P.; Hou, X.-L.; Cheng, Y.-F.; Huang, X.-J. The Prognosis of Haploidentical Hematopoietic Stem Cell Transplantation in Infants and Patients under 3 Years Old with Acute Leukemia. *Clin. Transplant.* **2024**, *38*, e15247. [CrossRef] [PubMed]
97. Mayumi, H.; Umesue, M.; Nomoto, K. Cyclophosphamide-Induced Immunological Tolerance: An Overview. *Immunobiology* **1996**, *195*, 129–139. [CrossRef] [PubMed]
98. Luznik, L.; O'Donnell, P.V.; Symons, H.J.; Chen, A.R.; Leffell, M.S.; Zahurak, M.; Gooley, T.A.; Piantadosi, S.; Kaup, M.; Ambinder, R.F.; et al. HLA-Haploidentical Bone Marrow Transplantation for Hematologic Malignancies Using Nonmyeloablative Conditioning and High-Dose, Posttransplantation Cyclophosphamide. *Biol. Blood Marrow Transplant.* **2008**, *14*, 641–650. [CrossRef] [PubMed]
99. Luznik, L.; Engstrom, L.W.; Iannone, R.; Fuchs, E.J. Posttransplantation Cyclophosphamide Facilitates Engraftment of Major Histocompatibility Complex-Identical Allogeneic Marrow in Mice Conditioned with Low-Dose Total Body Irradiation. *Biol. Blood Marrow Transplant.* **2002**, *8*, 131–138. [CrossRef]

100. O'Donnell, P.V.; Luznik, L.; Jones, R.J.; Vogelsang, G.B.; Leffell, M.S.; Phelps, M.; Rhubart, P.; Cowan, K.; Piantadosi, S.; Fuchs, E.J. Nonmyeloablative Bone Marrow Transplantation from Partially HLA-Mismatched Related Donors Using Posttransplantation Cyclophosphamide. *Biol. Blood Marrow Transplant.* **2002**, *8*, 377–386. [CrossRef] [PubMed]
101. Fuchs, E.J.; O'Donnell, P.V.; Eapen, M.; Logan, B.; Antin, J.H.; Dawson, P.; Devine, S.; Horowitz, M.M.; Horwitz, M.E.; Karanes, C.; et al. Double Unrelated Umbilical Cord Blood vs HLA-Haploidentical Bone Marrow Transplantation: The BMT CTN 1101 Trial. *Blood* **2021**, *137*, 420–428. [CrossRef]
102. Gagelmann, N.; Bacigalupo, A.; Rambaldi, A.; Hoelzer, D.; Halter, J.; Sanz, J.; Bonifazi, F.; Meijer, E.; Itälä-Remes, M.; Marková, M.; et al. Haploidentical Stem Cell Transplantation with Posttransplant Cyclophosphamide Therapy vs. Other Donor Transplantations in Adults with Hematologic Cancers. *JAMA. Oncol.* **2019**, *5*, 1739–1748. [CrossRef]
103. Sachdev, M.; Chakraborty, S.; Bansal, M.; Bhargava, R.; Dua, V. Encouraging Outcomes of Alternate Donor Hematopoietic Stem Cell Transplant in Pediatric High-Risk/Relapsed Leukemias: A Single Center Experience. *J. Pediatr. Hematol. Oncol.* **2021**, *43*, e1148–e1152. [CrossRef] [PubMed]
104. Xue, Y.-J.; Cheng, Y.-F.; Lu, A.-D.; Wang, Y.; Zuo, Y.-X.; Yan, C.-H.; Suo, P.; Zhang, L.-P.; Huang, X.-J. Efficacy of Haploidentical Hematopoietic Stem Cell Transplantation Compared With Chemotherapy as Postremission Treatment of Children With Intermediate-Risk Acute Myeloid Leukemia in First Complete Remission. *Clin. Lymphoma. Myeloma. Leuk* **2021**, *21*, e126–e136. [CrossRef] [PubMed]
105. Tannumsaeung, S.; Anurathapan, U.; Pakakasama, S.; Pongpitcha, P.; Songdej, D.; Sirachainan, N.; Andersson, B.S.; Hongeng, S. Effective T-Cell Replete Haploidentical Stem Cell Transplantation for Pediatric Patients with High-Risk Hematologic Disorders. *Eur. J. Haematol.* **2023**, *110*, 305–312. [CrossRef] [PubMed]
106. Song, Z.-L.; Liu, R.; Hu, T.; Li, J.-H.; Zhang, C.-X.; Zhang, L.; Zhong, D.-X.; Yue, M.; Shi, X.-D. Clinical Efficacy of Haplo-HSCT of ATG Combined with PTCy for Children with Myelodysplastic Syndrome. *Zhongguo Shi Yan Xue Ye Xue Za Zhi* **2022**, *30*, 516–521. [CrossRef] [PubMed]
107. Suo, P.; Wang, S.; Xue, Y.; Cheng, Y.; Kong, J.; Yan, C.; Zhao, X.; Chen, Y.; Han, W.; Xu, L.; et al. Unmanipulated Haploidentical Hematopoietic Stem Cell Transplantation for Children with Myelodysplastic Syndrome. *Pediatr. Transplant.* **2020**, *24*, e13864. [CrossRef] [PubMed]
108. Kohli, S.; Rastogi, N.; Nivargi, S.; Thakkar, D.; Katewa, S.; Yadav, S.P. Successful Haploidentical Stem Cell Transplant With Posttransplant Cyclophosphamide for Hemophagocytic Lymphohistiocytosis. *J. Pediatr. Hematol. Oncol.* **2019**, *41*, e158–e160. [CrossRef]
109. Swaminathan, V.V.; Uppuluri, R.; Meena, S.K.; Varla, H.; Chandar, R.; Ramakrishnan, B.; Jayakumar, I.; Raj, R. Treosulfan-Based Conditioning in Matched Family, Unrelated and Haploidentical Hematopoietic Stem Cell Transplantation for Genetic Hemophagocytic Lymphohistiocytosis: Experience and Outcomes over 10 Years from India. *Indian J. Hematol. Blood Transfus.* **2022**, *38*, 84–91. [CrossRef]
110. Fischer, A. Human Primary Immunodeficiency Diseases. *Immunity* **2007**, *27*, 835–845. [CrossRef] [PubMed]
111. Bousfiha, A.; Jeddane, L.; Picard, C.; Ailal, F.; Bobby Gaspar, H.; Al-Herz, W.; Chatila, T.; Crow, Y.J.; Cunningham-Rundles, C.; Etzioni, A.; et al. The 2017 IUIS Phenotypic Classification for Primary Immunodeficiencies. *J. Clin. Immunol.* **2018**, *38*, 129–143. [CrossRef]
112. Smith, A.R.; Gross, T.G.; Baker, K.S. Transplant Outcomes for Primary Immunodeficiency Disease. *Semin. Hematol.* **2010**, *47*, 79–85. [CrossRef]
113. Gragert, L.; Eapen, M.; Williams, E.; Freeman, J.; Spellman, S.; Baitty, R.; Hartzman, R.; Rizzo, J.D.; Horowitz, M.; Confer, D.; et al. HLA Match Likelihoods for Hematopoietic Stem-Cell Grafts in the U.S. Registry. *N. Engl. J. Med.* **2014**, *371*, 339–348. [CrossRef] [PubMed]
114. Gennery, A.R.; Slatter, M.A.; Grandin, L.; Taupin, P.; Cant, A.J.; Veys, P.; Amrolia, P.J.; Gaspar, H.B.; Davies, E.G.; Friedrich, W.; et al. Transplantation of Hematopoietic Stem Cells and Long-Term Survival for Primary Immunodeficiencies in Europe: Entering a New Century, Do We Do Better? *J. Allergy Clin. Immunol.* **2010**, *126*, 602–610.e1-11. [CrossRef] [PubMed]
115. Bethge, W.A.; Haegele, M.; Faul, C.; Lang, P.; Schumm, M.; Bornhauser, M.; Handgretinger, R.; Kanz, L. Haploidentical Allogeneic Hematopoietic Cell Transplantation in Adults with Reduced-Intensity Conditioning and CD3/CD19 Depletion: Fast Engraftment and Low Toxicity. *Exp. Hematol.* **2006**, *34*, 1746–1752. [CrossRef] [PubMed]
116. Locatelli, F.; Bauquet, A.; Palumbo, G.; Moretta, F.; Bertaina, A. Negative Depletion of α/B+ T Cells and of CD19+ B Lymphocytes: A Novel Frontier to Optimize the Effect of Innate Immunity in HLA-Mismatched Hematopoietic Stem Cell Transplantation. *Immunol. Lett.* **2013**, *155*, 21–23. [CrossRef] [PubMed]
117. Shah, R.M.; Elfeky, R.; Nademi, Z.; Qasim, W.; Amrolia, P.; Chiesa, R.; Rao, K.; Lucchini, G.; Silva, J.M.F.; Worth, A.; et al. T-Cell Receptor Aβ+ and CD19+ Cell-Depleted Haploidentical and Mismatched Hematopoietic Stem Cell Transplantation in Primary Immune Deficiency. *J. Allergy Clin. Immunol.* **2018**, *141*, 1417–1426.e1. [CrossRef] [PubMed]
118. Brettig, T.; Smart, J.; Choo, S.; Mechinaud, F.; Mitchell, R.; Raj, T.S.; Cole, T. Use of TCR A+β+/CD19+-Depleted Haploidentical Hematopoietic Stem Cell Transplant Is a Viable Option in Patients With Primary Immune Deficiency without Matched Sibling Donor. *J. Clin. Immunol.* **2019**, *39*, 505–511. [CrossRef] [PubMed]
119. Buckley, R.H.; Schiff, S.E.; Schiff, R.I.; Markert, L.; Williams, L.W.; Roberts, J.L.; Myers, L.A.; Ward, F.E. Hematopoietic Stem-Cell Transplantation for the Treatment of Severe Combined Immunodeficiency. *N. Engl. J. Med.* **1999**, *340*, 508–516. [CrossRef] [PubMed]

120. Buckley, R.H. Transplantation of Hematopoietic Stem Cells in Human Severe Combined Immunodeficiency: Longterm Outcomes. *Immunol. Res.* **2011**, *49*, 25–43. [CrossRef]
121. Neven, B.; Diana, J.-S.; Castelle, M.; Magnani, A.; Rosain, J.; Touzot, F.; Moreira, B.; Fremond, M.-L.; Briand, C.; Bendavid, M.; et al. Haploidentical Hematopoietic Stem Cell Transplantation with Post-Transplant Cyclophosphamide for Primary Immunodeficiencies and Inherited Disorders in Children. *Biol. Blood Marrow Transplant.* **2019**, *25*, 1363–1373. [CrossRef]
122. Holzer, U.; Döring, M.; Eichholz, T.; Ebinger, M.; Queudeville, M.; Turkiewicz, D.; Schwarz, K.; Handgretinger, R.; Lang, P.; Toporski, J. Matched versus Haploidentical Hematopoietic Stem Cell Transplantation as Treatment Options for Primary Immunodeficiencies in Children. *Transplant. Cell Ther.* **2021**, *27*, 71.e1–71.e12. [CrossRef]
123. Hassan, A.; Booth, C.; Brightwell, A.; Allwood, Z.; Veys, P.; Rao, K.; Hönig, M.; Friedrich, W.; Gennery, A.; Slatter, M.; et al. Outcome of Hematopoietic Stem Cell Transplantation for Adenosine Deaminase-Deficient Severe Combined Immunodeficiency. *Blood* **2012**, *120*, 3615–3624; quiz 3626. [CrossRef] [PubMed]
124. Sauer, A.V.; Mrak, E.; Jofra Hernandez, R.; Zacchi, E.; Cavani, F.; Casiraghi, M.; Grunebaum, E.; Roifman, C.M.; Cervi, M.C.; Ambrosi, A.; et al. ADA-Deficient SCID Is Associated with a Specific Microenvironment and Bone Phenotype Characterized by RANKL/OPG Imbalance and Osteoblast Insufficiency. *Blood* **2009**, *114*, 3216–3226. [CrossRef] [PubMed]
125. Bolaños-Meade, J.; Fuchs, E.J.; Luznik, L.; Lanzkron, S.M.; Gamper, C.J.; Jones, R.J.; Brodsky, R.A. HLA-Haploidentical Bone Marrow Transplantation with Posttransplant Cyclophosphamide Expands the Donor Pool for Patients with Sickle Cell Disease. *Blood* **2012**, *120*, 4285–4291. [CrossRef] [PubMed]
126. Morin-Zorman, S.; Loiseau, P.; Taupin, J.-L.; Caillat-Zucman, S. Donor-Specific Anti-HLA Antibodies in Allogeneic Hematopoietic Stem Cell Transplantation. *Front. Immunol.* **2016**, *7*, 307. [CrossRef] [PubMed]
127. Foell, J.; Schulte, J.H.; Pfirstinger, B.; Troeger, A.; Wolff, D.; Edinger, M.; Hofmann, P.; Aslanidis, C.; Lang, P.; Holler, E.; et al. Haploidentical CD3 or α/β T-Cell Depleted HSCT in Advanced Stage Sickle Cell Disease. *Bone Marrow Transplant.* **2019**, *54*, 1859–1867. [CrossRef] [PubMed]
128. Dallas, M.H.; Triplett, B.; Shook, D.R.; Hartford, C.; Srinivasan, A.; Laver, J.; Ware, R.; Leung, W. Long-Term Outcome and Evaluation of Organ Function in Pediatric Patients Undergoing Haploidentical and Matched Related Hematopoietic Cell Transplantation for Sickle Cell Disease. *Biol. Blood Marrow Transplant.* **2013**, *19*, 820–830. [CrossRef] [PubMed]
129. Wiebking, V.; Hütker, S.; Schmid, I.; Immler, S.; Feuchtinger, T.; Albert, M.H. Reduced Toxicity, Myeloablative HLA-Haploidentical Hematopoietic Stem Cell Transplantation with Post-Transplantation Cyclophosphamide for Sickle Cell Disease. *Ann. Hematol.* **2017**, *96*, 1373–1377. [CrossRef] [PubMed]
130. Xu, L.P.; Zhang, X.H.; Wang, F.R.; Mo, X.D.; Han, T.T.; Han, W.; Chen, Y.H.; Zhang, Y.Y.; Wang, J.Z.; Yan, C.H.; et al. Haploidentical Transplantation for Pediatric Patients with Acquired Severe Aplastic Anemia. *Bone Marrow Transplant.* **2017**, *52*, 381–387. [CrossRef] [PubMed]
131. Wang, Z.-K.; Yu, H.-J.; Cao, F.-L.; Liu, Z.-H.; Liu, Z.-Y.; Feng, W.-J.; Liu, X.-L.; Yu, Y.-Y.; Xiao, Y.; Li, L.-M.; et al. Donor-Derived Marrow Mesenchymal Stromal Cell Co-Transplantation Following a Haploidentical Hematopoietic Stem Cell Transplantation Trail to Treat Severe Aplastic Anemia in Children. *Ann. Hematol.* **2019**, *98*, 473–479. [CrossRef]
132. Jaiswal, S.R.; Bhakuni, P.; Zaman, S.; Bansal, S.; Bharadwaj, P.; Bhargava, S.; Chakrabarti, S. T Cell Costimulation Blockade Promotes Transplantation Tolerance in Combination with Sirolimus and Post-Transplantation Cyclophosphamide for Haploidentical Transplantation in Children with Severe Aplastic Anemia. *Transpl. Immunol.* **2017**, *43–44*, 54–59. [CrossRef]
133. Jaiswal, S.R.; Chatterjee, S.; Mukherjee, S.; Ray, K.; Chakrabarti, S. Pre-Transplant Sirolimus Might Improve the Outcome of Haploidentical Peripheral Blood Stem Cell Transplantation with Post-Transplant Cyclophosphamide for Patients with Severe Aplastic Anemia. *Bone Marrow Transplant.* **2015**, *50*, 873–875. [CrossRef] [PubMed]
134. Ayas, M.; Siddiqui, K.; Al-Jefri, A.; Al-Ahmari, A.; Ghemlas, I.; Al-Saedi, H.; Alanazi, A.; Jafri, R.; Ayas, M.F.; Al-Seraihi, A. Successful Outcome in Patients with Fanconi Anemia Undergoing T Cell-Replete Mismatched Related Donor Hematopoietic Cell Transplantation Using Reduced-Dose Cyclophosphamide Post-Transplantation. *Biol. Blood Marrow Transplant.* **2019**, *25*, 2217–2221. [CrossRef] [PubMed]
135. Gluckman, E.; Rocha, V.; Ionescu, I.; Bierings, M.; Harris, R.E.; Wagner, J.; Kurtzberg, J.; Champagne, M.A.; Bonfim, C.; Bittencourt, M.; et al. Results of Unrelated Cord Blood Transplant in Fanconi Anemia Patients: Risk Factor Analysis for Engraftment and Survival. *Biol. Blood Marrow Transplant.* **2007**, *13*, 1073–1082. [CrossRef] [PubMed]
136. Strocchio, L.; Pagliara, D.; Algeri, M.; Li Pira, G.; Rossi, F.; Bertaina, V.; Leone, G.; Pinto, R.M.; Andreani, M.; Agolini, E.; et al. HLA-Haploidentical TCRαβ+/CD19+-Depleted Stem Cell Transplantation in Children and Young Adults with Fanconi Anemia. *Blood Adv.* **2021**, *5*, 1333–1339. [CrossRef] [PubMed]
137. Sharma, A.; Rastogi, N.; Chatterjee, G.; Kapoor, R.; Nivargi, S.; Yadav, S.P. Haploidentical Stem Cell Transplantation With Post-Transplant Cyclophosphamide for Pediatric Acute Leukemia Is Safe and Effective. *J. Pediatr. Hematol. Oncol.* **2021**, *43*, e1033–e1036. [CrossRef] [PubMed]
138. Saglio, F.; Berger, M.; Spadea, M.; Pessolano, R.; Carraro, F.; Barone, M.; Quarello, P.; Vassallo, E.; Fagioli, F. Haploidentical HSCT with Post Transplantation Cyclophosphamide versus Unrelated Donor HSCT in Pediatric Patients Affected by Acute Leukemia. *Bone Marrow Transplant.* **2021**, *56*, 586–595. [CrossRef] [PubMed]

139. Srinivasan, A.; Raffa, E.; Wall, D.A.; Schechter, T.; Ali, M.; Chopra, Y.; Kung, R.; Chiang, K.-Y.; Krueger, J. Outcome of Haploidentical Peripheral Blood Allografts Using Post-Transplantation Cyclophosphamide Compared to Matched Sibling and Unrelated Donor Bone Marrow Allografts in Pediatric Patients with Hematologic Malignancies: A Single-Center Analysis. *Transplant. Cell Ther.* **2022**, *28*, 158.e1–158.e9. [CrossRef] [PubMed]
140. Maier, C.-P.; Klose, C.; Seitz, C.M.; Heubach, F.; Döring, M.; Meisel, R.; Schuster, F.R.; Gruhn, B.; Keller, F.; Rabsteyn, A.; et al. Influence of ATLG Serum Levels on CD3/CD19-Depleted Hematopoietic Grafts and on Immune Recovery in Pediatric Haplo-HSCT. *Blood Adv.* **2024**, *8*, 2160–2171. [CrossRef] [PubMed]
141. Yang, L.; Tan, Y.; Shi, J.; Zhao, Y.; Yu, J.; Hu, Y.; Lai, X.; Yang, Y.; Huang, H.; Luo, Y. Prophylactic Modified Donor Lymphocyte Infusion after Low-Dose ATG-F-Based Haploidentical HSCT with Myeloablative Conditioning in High-Risk Acute Leukemia: A Matched-Pair Analysis. *Bone Marrow Transplant.* **2021**, *56*, 664–672. [CrossRef]
142. Qi, S.-S.; Chen, Z.; Du, Y.; Sun, M.; Wang, Z.; Long, F.; Luo, L.; Xiong, H. Prophylactic Donor Lymphocyte Infusion after Haploidentical Hematopoietic Cell Transplantation and Post-Transplant Cyclophosphamide for Treatment of High-Risk Myeloid Neoplasms in Children: A Retrospective Study. *Pediatr. Blood Cancer* **2023**, *70*, e30659. [CrossRef]
143. Swaminathan, V.V.; Uppuluri, R.; Patel, S.; Sivashankaran, M.; Ravichandran, N.; Ramanan, K.M.; Ramakrishnan, B.; Vaidhyanathan, L.; Raj, R. Safety and Efficacy of Fresh Whole Blood Donor Lymphocyte Infusion in Children. *Bone Marrow Transplant.* **2019**, *54*, 1892–1897. [CrossRef] [PubMed]
144. Ruan, Y.; Luo, T.; Liu, Q.; Liu, X.; Chen, L.; Wen, J.; Xiao, Y.; Xie, D.; He, Y.; Wu, X.; et al. Features of Cytomegalovirus Infection and Evaluation of Cytomegalovirus-Specific T Cells Therapy in Children's Patients Following Allogeneic Hematopoietic Stem Cell Transplantation: A Retrospective Single-Center Study. *Front. Cell Infect. Microbiol.* **2022**, *12*, 1027341. [CrossRef] [PubMed]
145. Nishikawa, T. Human Leukocyte Antigen-Haploidentical Haematopoietic Stem Cell Transplantation Using Post-Transplant Cyclophosphamide for Paediatric Haematological Malignancies. *Cancers* **2024**, *16*, 600. [CrossRef] [PubMed]
146. Lin, A.; Flynn, J.; DeRespiris, L.; Figgins, B.; Griffin, M.; Lau, C.; Proli, A.; Devlin, S.; Cho, C.; Tamari, R.; et al. Letermovir for Prevention of Cytomegalovirus Reactivation in Haploidentical and Mismatched Adult Donor Allogeneic Hematopoietic Cell Transplantation with Post-Transplant Cyclophosphamide for Graft-versus-Host Disease Prophylaxis. *Transplant. Cell Ther.* **2021**, *27*, 85.e1–85.e6. [CrossRef] [PubMed]
147. Richert-Przygonska, M.; Jaremek, K.; Debski, R.; Konieczek, J.; Lecka, M.; Dziedzic, M.; Bogiel, T.; Styczynski, J.; Czyzewski, K. Letermovir Prophylaxis for Cytomegalovirus Infection in Children After Hematopoietic Cell Transplantation. *Anticancer Res.* **2022**, *42*, 3607–3612. [CrossRef]
148. Kuhn, A.; Puttkammer, J.; Madigan, T.; Dinnes, L.; Khan, S.; Ferdjallah, A.; Kohorst, M. Letermovir as Cytomegalovirus Prophylaxis in a Pediatric Cohort: A Retrospective Analysis. *Transplant. Cell Ther.* **2023**, *29*, 62.e1–62.e4. [CrossRef]

International Journal of
Molecular Sciences

MDPI

Opinion

The Current Landscape of Secondary Malignancies after CAR T-Cell Therapies: How Could Malignancies Be Prevented?

Stella Bouziana [1,*] and Dimitrios Bouzianas [2]

1 Department of Hematology, King's College Hospital, London SE59RS, UK
2 BReMeL, Biopharmaceutical and Regenerative Medicine Laboratories, 55534 Thessaloniki, Greece; dimbou55@gmail.com
* Correspondence: styliani.bouziana@nhs.net

Abstract: Chimeric antigen receptor (CAR) T-cell therapies have revolutionised the field of haematological malignancies by achieving impressive remission rates in patients with highly refractory haematological malignancies, improving overall survival. To date, six commercial anti-CD19 and anti-BCMA CAR T-cell products have been approved by the Food and Drug Administration (FDA) for the treatment of relapsed/refractory B-cell haematological malignancies and multiple myeloma. The indications for CAR T-cell therapies are gradually expanding, with these therapies being investigated in a variety of diseases, including non-malignant ones. Despite the great success, there are several challenges surrounding CAR T-cell therapies, such as non-durable responses and high-grade toxicities. In addition, a new safety concern was added by the FDA on 28 November 2023 following reports of T-cell malignancies in patients previously treated with either anti-CD19 or anti-BCMA autologous CAR T-cell therapies both in clinical trials and in the real-world setting. Since then, several reports have been published presenting the incidence and analysing the risks of other secondary malignancies after CAR T-cell therapies. In this opinion article, the current landscape of secondary malignancies after CAR T-cell therapies is presented, along with a proposed strategy for future research aiming at potentially diminishing or abrogating the risk of developing secondary malignancies after CAR T-cell therapies.

Keywords: CAR T-cell therapies; relapsed/refractory haematological malignancies; secondary T-cell lymphomas/leukaemias; secondary malignancies; viral vectors; genome editing; genotoxicity

1. Introduction: Current CAR T-Cell Treatment Landscape

The broad application of novel technologies and the advancement of genetic engineering have resulted in the development of chimeric antigen receptor (CAR) T-cell therapies, which have revolutionised the field of haematological malignancies. CAR T-cell therapies are engineered to selectively target and eliminate tumour cells while recruiting and activating host immune cells as scavengers in the battle against the killing of cancer cells [1]. T-cells are collected through leukapheresis, and a synthetic transgene is incorporated into the genome of T-cells ex vivo by a replication-defective self-inactivated viral vector to express a CAR on the surface of T-cells [2]. CARs comprise an antigen-binding extracellular immunoglobulin-derived single-chain variable fragment domain fused to a hinge and a transmembrane region. The latter binds to an intracellular costimulatory domain in second-generation products, either 4-1BB or CD28, followed by the CD3z T-cell receptor signalling chain. Currently, there are five generations of CAR T-cells under development [3,4]. CAR T-cells are infused after the administration of a lymphodepleting regimen that creates a favourable immune environment for CAR T-cells to proliferate and function. Once bound to the targeted antigen, CAR T-cells are activated and expanded in vivo to destroy cancer cells [3,5].

CAR T-cell therapies have proven extremely potent in inducing remission in patients with highly refractory and aggressive haematological malignancies, offering effective

disease control and improving overall survival [6–8]. To date, six commercial anti-CD19 and anti-BCMA CAR T-cell products have been approved by the Food and Drug Administration (FDA) with the indication of treating relapsed/refractory (R/R) high-grade and indolent B-cell non-Hodgkin lymphomas (B-NHLs), B-cell acute lymphoblastic leukaemia (B-ALL) and multiple myeloma [9]. Recently, the FDA granted accelerated approval to one of these products (lisocabtagene maraleucel) for the treatment of adult patients with R/R chronic lymphocytic leukaemia or small lymphocytic lymphoma [10] (Table 1).

Table 1. Summary of the currently approved CAR T-cell products by the FDA for commercial application.

CAR T-Cell Product	Brand Name	Company	Disease Indications (R/R)	Year Initially Approved	Target Antigen	Costimulatory Domain	Viral Vector
Tisagenlecleucel	Kymriah	Novartis	B-ALL (≤25 years) LBCL FL	2017	CD19	4-1BB	Lentiviral
Axicabtagene ciloleucel	Yescarta	Kite	LBCL FL	2017	CD19	CD28	Retroviral
Brexucabtagene autoleucel	Tecartus	Kite	B-ALL (>25 years) MCL	2020	CD19	CD28	Retroviral
Lisocabtagene maraleucel	Breyanzi	Juno/BMS	LBCL MCL FL CLL/SLL (AA)	2021	CD19	4-1BB	Lentiviral
Idecabtagene vicleucel	Abecma	Celgene/BMS	MM	2021	BCMA	4-1BB	Lentiviral
Ciltacabtagene autoleucel	Carvykti	Legend/J&J	MM	2022	BCMA	4-1BB	Lentiviral

Abbreviations: AA, accelerated approval; B-ALL, B-cell acute lymphoblastic leukaemia; BCMA, B-cell maturation antigen; BMS, Bristol-Myers Squibb; CAR, chimeric antigen receptor; CLL, chronic lymphocytic leukaemia; FDA, Food and Drug Administration; FL, follicular lymphoma; J&J, Johnson & Johnson; LBCL, large B-cell lymphoma; MCL, mantle cell lymphoma; MM, multiple myeloma; R/R, relapsed/refractory; SLL, small lymphocytic lymphoma.

Despite the startling initial disease responses, long-term durable remissions are seen only in a minority of CAR T-treated patients, although there are a few reported cases considered cured [6,11]. Disease recurrence is one of the major obstacles in the field of CAR T-cell therapies [12]. In order to achieve prolonged remissions, different scientific groups try to develop more efficacious products by exploiting the principles of genetic engineering or other sophisticated technologies [13–15]. In addition, several other challenges surround the administration of CAR T-cell therapies, including high-grade toxicities and life-threating infections that may lead to prolonged hospitalisations, increase the financial burden for health care and insurance systems and impair patients' quality of life or even lead to death [16,17].

Currently, there are no approved CAR T-cell products against solid tumours; however, multiple research teams across the globe are investigating the treatment potential of CAR T-cells in solid tumours, joining their forces to augment CAR T-cell efficacy in lethal and untreatable cancers [14,18]. In parallel, the potential of CAR T-cell therapies has been expanded beyond oncology in treating autoimmune diseases. Clinical data of the first-treated patients with a variety of autoimmune diseases is very impressive and promising [19,20]. Preclinical data deriving from other non-malignant conditions show the potential of CAR T-cells to change the treatment arena of a plethora of conditions, including chronic infections, cardiac fibrosis and senescence-associated diseases [21].

The potential of a broader applicability of CAR T-cell therapies has caused a lot of excitement. However, on 28 November 2023 the FDA announced reported cases of T-cell malignancies in patients previously treated with either anti-CD19- or anti-BCMA-directed autologous CAR T-cell therapies both in clinical trials and in the real-world setting, raising concerns about the safety of these promising therapies. The reports of T-cell malignancies were associated with serious outcomes, including hospitalisation and death [22]. In this opinion article, the current landscape of secondary malignancies after CAR T-cell therapies is presented, along with the risk of genotoxicity carried by gene delivery systems. In addition, a strategy for future research is proposed, aiming at potentially diminishing or abrogating the risk of developing secondary malignancies after CAR T-cell therapies.

2. Reports of Secondary Malignancies after CAR T-Cell Therapies and Potential Mechanistic Causes

In November 2023, the FDA released a statement regarding reports of malignancies of T-cell origin, both lymphomas and leukaemias, including CAR-positive cases, in patients who had been previously treated with either anti-CD19- or anti-BCMA-directed autologous CAR T-cell products. These reports derived from either clinical trials or post-marketing adverse event databases. The FDA has defined that the risk of T-cell malignancies concerns all the CAR T-cell products currently approved for commercial usage [22]. So far, 22 cases of secondary T-cell malignancies have been reported, with the majority (14 of 22 cases) occurring within 2 years after CAR T-cell administration (range 1 to 19 months) and one-third of cases manifesting in the first year. Further details on these cases are under investigation [23]. As more data are accumulated and more patients are treated with CAR T-cells under growing indications, this number may further increase. It is believed that the number of these reported cases may be an underestimation of the true incidence, as currently more than 34,400 patients have been treated with commercial CAR T-cell therapies and only 8000 cases have officially been reported in the FDA Adverse Events Reporting System (FAERS) database [24]. It is noteworthy that 8 of the 17 reported secondary T-cell lymphomas after CAR T therapy in the FAERS database reported death; it was unclear whether these patients died from the primary disease or the secondary T-cell lymphoma, as the FAERS reporting system does not allow the establishment of causal relationships [25]. The genetically modified CAR T-cell products, which have been recently introduced into clinical care, have been approved with the mandatory requirement of following up treated patients for 15 years in a post-authorisation safety framework to monitor for long-term adverse events, including the possibility of genotoxicity. Since November 2023, the FDA has announced that the safety observation for future malignancies will extend to a life-long requirement, whilst adding class-wide boxed warnings to all CAR T-cell therapies, which represents the highest safety-related caution for medical treatments [26].

The published data concerning these rare cases reported to the FDA are scant, and the exact mechanistic cause driving the development of secondary T-cell malignancies is unclear. So far, data derive from published anecdotal cases and retrospective cohorts. Importantly, of the 22 reported cases of T-cell malignancies, the CAR transgene has been identified in the malignant clones by genetic sequencing in only 3 of these cases [23]. The CAR transgene has been identified within the 3′ untranslated region of PBX2, a gene related to the development of lymphomas, in a secondary T-cell lymphoma case previously treated with ciltacabtagene autoleucel, a commercial anti-BCMA product. It was unclear whether the CAR integration contributed to the T-cell malignant transformation, because genetic mutations within the T-cells predated the CAR T-cell manufacturing and infusion [27]. It is believed that the disruption either of tumour suppressor genes or the activation of protooncogenes or other crucial genetic loci orchestrating transcription, translation regulation or cell activation could be the leading cause of lymphomagenesis [28]. Pre-existing T-cell clones with a malignant potential used for CAR T-cell manufacturing may be another contributing mechanism to oncogenesis. In these cases, the CAR transgene will inevitably be identified within the tumour cells and biopsies [27,29]. However, the number of CAR transgene copies identified in the tumour biopsies plays a significant role in interpreting the results, as very low levels may represent infiltrating CAR T-cells rather than the neoplastic T-cells, reflecting a case of a CAR-negative T-cell malignancy [29]. It is also believed that the continuous and prolonged stimulation of T-cells through the CAR or endogenous T-cell receptor may lead to secondary mutational events and progression to overt malignancies, serving as an additional driving mechanism [30].

In other cases, the CAR transgene has not been identified within the tumour cells, and secondary T-cell malignancies have not been associated with the CAR T-cell treatment as a causative factor [31–33]. Interestingly, patients with B-NHLs have a fivefold higher risk than the general healthy population of developing secondary T-cell lymphomas [34]. Similarly, secondary T-cell lymphomas have been reported after treatment with immune checkpoint inhibitors with a low incidence of 0.02%, while the rate currently reported for CAR T-cell therapies reaches up to 0.06% (22 out of 34,400 cases) [24]. It has been found that PD-1 has an additional role of being a tumour suppressor, and loss of PD-1 tumour suppressor function can lead to T-cell lymphomagenesis [35]. It is possible that the combination of previous multiple lines of treatment with chemoimmunotherapy, radiation or even autologous or allogeneic transplant, along with the immune dysregulation and inflammation induced by CAR T-cells, may drive the occurrence of CAR-negative T-cell malignancies as a multi-hit mechanism. These CAR-negative malignancies may represent the evolution of new emerging T-cell clones or pre-existing malignant clones that failed CAR transduction, and they were further stimulated by T-cell activation during CAR T-cell manufacturing and the subsequent inflammation caused by post-infusion CAR T-cells [29,33] (Figure 1).

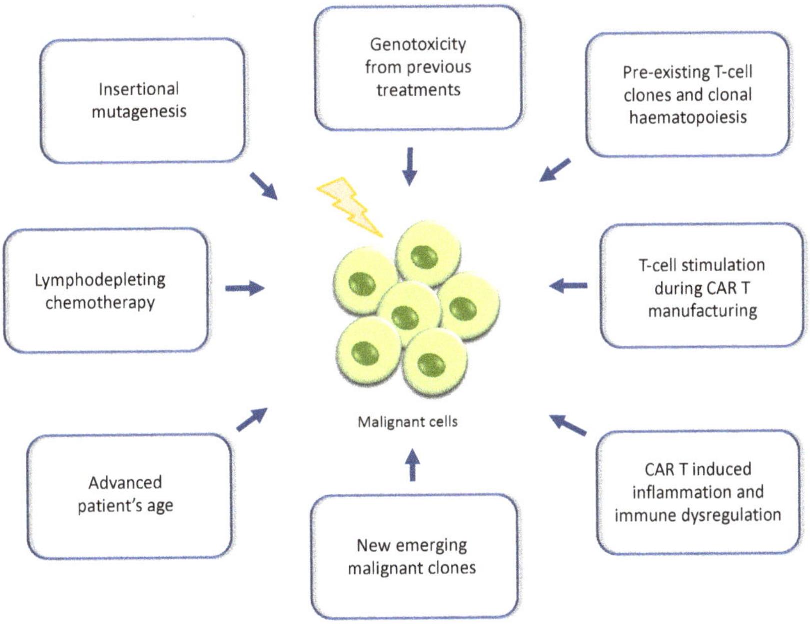

Figure 1. Potential mechanisms contributing to the development of secondary malignancies after CAR T-cell therapies: The exact mechanisms driving the occurrence of secondary malignancies, including T-cell malignancies after treatment with CAR T-cell therapies, are not well understood and remain a field under investigation. It is believed that these malignancies represent the result of multiple hits or combinatorial causative factors culminating in the emergence of malignant clones and overt oncogenesis.

Since the FDA announcement of the secondary T-cell malignancies after CAR T-cell therapy, a handful of reports have been published. They present the incidence of other secondary malignancies occurring after CAR T-cell therapies, as reported in the FAERS database or captured by the Center for International Blood and Marrow Transplant Research (CIBMTR) or by retrospective cohorts. Of note, most of the pivotal CAR T clinical trials also reported the incidence of secondary malignancies [25,36,37]. The relevant incidence reported in the FAERS database is 4.3% (536 of 12,394) out of all adverse event reports following CAR T-cell therapies, with axicabtagene ciloleucel and tisagenlecleucel comprising most of the secondary malignancy reports (51.7% and 33.0%, respectively) [25]. Real-world data report an incidence of secondary malignancies after commercial CAR T-cells ranging from 2.2% to 4.5%, varying between paediatric and adult reports and not being higher than expected in this population of patients previously exposed to cytotoxic therapies [25,29,38,39]. These neoplasms refer mainly to haematological myeloid malignancies, but they also include solid tumours, with a median time of presentation from CAR T infusion being 9 months [24]. The first category predominantly comprises myelodysplastic syndromes (MDS) and acute myeloid leukaemia. According to the FAERS database, the corresponding incidence is 38.8% and 19.8% out of all reported secondary malignancies [25]. Clinical trials with long-term follow-up have reported an incidence of secondary myeloid malignancies ranging from 4 to 16% of CAR T-treated patients [36,37,40]. Among the solid tumours, the most common are non-melanomatous skin cancers (7.8% of all reported secondary neoplasms in the FAERS database) [25]. A retrospective study performed by the University of Pennsylvania estimated that the 5-year incidence of secondary malignancies was 15.2% for solid cancers and 2.3% for haematological cancers [29]. Another single-centre retrospective study identified 25 cases of secondary solid cancers, excluding non-melanoma skin cancers, and 14 secondary haematological cancers, including 1 case of T-cell lymphoma, out of 724 patients treated with CAR T-cell therapies for either haematological malignancies or solid tumours who had a median follow-up of 15 months [33].

Multifactorial drivers are believed to play a role in the development of such secondary malignancies, especially the myeloid ones, including advanced age and the pre-existence of clonal haematopoiesis before CAR T-cell treatment potentially resulting from the exposure to previous intensive treatments. Indeed, a high proportion of patients ranging from 20% to 60% have been found to have clonal haematopoiesis of indeterminate potential at baseline before receiving CAR T-cells [41,42]. In addition, the CAR T-related inflammation developing after the infusion and onwards, especially by the CAR T-cells residing in the bone marrow, may accelerate the progression of abnormal haematopoietic clones to malignancies or the generation of new mutated clones in heavily pre-treated patients [43–47]. The lymphodepleting chemotherapy before CAR T may also play a contributing role by either suppressing a crucial subset of the cellular antitumour immunity or causing genotoxicity [48] (Figure 1).

Despite these reports, FDA has not pulled CAR T-cell therapies off the market, as the reported rate and risk of secondary malignancies, particularly T-cell malignancies, appears low compared with other cancer treatments. In addition, investigations on the driving mechanisms are still underway, and researchers are waiting for emerging data to enlighten the field to reach a consensus [23,24]. The true risk of potential insertional mutagenesis remains unknown given the high disease refractoriness of patients receiving CAR T-cell therapies. In addition, the principle of immortal time bias should also be taken into account, as patients receiving CAR T therapies currently achieve longer survival, which may translate to a higher cumulative risk of secondary malignancies in the background of R/R disease [49]. However, reports of T-cell and other malignancies after CAR T-cell therapy should prompt continued long-term investigations [22]. In alignment with the FDA, leading global organisations such as the American Society for Transplantation and Cellular Therapy, the European Society for Blood and Marrow Transplantation, the International Society for Cell and Gene Therapy and the CIBMTR recommend that CAR T-cells should be continued to be administered, as currently the benefits far outweigh the small and uncertain risks, which are much lower compared with other established cancer treatments [24]. However, strict surveillance and safety reporting to regulatory authorities are highly recommended, in addition to health care professionals being alert while monitoring CAR T-treated patients [22,24]. In the meantime, different research groups are trying to validate the significance of models incorporating established scoring

systems, such as the CAR-HEMATOTOX and the Clonal Haematopoiesis Risk Score, in predicting the risk of developing secondary myeloid malignancies after CAR T-cell therapy and stratifying patients according to the relevant risk. This clinical stratification seems necessary in order to identify a subgroup of high-risk patients who will benefit most from closer surveillance after CAR T-cell therapy and potential additional screening before CAR T treatment [50,51].

3. Viral Vectors and Genetic Engineering Technologies in Gene Therapy and CAR T-Cell Manufacturing

The use of viruses as vectors in transferring transgenes has been the mainstay of transduction methods in gene therapy. The ability of certain viruses to integrate transgenes into the genome has been exploited in CAR T-cell manufacturing technology [52]. Vector integration into the host genome has always been a matter of concern in terms of the potential alteration of gene expression or the promotion of neoplastic transformation. Mechanisms include vector insertion into the gene enhancer or the promoter mediating gene overexpression or integration causing gene inactivation [53]. Currently, lentiviruses (LVs) and retroviruses constitute the most commonly used viral vectors in gene therapy. In the past, conventional retro-gamma viruses and adenoviruses were used as delivery machines in gene therapy. However, the initial triumph was overshadowed by reports of insertional mutagenesis resulting in leukaemia and MDS in patients treated with gene therapy using retro-gamma viruses for X-linked severe combined immunodeficiency, chronic granulomatous disease and Wiskott–Aldrich syndrome [54–56]. On the other hand, adenoviruses are strongly immunogenic, and they caused undesired immune responses in treated subjects [57]. Since then, viral vector technology has been massively refined to develop safer next-generation non-replication-competent viral vectors, including self-inactivating (SIN) vectors, enhancer-blocking insulators and microRNA targeting of vectors. There are multiple factors influencing vector-mediated genotoxicity, such as virus type, integration target site and target cell type, while non-viral factors such as patient age, disease type and dose are equally important. [58,59].

SIN LVs are currently preferably utilised, as they permit long-term transgene expression, have high packaging capacity and are deemed safer in integrating transgenes in specific genetic loci into the genome, confining random integration [53,60]. In addition, they have the advantage of enabling efficient transduction of nondividing or slowly dividing cells, surpassing the need for extra activating of the host cells [58]. On the downside, production with LVs is more costly, lengthy and cumbersome. However, SIN LV vectors may still be genotoxic, as despite integrating in a semirandom fashion, they tend toward genomic areas with active gene expression, including cancer-related genes [60]. Both in vitro and in vivo preclinical studies have shown that SIN LV integration caused aberrant splicing and premature termination of transcripts and tumour acceleration by disruption of tumour suppression genes or oncogene activation [61,62]. Notably, although initial concerns regarding the risk of potential insertional mutagenesis were regarded as more relevant in the transduction of hematopoietic stem cells, the recent FDA report on T-cell malignancies brings to light the risk of insertional mutagenesis in differentiated cells [63].

Although the FDA has not related any of the recently reported cases to vector-mediated oncogenicity so far, previously published cases have highlighted the possibility of clonal CAR T-cell expansion in anti-CD19 and anti-CD22 CAR T-cell therapies. This occurred via the integration of an LV either in the TET2 gene, which regulates haematopoiesis and T-cell differentiation, or in the CBL gene, which regulates T-cell responses [64,65]. These cases did not result in the development of neoplasms but demonstrate the risk of insertional mutagenesis. Of note, the clonal expansion of a myeloid-biased cell clone has also been reported in an adult patient with severe β-thalassaemia treated with LV β-globin gene transfer, in whom the integrated vector caused enhancer-mediated transcriptional activation of the HMGA2 gene with increased expression of a truncated HMGA2 mRNA insensitive to degradation [66]. In a clinical trial investigating hematopoietic stem-cell gene therapy for cerebral adrenoleukodystrophy, the top abundant integration sites of SIN LVs were genes involved in cell cycle regulation, cell division and oncogenesis; such genes included SGM6, CCND2 and MECOM, leading to clonal expansion and subsequent reports of MDS cases related to the viral insertion [67,68]. Rare cases of myeloid malignancies have been reported after hematopoietic stem-cell gene therapy in sickle cell disease. However, it is likely that the myeloablative conditioning chemotherapy previously administered resulted in the development of driver mutations associated with myeloid neoplasms or created positive selection pressure resulting in the progression of a pre-existing clone. It is well known that sickle cell patients harbour an inherently higher risk of developing clonal haematopoiesis and malignancies compared to the general population [69–71]. None of these cases have been explicitly related to random insertional mutagenesis caused by the viral vector [70,71].

Adeno-associated viruses (AAVs) are another vector option deemed safer than lentiviruses for gene therapy because they are not designed to insert their cargo into a cell's genome but rather remain as an episome in the nucleus of the transduced cells. However, although an AAV is considered a non-integrated vector, integrational events have been observed with a low frequency of 0.1–3% [53]. A phase 3 gene therapy trial for haemophilia using an AAV vector was halted by the FDA because a patient developed a liver tumour, although it was thought highly unlikely to be related to the gene therapy [72]. However, animal models have shown increased incidence of hepatocellular carcinoma after AAV liver gene transfer, which is alarming for potential vector-related tumourogenesis [73,74]. In addition, AAV type 2 has been associated with oncogenic insertional mutagenesis in humans with hepatocellular carcinomas through integrations in known cancer driver genes, such as CCNA2, TERT, CCNE1, TNFSF10 and KMT2B, leading to overexpression of the target genes [75].

Genetic engineering has massively changed the field of cell and gene therapy, allowing alternative, more precise technologies to achieve genetic manipulation, minimising the complexity and the risks of genotoxicity associated with viral vectors. Currently implemented methods of gene editing include non-viral delivery systems, such as CRISPR-Cas9, transposons, zinc-finger nucleases, transcription-activator-like effector nucleases and meganucleases [76]. These methods are being exploited in several research platforms to generate safer and more potent CAR T-cell therapies, while commercial products developed by harnessing gene-editing techniques (CRISPR-Cas9-based products) have been approved as gene therapy treatments for sickle cell and transfusion-dependent β-thalassemia patients [13,77,78]. However, genome editing is not always precise, resulting in off-target effects with mutations, genomic disruption and chromosome rearrangement with unknown biological and clinical significance [79–81]. More importantly, cases of secondary T-cell lymphoma have been reported after applying piggyBac, a transposon system for CAR gene delivery in the manufacturing of CAR T-cells. The lymphomagenesis was related to high transgene insertion copy numbers, but it was thought that the widespread genomic copy number variations found within the genome of lymphoma cells was the dominant driver of carcinogenesis [30,82]. Notably, in this phase 1 trial, it was found that 7% of the transgene integration sites occurred within cancer-related genes, but these were not different than those previously reported with similar gene delivery methods. This trial was suspended by the FDA after the occurrence of these CAR-positive T-cell lymphoma cases [30]. The high insertion copy numbers are in line with the importance of the vector copy number in the use of viral vectors. The vector copy number reflects the number of integrated transgene copies within a CAR T-cell product and remains one of the FDA's quality and safety requirements (less than five vector copies per transduced cell), as it correlates with the product potency, but it may also reflect the oncogenic potential, as greater copy numbers are associated with a greater risk of random vector integration into the host genome [83].

Base editing is a novel technology editing only targeted single DNA bases rather than removing, adding or altering sections of the DNA sequence; therefore, it is deemed safer in terms of genotoxicity. However, despite being more accurate, base editing has been found to trigger mutations at random sites in the genome beyond the target site [84,85]. Ongoing research may lead to the identification of genomic safe harbours in parallel with the development of new strategies that target the insertion of the CAR construct to these specific loci within the genome, avoiding the risk of oncogenesis [86].

4. A Proposed Strategy for Future Research Aiming to Mitigate the Risk of Secondary Malignancies

Due to the theoretical risk of insertional mutagenesis, all CAR T-cell-treated patients have been under long-term surveillance. Therefore, the FDA announcement of secondary T-cell malignancies after CAR T-cell therapies came as a surprise to the scientific community. The confirmation of these allegations has raised concerns about the future of CAR T-cell therapies and cell and gene therapies in general, as different genetically manipulated products are underway to be applied in the clinical setting for various disease types, both malignant and non-malignant. The exact causes driving the development of secondary malignancies after CAR T-cell therapies are unclear. Regarding the T-cell malignancies, none of the 22 reported cases of secondary T-cell malignancies have been explicitly related to vector-mediated insertional oncogenicity. This number could be an underestimation of the true incidence, as more than 34,400 patients have been treated with commercial CAR T-cell therapies and only 8000 cases have been officially reported with adverse events [24]. Apparently, the decoding of the triggering mechanisms of secondary T-cell and other malignancies requires the wider study of further potentially unreported cases. This is a laborious and lengthy follow-up process and is consistent with the advance of genetic engineering.

Based on the reported scientific evidence characterising the nascent and unclear current landscape of secondary malignancies after CAR T-cell infusion and the potential mechanisms of their development, a composite set of six proposals is presented for future research. If this suggestive strategy is confirmed, it can potentially contribute to mitigating or preventing the risks of developing secondary malignancies either by avoiding genotoxicity or reducing CAR T-associated inflammation and the immunosuppressive microenvironment (Figure 2):

A. Exploitation of mRNA technologies instead of viral vectors or gene-editing techniques for the CAR introduction to avoid random transgene integration into the host cells and subsequent genotoxicity. mRNA technologies have been proven very efficient in translating the CAR protein. Preliminary results from experimental CAR T-cell platforms harnessing mRNA techniques have shown promising safety and efficacy in eliminating tumour cells [87,88] (Figure 2A).

B. Short CAR T-cell persistence to reduce the period of overt and subclinical inflammation and immune dysregulation, which may drive the occurrence of abnormal clonal haematopoiesis, the clonal evolution of already pre-existing aberrant clones to malignancies and the development of secondary lymphomas (Figure 2B).

C. Infusion of high cell doses with defined cell compositions in fractions, as it seems that doses with high cell numbers have the ability to randomly eliminate malignancies early after infusion and offer a cure [89,90]. In this perspective, long-term CAR T-cell persistence does not seem to be necessary but rather augments the risk of further adverse events and toxicities (Figure 2C).

D. Move of CAR T-cell therapies to earlier lines of treatment to avoid the accumulation of chemotherapy or radiotherapy-related genotoxicity and the development of pre-malignant clones (Figure 2D).

E. Effective control of disease burden prior to infusion to reduce the subsequent generation of excessive CAR T-cell-related inflammation and the potential detrimental effects of inflammation (Figure 2E).

F. Promotion of automated in-house CAR T-cell manufacturing to reduce production time and complexity as a measure to prevent disease progression and an increase in the disease burden prior to CAR T-cell infusion (Figure 2F).

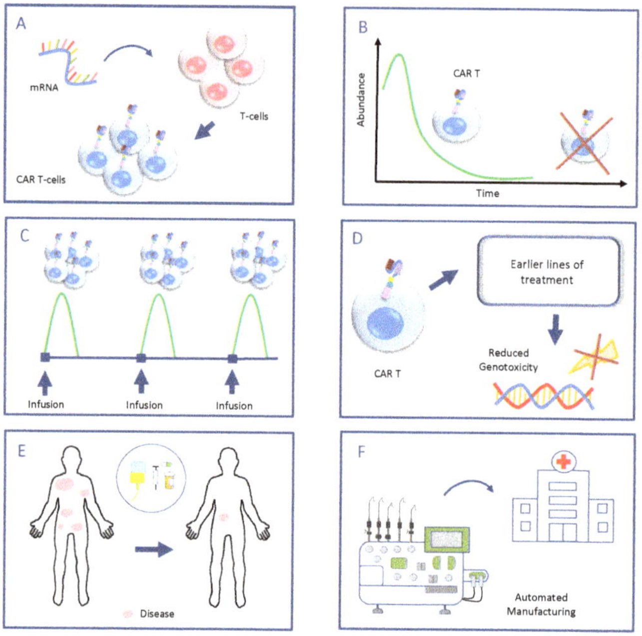

Figure 2. A proposed strategy for future research aiming to mitigate the risks of developing secondary malignancies after CAR T-cell therapies: (**A**) harnessing of mRNA technologies for the CAR introduction to avoid genotoxicity caused by viral vectors or gene editing; (**B**) short CAR T-cell persistence to diminish immune dysregulation, which may drive clonal evolution and the development of secondary malignancies; (**C**) infusion of high cell doses with defined cell compositions in fractions, which can increase the likelihood of early disease eradication, making unnecessary CAR T-cell persistence; (**D**) move of CAR T-cell therapies to earlier lines of treatment to avoid accumulated genotoxicity caused by previous intense treatments; (**E**) effective control of disease burden prior to infusion to reduce the detrimental effects of subsequent inflammation; (**F**) promotion of automated in-house CAR T-cell manufacturing to reduce the production time and the risk of disease progression with high tumour burden.

5. Conclusions

The announcement on 28 November 2023 by the FDA concerning the occurrence of rare secondary T-malignancies after CAR T-cell therapies should in no way act as a brake on the further clinical use of CAR T-cells. Given the expanding indications of treating diseases with the CAR T-cell technology, this type of cell therapy seems to enclose the potential to be converted into the "cellular penicillin" of the 21st century, a lifesaving and survival-prolonging treatment. Therefore, it seems imperative to render CAR T-cell therapies a safer treatment modality. The abovementioned strategy can pave the way for extensive research and bridge the existing therapeutic gap in CAR T-cell therapies in order to turn CAR T-cell therapies into a treatment with a higher curative potential and sparing toxic or even life-threatening side effects.

Author Contributions: Conceptualization, S.B. and D.B.; visualization, S.B.; writing—original draft preparation, S.B.; writing—review and editing, D.B. All authors have read and agreed to the published version of the manuscript.

Funding: This research received no external funding.

Conflicts of Interest: The authors declare no conflicts of interest.

References

1. Guerra, E.; Di Pietro, R.; Basile, M.; Trerotola, M.; Alberti, S. Cancer-Homing CAR-T Cells and Endogenous Immune Population Dynamics. *Int. J. Mol. Sci.* **2022**, *23*, 405. [CrossRef] [PubMed]
2. Ayala Ceja, M.; Khericha, M.; Harris, C.M.; Puig-Saus, C.; Chen, Y.Y. CAR-T cell manufacturing: Major process parameters and next-generation strategies. *J. Exp. Med.* **2024**, *221*, e20230903. [CrossRef] [PubMed]
3. Mitra, A.; Barua, A.; Huang, L.; Ganguly, S.; Feng, Q.; He, B. From bench to bedside: The history and progress of CAR T cell therapy. *Front. Immunol.* **2023**, *14*, 1188049. [CrossRef] [PubMed]
4. Asmamaw Dejenie, T.; Tiruneh G/Medhin, M.; Dessie Terefe, G.; Tadele Admasu, F.; Wale Tesega, W.; Chekol Abebe, E. Current updates on generations, approvals, and clinical trials of CAR T-cell therapy. *Hum. Vaccin. Immunother.* **2022**, *18*, 2114254. [CrossRef]
5. Korell, F.; Berger, T.R.; Maus, M.V. Understanding CAR T cell-tumor interactions: Paving the way for successful clinical outcomes. *Med* **2022**, *3*, 538–564. [CrossRef]
6. Neelapu, S.S.; Jacobson, C.A.; Ghobadi, A.; Miklos, D.B.; Lekakis, L.J.; Oluwole, O.O.; Lin, Y.; Braunschweig, I.; Hill, B.T.; Timmerman, J.M.; et al. Five-year follow-up of ZUMA-1 supports the curative potential of axicabtagene ciloleucel in refractory large B-cell lymphoma. *Blood* **2023**, *141*, 2307–2315. [PubMed]
7. Laetsch, T.W.; Maude, S.L.; Rives, S.; Hiramatsu, H.; Bittencourt, H.; Bader, P.; Baruchel, A.; Boyer, M.; De Moerloose, B.; Qayed, M.; et al. Three-Year Update of Tisagenlecleucel in Pediatric and Young Adult Patients With Relapsed/Refractory Acute Lymphoblastic Leukemia in the ELIANA Trial. *J. Clin. Oncol.* **2023**, *41*, 1664–1669. [CrossRef]
8. Martin, T.; Usmani, S.Z.; Berdeja, J.G.; Agha, M.; Cohen, A.D.; Hari, P.; Avigan, D.; Deol, A.; Htut, M.; Lesokhin, A.; et al. Ciltacabtagene Autoleucel, an Anti–B-cell Maturation Antigen Chimeric Antigen Receptor T-Cell Therapy, for Relapsed/Refractory Multiple Myeloma: CARTITUDE-1 2-Year Follow-Up. *J. Clin. Oncol.* **2023**, *41*, 1265–1274. [CrossRef]
9. Approved Cellular and Gene Therapy Products. US Food & Drug Administration. Available online: https://www.fda.gov/vaccines-blood-biologics/cellular-gene-therapy-products/approved-cellular-and-gene-therapy-products (accessed on 26 April 2024).
10. U.S. FDA Approves Bristol Myers Squibb's Breyanzi as the First and Only CAR T Cell Therapy for Adults with Relapsed or Refractory Chronic Lymphocytic Leukemia (CLL) or Small Lymphocytic Lymphoma (SLL). Available online: https://news.bms.com/news/details/2024/U.S.-FDA-Approves-Bristol-Myers-Squibbs-Breyanzi--as-the-First-and-Only-CAR-T-Cell-Therapy-for-Adults-with-Relapsed-or-Refractory-Chronic-Lymphocytic-Leukemia-CLL-or-Small-Lymphocytic-Lymphoma-SLL/default.aspx (accessed on 3 March 2024).
11. Melenhorst, J.J.; Chen, G.M.; Wang, M.; Porter, D.L.; Chen, C.; Collins, M.A.; Gao, P.; Bandyopadhyay, S.; Sun, H.; Zhao, Z.; et al. Decade-long leukemia remissions with the persistence of CD4+ CAR T cells. *Nature* **2022**, *602*, 503–509. [CrossRef]
12. Bouziana, S.; Bouzianas, D. Anti-CD19 CAR-T cells: Digging in the dark side of the golden therapy. *Crit. Rev. Oncol. Hematol.* **2021**, *157*, 103096. [CrossRef] [PubMed]
13. Dimitri, A.; Herbst, F.; Fraietta, J.A. Engineering the next-generation of CAR T-cells with CRISPR-Cas9 gene editing. *Mol. Cancer.* **2022**, *21*, 78. [CrossRef]
14. Young, R.M.; Engel, N.W.; Uslu, U.; Wellhausen, N.; June, C.H. Next-Generation CAR T-cell Therapies. *Cancer Discov.* **2022**, *12*, 1625–1633. [CrossRef]
15. Benjamin, R.; Jain, N.; Maus, M.V.; Boissel, N.; Graham, C.; Jozwik, A.; Yallop, D.; Konopleva, M.; Frigault, M.J.; Teshima, T.; et al. UCART19, a first-in-class allogeneic anti-CD19 chimeric antigen receptor T-cell therapy for adults with relapsed or refractory B-cell acute lymphoblastic leukaemia (CALM): A phase 1, dose-escalation trial. *Lancet Haematol.* **2022**, *9*, e833–e843. [CrossRef] [PubMed]
16. Spiegel, J.Y.; Jain, M.D.; Nastoupil, L.J.; Tamaresis, J.; Ghobadi, A.; Lin, Y.; Lekakis, L.J.; Reagan, P.M.; Oluwole, O.O.; McGuirk, J.P.; et al. Five year outcomes of patients with large B-Cell lymphoma treated with standard-of-care Axicabtagene Ciloleucel: Results from the US lymphoma CAR-T cell consortium. *Blood* **2023**, *142* (Suppl. S1), 1032. [CrossRef]
17. Brudno, J.N.; Kochenderfer, J.N. Current understanding and management of CAR T cell-associated toxicities. *Nat. Rev. Clin. Oncol.* **2024**, *21*, 501–521. [CrossRef] [PubMed]
18. Zhong, W.; Xiao, Z.; Qin, Z.; Yang, J.; Wen, Y.; Yu, Z.; Li, Y.; Sheppard, N.C.; Fuchs, S.Y.; Xu, X.; et al. Tumor-Derived Small Extracellular Vesicles Inhibit the Efficacy of CAR T Cells against Solid Tumors. *Cancer Res.* **2023**, *83*, 2790–2806. [CrossRef] [PubMed]
19. Mackensen, A.; Müller, F.; Mougiakakos, D.; Böltz, S.; Weilhem, A.; Aigner, M.; Völkl, S.; Simon, D.; Kleyer, A.; Munoz, L.; et al. Anti-CD19 CAR T cell therapy for refractory systemic lupus erythematosus. *Nat. Med.* **2022**, *28*, 2124–2132. [CrossRef]
20. Müller, F.; Taubmann, J.; Bucci, L.; Wilhelm, A.; Bergmann, C.; Völkl, S.; Aigner, M.; Rothe, T.; Minopoulou, I.; Tur, C.; et al. CD19 CAR T-Cell Therapy in Autoimmune Disease—A Case Series with Follow-up. *N. Engl. J. Med.* **2024**, *390*, 687–700. [CrossRef] [PubMed]
21. Baker, D.J.; Arany, Z.; Baur, J.A.; Epstein, J.A.; June, C.H. CAR T therapy beyond cancer: The evolution of a living drug. *Nature* **2023**, *619*, 707–715. [CrossRef]

22. FDA Investigating Serious Risk of T-cell Malignancy Following BCMA-Directed or CD19-Directed Autologous Chimeric Antigen Receptor (CAR) T cell Immunotherapies. US Food & Drug Administration. Available online: https://www.fda.gov/vaccines-blood-biologics/safety-availability-biologics/fda-investigating-serious-risk-t-cell-malignancy-following-bcma-directed-or-cd19-directed-autologous (accessed on 28 November 2023).
23. Verdun, N.; Marks, P. Secondary Cancers after Chimeric Antigen Receptor T-Cell Therapy. *N. Engl. J. Med.* **2024**, *390*, 584–586. [CrossRef]
24. Levine, B.L.; Pasquini, M.C.; Connolly, J.E.; Porter, D.L.; Gustafson, M.P.; Boelens, J.J.; Horwitz, E.M.; Grupp, S.A.; Maus, M.V.; Locke, F.L.; et al. Unanswered questions following reports of secondary malignancies after CAR-T cell therapy. *Nat. Med.* **2024**, *30*, 338–341. [CrossRef]
25. Elsallab, M.; Ellithi, M.; Lunning, M.A.; D'Angelo, C.; Ma, J.; Perales, M.A.; Frigault, M.; Maus, M.V. Second Primary Malignancies After Commercial CAR T Cell Therapy: Analysis of FDA Adverse Events Reporting System (FAERS). *Blood* **2024**, *143*, 2099–2105. [CrossRef] [PubMed]
26. FDA Requires Boxed Warning for T cell Malignancies Following Treatment with BCMA-Directed or CD19-Directed Autologous Chimeric Antigen Receptor (CAR) T cell Immunotherapies. US Food & Drug Administration. Available online: https://www.fda.gov/vaccines-blood-biologics/safety-availability-biologics/fda-requires-boxed-warning-t-cell-malignancies-following-treatment-bcma-directed-or-cd19-directed (accessed on 18 April 2024).
27. Harrison, S.J.; Nguyen, T.; Rahman, M.; Er, J.; Li, J.; Li, K.; Lendvai, N.; Schecter, J.M.; Banerjee, A.; Roccia, T.; et al. CAR+ T-Cell Lymphoma Post Ciltacabtagene Autoleucel Therapy for Relapsed Refractory Multiple Myeloma. *Blood* **2023**, *142* (Suppl. S1), 6939. [CrossRef]
28. Heinrich, T.; Rengstl, B.; Muik, A.; Petkova, M.; Schmid, F.; Wistinghausen, R.; Warner, K.; Crispatzu, G.; Hansmann, M.L.; Herling, M.; et al. Mature T-cell lymphomagenesis induced by retroviral insertional activation of Janus kinase 1. *Mol. Ther.* **2013**, *21*, 1160–1168. [CrossRef] [PubMed]
29. Ghilardi, G.; Fraietta, J.A.; Gerson, J.N.; Van Deerlin, V.M.; Morrissette, J.J.D.; Caponetti, G.C.; Paruzzo, L.; Harris, J.C.; Chong, E.A.; Susanibar Adaniya, S.P.; et al. T-cell Lymphoma and Secondary Primary Malignancy Risk After Commercial CAR T-cell Therapy. *Nat. Med.* **2024**, *30*, 984–989. [CrossRef]
30. Bishop, D.C.; Clancy, L.E.; Simms, R.; Burgess, J.; Mathew, G.; Moezzi, L.; Street, J.A.; Sutrave, G.; Atkins, E.; McGuire, H.M.; et al. Development of CAR T-cell lymphoma in 2 of 10 patients effectively treated with piggyBac-modified CD19 CAR T cells. *Blood* **2021**, *138*, 1504–1509. [CrossRef] [PubMed]
31. Li, P.; Yu, W.J.; Zhou, L.; Yang, M.; Ye, S.; Zhu, J.; Huang, J.; Zhang, Y.; Li, L.; Zhao, J.; et al. C-CAR039, a Novel Anti-CD20/CD19 Bi-Specific CAR T-Cell Therapy Shows Deep and Durable Clinical Benefits in Patients with Relapsed or Refractory (r/r) B-Cell Non-Hodgkin Lymphoma (B-NHL) in Long Term Follow up. *Blood* **2023**, *142* (Suppl. S1), 1025. [CrossRef]
32. Steffin, D.H.M.; Muhsen, I.N.; Hill, L.C.; Ramos, C.A.; Ahmed, N.; Hegde, M.; Wang, T.; Wu, M.; Gottschalk, S.; Whittle, S.B.; et al. Long-term follow-up for the development of subsequent malignancies in patients treated with genetically modified IECs. *Blood* **2022**, *140*, 16–24. [CrossRef]
33. Hamilton, M.P.; Sugio, T.; Noordenbos, T.; Shi, S.; Bulterys, P.L.; Liu, C.L.; Kang, X.; Olsen, M.N.; Good, Z.; Dahiya, S.; et al. Risk of Second Tumors and T-Cell Lymphoma after CAR T-Cell Therapy. *N. Engl. J. Med.* **2024**, *390*, 2047–2060. [CrossRef]
34. Chihara, D.; Dores, G.M.; Flowers, C.R.; Morton, L.M. The bidirectional increased risk of B-cell lymphoma and T-cell lymphoma. *Blood* **2021**, *138*, 785–789. [CrossRef]
35. Wartewig, T.; Kurgyis, Z.; Keppler, S.; Pechloff, K.; Hameister, E.; Öllinger, R.; Maresch, R.; Buch, T.; Steiger, K.; Winter, C.; et al. PD-1 is a haploinsufficient suppressor of T cell lymphomagenesis. *Nature* **2017**, *552*, 121–125. [CrossRef] [PubMed]
36. Chong, E.A.; Ruella, M.; Schuster, S.J. Lymphoma Program Investigators at the University of Pennsylvania. Five-year outcomes for refractory B-cell lymphomas with CAR T-cell therapy. *N. Engl. J. Med.* **2021**, *384*, 673–674. [CrossRef]
37. Cordeiro, A.; Bezerra, E.D.; Hirayama, A.V.; Hill, J.A.; Wu, Q.V.; Voutsinas, J.; Sorror, M.L.; Turtle, C.J.; Maloney, D.G.; Bar, M. Late events after treatment with CD19-targeted chimeric antigen receptor modified T cells. *Biol. Blood Marrow Transpl.* **2020**, *26*, 26–33. [CrossRef]
38. Tward, J.D.; Wendland, M.M.; Shrieve, D.C.; Szabo, A.; Gaffney, D.K. The risk of secondary malignancies over 30 years after the treatment of non-Hodgkin lymphoma. *Cancer* **2006**, *107*, 108–115. [CrossRef] [PubMed]
39. Hsieh, E.M.; Myers, R.M.; Yates, B.; Annesley, C.; John, S.; Taraseviciute, A.; Steinberg, S.M.; Sheppard, J.; Chung, P.; Chen, L.; et al. Low rate of subsequent malignant neoplasms after CD19 CAR T-cell therapy. *Blood Adv.* **2022**, *6*, 5222–5226. [CrossRef]
40. Strati, P.; Varma, A.; Adkins, S.; Nastoupil, L.J.; Westin, J.; Hagemeister, F.B.; Fowler, N.H.; Lee, H.J.; Fayad, L.E.; Samaniego, F.; et al. Hematopoietic recovery and immune reconstitution after axicabtagene ciloleucel in patients with large b-cell lymphoma. *Haematologica* **2021**, *106*, 2667–2672. [CrossRef]
41. Panagiota, V.; Kerschbaum, J.F.; Penack, O.; Stein, C.M.; Arends, C.M.; Koenecke, C.; Strzelecka, P.M.; Kloos, A.; Wiegand, L.; Lasch, A.; et al. Clinical implications and dynamics of clonal hematopoiesis in anti- CD19 CAR T-cell treated patients. *Hemasphere* **2023**, *7*, e957. [CrossRef] [PubMed]
42. Teipel, R.; Kroschinsky, F.; Kramer, M.; Kretschmann, T.; Egger-Heidrich, K.; Krüger, T.; Ruhnke, L.; Herold, S.; Stasik, S.; Sockel, K.; et al. Prevalence and variation of CHIP in patients with aggressive lymphomas undergoing CD19-directed CAR T-cell treatment. *Blood Adv.* **2022**, *6*, 1941–1946. [CrossRef] [PubMed]

43. Hamilton, M.P.; Sworder, B.J.; Alig, S.K.; Good, Z.; Boegeholz, J.; Schroers-Martin, J.; Tamaresis, J.; Shahrokh Esfahani, M.; Lu, Y.; Olsen, M.; et al. CAR19 Therapy Drives Expansion of Clonal Hematopoiesis and Associated Cytopenias. *Blood* **2023**, *142* (Suppl. S1), 360. [CrossRef]
44. Alkhateeb, H.B.; Mohty, R.; Greipp, P.; Bansal, R.; Hathcock, M.; Rosenthal, A.; Murth, H.; Kharfan-Dabaja, M.; Bisneto Villasboas, J.C.; Bennani, N.; et al. Therapy-related myeloid neoplasms following chimeric antigen receptor T-cell therapy for Non-Hodgkin Lymphoma. *Blood Cancer J.* **2022**, *12*, 113. [CrossRef] [PubMed]
45. Miller, P.G.; Sperling, A.S.; Brea, E.J.; Leick, M.B.; Fell, G.G.; Jan, M.; Gohil, S.H.; Tai, Y.T.; Munshi, N.C.; Wu, C.J.; et al. Clonal hematopoiesis in patients receiving chimeric antigen receptor T-cell therapy. *Blood Adv.* **2021**, *5*, 2982–2986. [CrossRef] [PubMed]
46. Ahmadreza, A.; Srikanthan, J.; Khelil, M.B.; Marcos-Kovandzik, L.; Amine-Hneineh, R.; Sabourin-Cousin, M.; Quivoron, C.; Christophe, M.; Baptiste Micol, J.; Zitvogel, L.; et al. CAR T cells reside in the bone marrow and inhibit hematopoiesis. *HemaSphere* **2024**, *8* (Suppl. S1), 2620.
47. Zhao, A.; Zhao, M.; Qian, W.; Liang, A.; Li, P.; Liu, H. Secondary myeloid neoplasms after CD19 CAR T therapy in patients with refractory/relapsed B-cell lymphoma: Case series and review of literature. *Front. Immunol.* **2023**, *13*, 1063986. [CrossRef]
48. Sacchi, S.; Marcheselli, L.; Bari, A.; Marcheselli, R.; Pozzi, S.; Luminari, S.; Lombardo, M.; Buda, G.; Lazzaro, A.; Gobbi, P.G.; et al. Secondary malignancies after treatment for indolent non-Hodgkin's lymphoma: A 16-year follow-up study. *Haematologica* **2008**, *93*, 398–404. [CrossRef]
49. Banerjee, R.; Poh, C.; Hirayama, A.V.; Gauthier, J.; Cassaday, R.D.; Shadman, M.; Cowan, A.J.; Till, B.G.; Green, D.J.; Kiem, H.P.; et al. Answering the "Doctor, can CAR-T therapy cause cancer?" question in clinic. *Blood Adv.* **2024**, *8*, 895–898. [CrossRef] [PubMed]
50. Gurney, M.; Alkhateeb, H.; Shah, S.; Bansal, R.; Hathcock, M.; Rosenthal, A.; Kharfan-Dabaja, M.; Kourelis, T.; Patnaik, M.; Chen, D.; et al. Cytopenias, age and CAR-HEMATOTOX score predict the development of post CAR T-cell therapy-related myeloid neoplasms. *Hemasphere* **2023**, *7* (Suppl. S3), e6718317. [CrossRef]
51. Galli, E.; Rossi, M.; Pansini, I.; Viscovo, M.; Malara, T.; Colangelo, M.; Alma, E.; Hohaus, S.; Sica, S.; Sorà, F.; et al. Predicting therapy-related myeloid neoplasms after CAR-T: Validation of the clonal hematopoiesis risk score (CHRS). *HemaSphere* **2024**, *8* (Suppl. S1), 398.
52. Levine, B.L.; Miskin, J.; Wonnacott, K.; Keir, C. Global Manufacturing of CAR T Cell Therapy. *Mol. Ther. Methods Clin. Dev.* **2016**, *4*, 92–101. [CrossRef]
53. Bulcha, J.T.; Wang, Y.; Ma, H.; Tai, P.W.L.; Gao, G. Viral vector platforms within the gene therapy landscape. *Signal Transduct. Target. Ther.* **2021**, *6*, 53. [CrossRef]
54. Howe, S.J.; Mansour, M.R.; Schwarzwaelder, K.; Bartholomae, C.; Hubank, M.; Kempski, H.; Brugman, M.H.; Pike-Overzet, K.; Chatters, S.J.; de Ridder, D.; et al. Insertional mutagenesis combined with acquired somatic mutations causes leukemogenesis following gene therapy of SCID-X1 patients. *J. Clin. Investig.* **2008**, *118*, 3143–3150. [CrossRef]
55. Stein, S.; Ott, M.G.; Schultze-Strasser, S.; Jauch, A.; Burwinkel, B.; Kinner, A.; Schmidt, M.; Krämer, A.; Schwäble, J.; Glimm, H.; et al. Genomic instability and myelodysplasia with monosomy 7 consequent to EVI1 activation after gene therapy for chronic granulomatous disease. *Nat. Med.* **2010**, *16*, 198–204. [CrossRef]
56. Braun, C.J.; Boztug, K.; Paruzynski, A.; Witzel, M.; Schwarzer, A.; Rothe, M.; Modlich, U.; Beier, R.; Göhring, G.; Steinemann, D.; et al. Gene therapy for Wiskott-Aldrich Syndrome—Long-term reconstitution and clinical benefits, but increased risk for leukemogenesis. *Sci. Transl. Med.* **2014**, *6*, 227ra33. [CrossRef] [PubMed]
57. Crystal, R.G. Adenovirus: The first effective in vivo gene delivery vector. *Hum. Gene Ther.* **2014**, *25*, 3–11. [CrossRef]
58. Cooray, S.; Howe, S.J.; Thrasher, A.J. Retrovirus and lentivirus vector design and methods of cell conditioning. *Methods Enzymol.* **2012**, *507*, 29–57.
59. David, R.M.; Doherty, A.T. Viral Vectors: The Road to Reducing Genotoxicity. *T Toxicol. Sci.* **2017**, *155*, 315–325. [CrossRef]
60. Labbé, R.P.; Vessillier, S.; Rafiq, Q.A. Lentiviral vectors for T cell engineering: Clinical applications, bioprocessing and future perspectives. *Viruses* **2021**, *13*, 1528. [CrossRef] [PubMed]
61. Moiani, A.; Paleari, Y.; Sartori, D.; Mezzadra, R.; Miccio, A.; Cattoglio, C.; Cocchiarella, F.; Lidonnici, M.R.; Ferrari, G.; Mavilio, F. Lentiviral vector integration in the human genome induces alternative splicing and generates aberrant transcripts. *J. Clin. Investig.* **2012**, *122*, 1653–1666. [CrossRef] [PubMed]
62. Cesana, D.; Ranzani, M.; Volpin, M.; Bartholomae, C.; Duros, C.; Artus, A.; Merella, S.; Benedicenti, F.; Sergi Sergi, L.; Sanvito, F.; et al. Uncovering and dissecting the genotoxicity of self-inactivating lentiviral vectors in vivo. *Mol. Ther.* **2014**, *22*, 774–785. [CrossRef] [PubMed]
63. Schubert, M.L.; Schmittl, M.; Wang, L.; Ramos, C.A.; Jordan, K.; Müller-Tidow, C.; Dreger, P. Side-effect management of chimeric antigen receptor (CAR) T-cell therapy. *Ann. Oncol.* **2021**, *32*, 34–48. [CrossRef]
64. Fraietta, J.A.; Nobles, C.L.; Sammons, M.A.; Lundh, S.; Carty, S.A.; Reich, T.J.; Cogdill, A.P.; Morrissette, J.J.D.; DeNizio, J.E.; Reddy, S.; et al. Disruption of TET2 promotes the therapeutic efficacy of CD19-targeted T cells. *Nature* **2018**, *558*, 307–312. [CrossRef] [PubMed]
65. Shah, N.N.; Qin, H.; Yates, B.; Su, L.; Shalabi, H.; Raffeld, M.; Ahlman, M.A.; Stetler-Stevenson, M.; Yuan, C.; Guo, S.; et al. Clonal expansion of CAR T cells harboring lentivector integration in the CBL gene following anti-CD22 CAR T-cell therapy. *Blood Adv.* **2019**, *3*, 2317–2322. [CrossRef]

66. Cavazzana-Calvo, M.; Payen, E.; Negre, O.; Wang, G.; Hehir, K.; Fusil, F.; Down, J.; Denaro, M.; Brady, T.; Westerman, K.; et al. Transfusion independence and HMGA2 activation after gene therapy of human β-thalassaemia. *Nature* **2010**, *467*, 318–322. [CrossRef]
67. Eichler, F.; Duncan, C.; Musolino, P.L.; Orchard, P.J.; De Oliveira, S.; Thrasher, A.J.; Armant, M.; Dansereau, C.; Lund, T.C.; Miller, W.P.; et al. Hematopoietic Stem-Cell Gene Therapy for Cerebral Adrenoleukodystrophy. *N. Engl. J. Med.* **2017**, *377*, 1630–1638. [CrossRef] [PubMed]
68. Gupta, A.O.; Raymond, G.; Pierpont, E.I.; Kemp, S.; McIvor, R.S.; Rayannavar, A.; Miller, B.; Lund, T.C.; Orchard, P.J. Treatment of cerebral adrenoleukodystrophy: Allogeneic transplantation and lentiviral gene therapy. *Exp. Opin. Biol. Ther.* **2022**, *22*, 1151–1162. [CrossRef] [PubMed]
69. Brunson, A.; Keegan, T.H.M.; Bang, H.; Mahajan, A.; Paulukonis, S.; Wun, T. Increased risk of leukemia among sickle cell disease patients in California. *Blood* **2017**, *130*, 1597–1599. [CrossRef]
70. Goyal, S.; Tisdale, J.; Schmidt, M.; Kanter, J.; Jaroscak, J.; Whitney, D.; Bitter, H.; Gregory, P.D.; Parsons, G.; Foos, M.; et al. Acute myeloid leukemia case after gene therapy for sickle cell disease. *N. Engl. J. Med.* **2022**, *386*, 138–147. [CrossRef] [PubMed]
71. Hsieh, M.M.; Bonner, M.; Pierciey, F.J.; Uchida, N.; Rottman, J.; Demopoulos, L.; Schmidt, M.; Kanter, J.; Walters, M.C.; Thompson, A.A.; et al. Myelodysplastic syndrome unrelated to lentiviral vector in a patient treated with gene therapy for sickle cell disease. *Blood Adv.* **2020**, *4*, 2058–2063. [CrossRef] [PubMed]
72. Global Newswire Uniqure Announces Findings from Reported Case of Hepatocellular Carcinoma (HCC) in Hemophilia B Gene Therapy Program. Available online: https://www.globenewswire.com/news-release/2021/03/29/2200653/0/en/uniQure-Announces-Findings-from-Reported-Case-of-Hepatocellular-Carcinoma-HCC-in-Hemophilia-B-Gene-Therapy-Program.html (accessed on 29 March 2021).
73. Chandler, R.J.; LaFave, M.C.; Varshney, G.K.; Trivedi, N.S.; Carrillo-Carrasco, N.; Senac, J.S.; Wu, W.; Hoffmann, V.; Elkahloun, A.G.; Burgess, S.M.; et al. Vector design influences hepatic genotoxicity after adeno-associated virus gene therapy. *J. Clin. Investig.* **2015**, *125*, 870–880. [CrossRef] [PubMed]
74. Nguyen, G.N.; Everett, J.K.; Kafle, S.; Roche, A.M.; Raymond, H.E.; Leiby, J.; Wood, C.; Assenmacher, C.A.; Merricks, E.P.; Long, C.T.; et al. A long-term study of AAV gene therapy in dogs with hemophilia A identifies clonal expansions of transduced liver cells. *Nat. Biotechnol.* **2021**, *39*, 47–55. [CrossRef]
75. Nault, J.C.; Datta, S.; Imbeaud, S.; Franconi, A.; Mallet, M.; Couchy, G.; Letouzé, E.; Pilati, C.; Verret, B.; Blanc, J.F.; et al. Recurrent AAV2-related insertional mutagenesis in human hepatocellular carcinomas. *Nat. Genet.* **2015**, *47*, 1187–1193. [CrossRef] [PubMed]
76. Li, H.; Yang, Y.; Hong, W.; Huang, M.; Wu, M.; Zhao, X. Applications of genome editing technology in the targeted therapy of human diseases: Mechanisms, advances and prospects. *Signal Transduct. Target. Ther.* **2020**, *5*, 1. [CrossRef] [PubMed]
77. FDA Approves First Gene Therapies to Treat Patients with Sickle Cell Disease. US Food & Drug Administration. Available online: www.fda.gov/news-events/press-announcements/fda-approves-first-gene-therapies-treat-patients-sickle-cell-disease (accessed on 8 December 2023).
78. Liu, X.; Zhang, Y.; Cheng, C.; Cheng, A.W.; Zhang, X.; Li, N.; Xia, C.; Wei, X.; Liu, X.; Wang, H. CRISPR-Cas9-mediated multiplex gene editing in CAR-T cells. *Cell Res.* **2017**, *27*, 154–157. [CrossRef] [PubMed]
79. Tsuchida, C.A.; Brandes, N.; Bueno, R.; Trinidad, M.; Mazumder, T.; Yu, B.; Hwang, B.; Chang, C.; Liu, J.; Sun, Y.; et al. Mitigation of chromosome loss in clinical CRISPR-Cas9-engineered T cells. *Cell* **2023**, *186*, 4567–4582. [CrossRef] [PubMed]
80. Höijer, I.; Emmanouilidou, A.; Östlund, R.; van Schendel, R.; Bozorgpana, S.; Tijsterman, M.; Feuk, L.; Gyllensten, U.; den Hoed, M.; Ameur, A. CRISPR-Cas9 induces large structural variants at on-target and off-target sites in vivo that segregate across generations. *Nat. Commun.* **2022**, *13*, 627. [CrossRef]
81. Lemmens, M.; Dorsheimer, L.; Zeller, A.; Dietz-Baum, Y. Non-clinical safety assessment of novel drug modalities: Genome safety perspectives on viral-, nuclease- and nucleotide-based gene therapies. *Mutat. Res. Genet. Toxicol. Environ. Mutagen.* **2024**, *896*, 503767. [CrossRef]
82. Micklethwaite, K.P.; Gowrishankar, K.; Gloss, B.S.; Li, Z.; Street, J.A.; Moezzi, L.; Mach, M.A.; Sutrave, G.; Clancy, L.E.; Bishop, D.C.; et al. Investigation of product-derived lymphoma following infusion of piggyBac-modified CD19 chimeric antigen receptor T cells. *Blood* **2021**, *138*, 1401–1415. [CrossRef]
83. Murphy, L.A.; Marians, R.C.; Miller, K.; Brenton, M.D.; Mallo, R.L.V.; Kohler, M.E.; Fry, T.J.; Winters, A.C. Digital polymerase chain reaction strategies for accurate and precise detection of vector copy number in CAR T cell products. *Cytotherapy* **2023**, *25*, 94–102. [CrossRef]
84. Yan, N.; Feng, H.; Sun, Y.; Xin, Y.; Zhang, H.; Lu, H.; Zheng, J.; He, C.; Zuo, Z.; Yuan, T.; et al. Cytosine base editors induce off-target mutations and adverse phenotypic effects in transgenic mice. *Nat. Commun.* **2023**, *14*, 1784. [CrossRef]
85. Slesarenko, Y.S.; Lavrov, A.V.; Smirnikhina, S.A. Off-target effects of base editors: What we know and how we can reduce it. *Curr. Genet.* **2022**, *68*, 39–48. [CrossRef]
86. Odak, A.; Yuan, H.; Feucht, J.; Cantu, V.A.; Mansilla-Soto, J.; Kogel, F.; Eyquem, J.; Everett, J.; Bushman, F.D.; Leslie, C.S.; et al. Novel extragenic genomic safe harbors for precise therapeutic T-cell engineering. *Blood* **2023**, *141*, 2698–2712. [CrossRef]
87. Metzloff, A.E.; Padilla, M.S.; Gong, N.; Billingsley, M.M.; Han, X.; Merolle, M.; Mai, D.; Figueroa-Espada, C.G.; Thatte, A.S.; Haley, R.M.; et al. Antigen Presenting Cell Mimetic Lipid Nanoparticles for Rapid mRNA CAR T Cell Cancer Immunotherapy. *Adv. Mater.* **2024**, *36*, e2313226. [CrossRef] [PubMed]

88. Wu, J.; Wu, W.; Zhou, B.; Li, B. Chimeric antigen receptor therapy meets mRNA technology. *Trends Biotech.* **2024**, *42*, 228–240. [CrossRef] [PubMed]
89. Bouzianas, D.; Bouziana, S. A decade of CD4+ chimeric antigen receptor T-cell evolution in two chronic lymphocytic leukemia patients: Were chronic lymphocytic leukemia cells present? *Explor. Target. Antitumor Ther.* **2023**, *4*, 1128–1135. [CrossRef] [PubMed]
90. Bouzianas, D.; Bouziana, S. First pediatric B-acute lymphoblastic leukemia patient treated with anti-CD19 chimeric antigen receptor T-cell therapy: Long-term remission or early cure? *Hum. Vaccines Immunother.* **2024**, *20*, 2321678. [CrossRef] [PubMed]

International Journal of
Molecular Sciences

MDPI

Case Report

ETV6::ABL1-Positive Myeloid Neoplasm: A Case of a Durable Response to Imatinib Mesylate without Additional or Previous Treatment

Maria Teresa Bochicchio [1,*], Giovanni Marconi [2], Carmen Baldazzi [3], Lorenza Bandini [3], Francesca Ruggieri [1,4], Alessandro Lucchesi [2], Claudio Agostinelli [4,5], Elena Sabattini [5], Agnese Orsatti [5], Anna Ferrari [1], Giorgia Capirossi [1], Chiara Servili [1], Andrea Ghelli Luserna di Rorà [6], Giovanni Martinelli [7], Giorgia Simonetti [1] and Gianantonio Rosti [2,*]

1 Biosciences Laboratory, IRCCS Istituto Scientifico Romagnolo per lo Studio e la Cura dei Tumori (IRST) "Dino Amadori", 47014 Meldola, FC, Italy; francesca.ruggieri@irst.emr.it (F.R.); anna.ferrari@irst.emr.it (A.F.); giorgia.capirossi@studio.unibo.it (G.C.); chiara.servili@irst.emr.it (C.S.); giorgia.simonetti@irst.emr.it (G.S.)
2 Hematology Unit, IRCCS Istituto Scientifico Romagnolo per lo Studio e la Cura dei Tumori (IRST) "Dino Amadori", 47014 Meldola, FC, Italy; giovanni.marconi@irst.emr.it (G.M.); alessandro.lucchesi@irst.emr.it (A.L.)
3 Istituto di Ematologia "Seràgnoli", IRCCS Azienda Ospedaliero-Universitaria di Bologna, 40138 Bologna, BO, Italy; carmen.baldazzi@gmail.com (C.B.); lorenza.bandini.92@gmail.com (L.B.)
4 Department of Medical and Surgical Sciences (DIMEC), University of Bologna, 40100 Bologna, BO, Italy; claudio.agostinelli@unibo.it
5 Haematopathology Unit, IRCCS Azienda Ospedaliero-Universitaria di Bologna, 40138 Bologna, BO, Italy; elena.sabattini@aosp.bo.it (E.S.); agnese.orsatti@studio.unibo.it (A.O.)
6 Fondazione Pisana per la Scienza ONLUS, 56017 San Giuliano Terme, PI, Italy; a.ghelli@fpscience.it
7 Scientific Directorate, IRCCS Istituto Scientifico Romagnolo per lo Studio e la Cura dei Tumori (IRST) "Dino Amadori", 47014 Meldola, FC, Italy; giovanni.martinelli@irst.emr.it
* Correspondence: teresa.bochicchio@irst.emr.it (M.T.B.); gianantonio.rosti@irst.emr.it (G.R.)

Abstract: *ETV6::ABL1* rearranged neoplasms are rare hematological diseases. To date, about 80 cases have been reported, including myeloid and lymphoid leukemias. The *ETV6* gene codes for an ETS family transcription factor and several fusion partners have been described. When translocated, *ETV6* causes the constitutive activation of the partner genes. Here, we report the case of a 54-year-old woman with a cryptic insertion of the 3′ region of *ABL1* in the *ETV6* gene. The patient was first diagnosed with idiopathic hypereosinophilic syndrome, according to the clinical history, conventional cytogenetics, standard molecular analyses and pathologist description. Next generation sequencing of diagnosis samples unexpectedly detected both *ETV6::ABL1* type A and B fusion transcripts, which were then confirmed by FISH. The diagnosis was Myeloid/Lymphoid neoplasm with *ETV6::ABL1* fusion, and the patient received imatinib mesylate treatment. In a follow-up after more than one year, the patient still maintained the molecular and complete hematological responses. This case highlights the importance of timely and proper diagnostics and prompt tyrosine kinase inhibitor treatment.

Keywords: myeloid/lymphoid neoplasm; *ETV6::ABL1*; fusion genes; imatinib mesylate; next generation sequencing; diagnostic RNA panels

1. Introduction

ETV6::ABL1 (also known as *TEL::ABL1*) is a rare fusion that has been found in different types of hematological diseases. To date, about 80 cases of hematological neoplasms (more frequently, acute lymphoblastic leukemia (ALL), myeloproliferative neoplasms (MPNs), Philadelphia-negative chronic myeloid leukemia (CML) [1], atypical (a)CML and chronic myelomonocytic leukemia (CMML)) carrying *ETV6::ABL1* translocation have been reported [2–6]. ETV6::ABL1 chimeric protein has been found in less than 1% of ALL cases; however, due to the lack of a systematic screening for this fusion transcript, its overall incidence in hematological neoplasms cannot be precisely defined [2]. The *ETV6* (ETS variant 6) gene encodes for an ETS family transcription factor containing two functional domains: the N-terminus PNT (exons 3–4) and the C-terminus ETS (exons 6–7) domains, flanking the central domain coded by the exon 5 [7]. ETV6 is involved in the maintenance of the vascular network, hematogenesis, embryogenesis and development of different tissues [7]. The *ABL1* gene encodes for a non-receptor tyrosine kinase containing different structural domains, including SRC-homology domains (SH1, SH2 and SH3) responsible for the regulation of their own activity, DNA-binding (DB) domains and actin-binding (AB) domains, in addition to a nuclear translocation signal (NTS) sequence, sites for phosphorylation by protein kinase C (PKC) and a proline-rich sequence [8]. Two types of *ETV6::ABL1* in-frame fusion isoforms have been described: the so-called "type A", involving exon 4 of *ETV6* and exon 2 of *ABL1*, and the "type B" translocation, involving exon 5 of *ETV6* and exon 2 of *ABL1*. The ETV6::ABL1 fusion protein retains both the SH domains and the tyrosine kinase domain of ABL1 [9], leading to the loss of ABL1 autoinhibitory activity, thus resulting in a constitutive active enzyme. Both transcripts encode for a chimeric non-receptor tyrosine kinase resembling the *BCR::ABL1* structure. Moreover, in vitro studies have demonstrated that ETV6::ABL1 phosphorylates the same substrates activated by BCR::ABL1 chimeric proteins, suggesting that ETV6 may replace the BCR role and activate ABL1 [10], and explaining why patients harboring *ETV6::ABL1* translocation are sensitive to TKI treatment [9]. Here, we present the case of a patient who received a diagnosis of Myeloid/Lymphoid neoplasm with *ETV6::ABL1* fusion and reached a durable response by imatinib mesylate treatment.

2. Case Description

In January 2019, a 54-year-old Caucasian woman was referred to our institution for leukocytosis. She had a mild increase in white blood cell (WBC) count over one year (mean WBC 12 $\times$ 10^9/L, mean neutrophils 8 $\times$ 10^9/L), basophilia (5%) and eosinophilia (14%). *JAK2*, *CALR* and *MPL* mutations and *BCR::ABL1* rearrangements were negative (peripheral blood). The patient was asymptomatic and was not receiving any chronic treatment. She had no significant medical history, no history of smoking, no ongoing infections, negative inflammation markers, a normal chest and abdomen examination, and a normal abdomen ultrasonography (US). The patient underwent a regular follow-up (every 4 months) and did not receive any treatment. In the following 18 months, the WBC counts fluctuated around 11–13 $\times$ 10^9/L and the clinical patients' conditions were stable. In June 2020, the WBC count was raised to 32 $\times$ 10^9/L (basophilia 4%, eosinophilia 11%), while hemoglobin and platelets count were within the normal range, spleen was not palpable and the abdomen US results were normal. *BCR-ABL1* translocation and *JAK2*, *CALR*, and *MPL* mutations were confirmed to be negative (peripheral blood). Furthermore, no *PDGFRA*, *PDGFRB* or *FGFR1* rearrangements were detected. A trephine biopsy showed hypercellular bone marrow (95%) with a diffuse eosinophilic infiltration, slightly reduced erythropoiesis, normal $CD34^+$ cells and mastocytes (Figure 1). Cytogenetic examination showed a unique clone characterized by 47, XX, +12 (on 20 metaphases, Figure 2A). Chest X-ray and heart US excluded any significant organ involvement. Therefore, the patient was disagosed with idiopathic hypereosinophilic syndrome.

Next generation sequencing (NGS) was performed on the diagnosis peripheral blood sample, on both DNA and RNA, using the Oncomine Myeloid Assay (Thermo Fisher Scientific, Waltham, MA, USA), surprisingly revealing the presence of both *ETV6::ABL1* type A and B fusion transcripts (Figure 2B and Table S1), while confirming the absence of the Philadelphia chromosome. The *ETV6::ABL1* fusions were confirmed by RT-PCR (Figure 2C) and Sanger sequencing (Figure 2D,E). No additional DNA variants were found. Further information on the sample collection, nucleic acids isolation, library preparation and RT-PCR are reported in the Supplementary Methods. The variants and fusions tested are reported in Tables S2–S4.

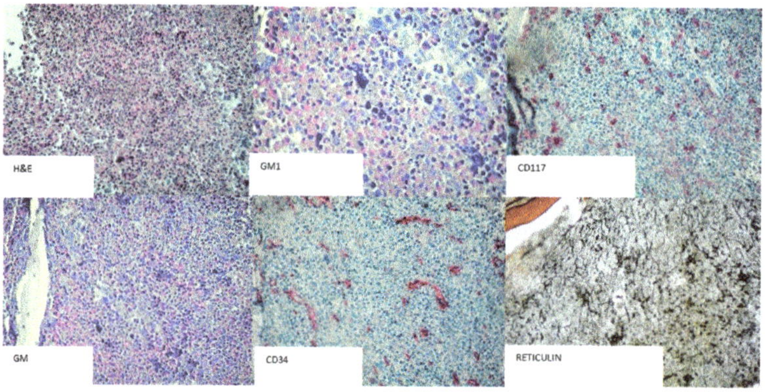

Figure 1. Morphological characterization. Hematoxylin and eosin (H&E, 200×) and Giemsa stain (GM, magnification 200×; GM1, magnification 400×); immunohistochemistry (IHC) stains for CD34 and CD117 (magnification 200×) and Gomori stain for reticulin fibers (Reticulin, magnification 200×).

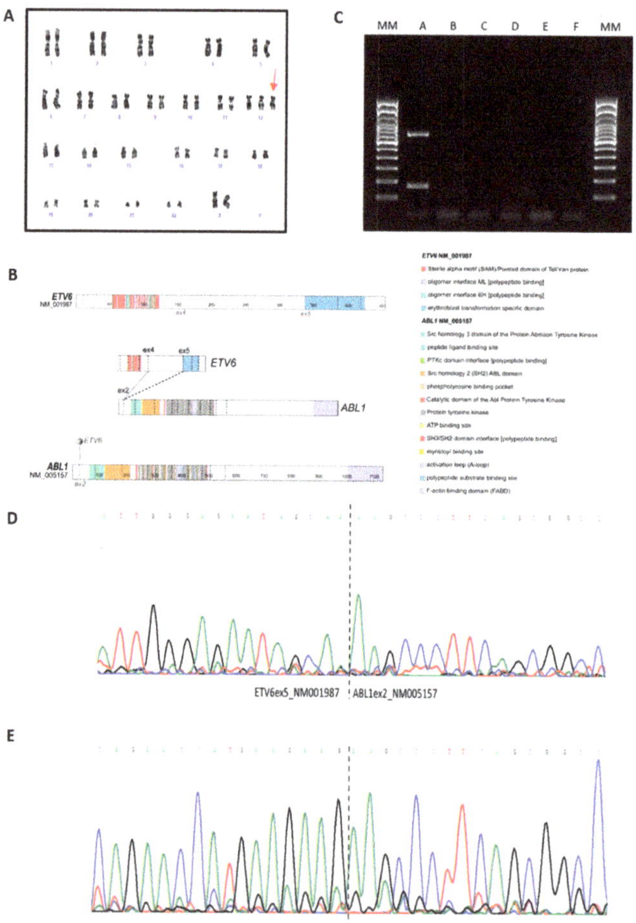

Figure 2. Cytogenetic and molecular characterization. (**A**) G-banded karyotype with trisomy involv-

ing the chromosome 12 (red arrow). (**B**) Overview of the *ETV6::ABL1* fusion transcripts detected by NGS and involving exon 5 of *ETV6* and exon 2 of *ABL1*, or exon 4 of *ETV6* and exon 2 of *ABL1*, respectively. (**C**) RT-PCR revealing the 706 bp *ETV6exon5::ABL1exon2* fusion transcript (upper band) and the 160 bp *ETV6exon4::ABL1exon2* fusion transcript (lower band). A 100 bp molecular weight marker was used. (**D**,**E**) Electropherograms of the sequences spanning the breakpoint confirming in-frame fusions involving *ETV6* exon 5 or *ETV6* exon 4 and *ABL1* exon 2. The dashed lines indicate the breakpoint regions. Each peak represents a single nucleotide in the DNA sequence, and each nucleotide has a different colour; A is green, T is red, C is blue and G is black. MM: Molecular Marker; A: diagnosis; B: 3 months follow-up; C: 6 months follow-up; D: 12 months follow-up; E: RT negative; F: PCR negative.

In order to confirm the fusion transcripts revealed by NGS, we performed fluorescent in situ hybridization (FISH). FISH analysis using an *ETV6* break-apart probe revealed three copies of the *ETV6* gene without evidence of *ETV6* rearrangement (Figure 3A). On the contrary, FISH analysis with a *BCR::ABL1* Tricolor Color Dual Fusion (TCDF) probe confirmed the presence of the *ABL1* rearrangement with *ABL* located on one chromosome 12 (Figure 3B). In order to confirm the *ETV6::ABL1* fusion, we performed FISH analysis combining *ETV6::RUNX1* ES Dual Color Dual Fusion and *BCR::ABL1* TCDF. FISH analysis showed the presence of the *ETV6::ABL1* fusion on chromosome 12 (Figure 3C). Therefore, we concluded that the *ETV6::ABL1* fusion was the result of a cryptic insertion of the 3′ of *ABL1* (q34) into the *ETV6* locus (12p13). Details on chromosome banding analysis (CBA) and FISH are described in the Supplementary Methods. Based on the results, the diagnosis was modified to Myeloid/Lymphoid neoplasm with *ETV6::ABL1* fusion, and the patient started imatinib mesylate treatment at the dose of 200 mg QD (8 September 2020).

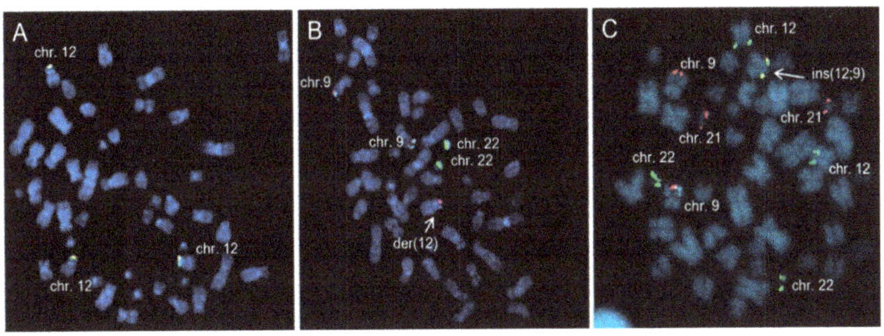

Figure 3. FISH analyses (100× magnification). (**A**) FISH analysis with *ETV6* break-apart on previously G-banded metaphase showing 3 fusion signals on 3 chromosomes 12, indicating 3 copies of *ETV6*. (**B**) FISH analysis with *BCR-ABL1* TCDF probes on previously G-banded metaphase showing 2 green signals on chromosome 22, two blue/red signals on chromosome 9 and an extra red signal on the short arm of chromosome 12, indicating *ABL1* rearrangement. (**C**) FISH analysis combining *ETV6-RUNX1* DCDF and *BCR-ABL1* TCDF probes on metaphase showing a fusion between *ETV6* marked in spectrum green and *ABL1* marked in spectrum orange on derivative chromosome 12, confirming *ETV6::ABL1* rearrangement. The arrows indicate the derivatives chromosome.

We monitored the most abundant fusion transcript, *ETV6*exon5::*ABL1* exon2, using both RT-PCR and Nested PCR. Follow-up peripheral blood samples were collected and analyzed at 3 months (time point B), at 6 months (time point C), at 12 months (time point D) and at 18 months (time point E) of therapy, according to clinical practice. RT-PCR results were negative in all the follow-up samples (Figure 4A). Negativity was confirmed by NGS at time points B and C using the Myeloid Plus Solution panel (Sophia Genetics). Nested-PCR negativity was reached at time point D, while samples at time points B and C were still weakly positive (1/2 replicates, Figure 4B). The complete hematological response was assessed by blood count, revealing all the parameters to be within the normal range.

The last evaluation—after 3 years of imatinib mesylate treatment—showed a WBC count of around $5 \times 10^9/L$ and a neutrophils count of $3.70 \times 10^9/L$ (basophilia 0.6%, eosinophilia 2.4%). The main clinical and laboratory information are summarized in Figure 5.

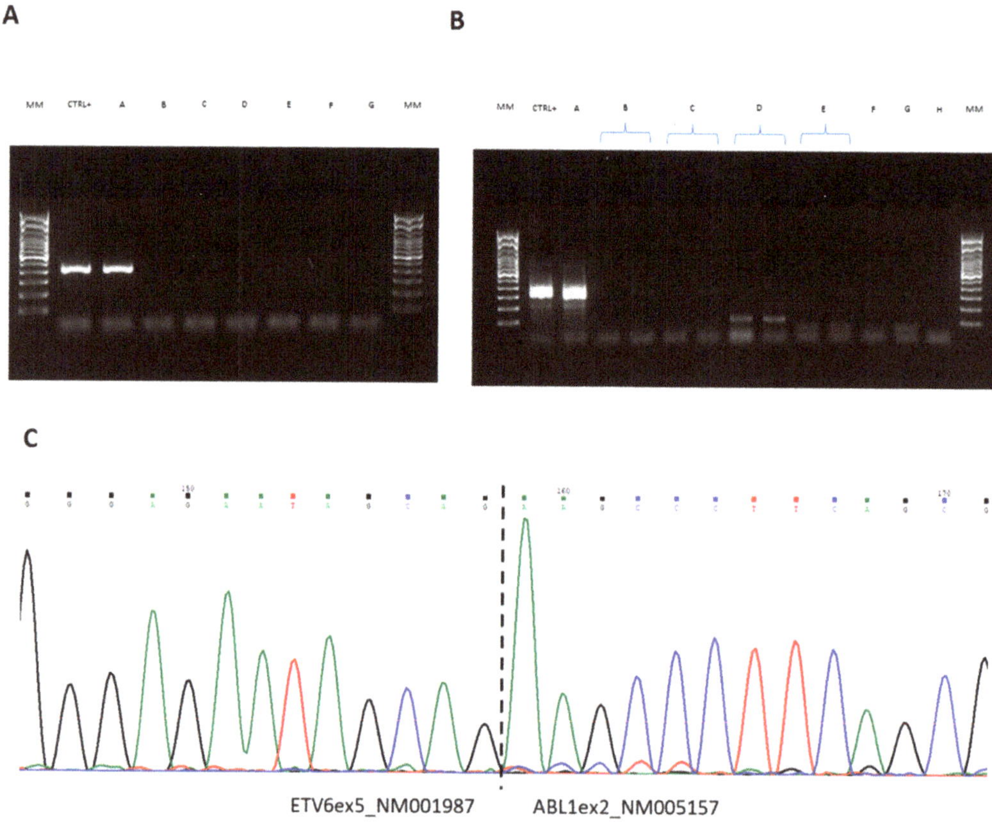

Figure 4. Monitoring of *ETV6*exon5::*ABL1*exon2 fusion overtime on peripheral blood samples. (**A**) RT-PCR revealing the 421-bp *ETV6*exon5-*ABL1*exon2 fusion transcript. (**B**) Nested PCR revealing the 321-bp *ETV6*exon5::*ABL1*exon2 fusion transcript. A 100 bp molecular weight marker was used. (**C**) Electropherogram of the sequence spanning the breakpoint that confirmed in-frame fusion involving *ETV6* exon 5 and *ABL1* exon 2. The dashed lines indicate the breakpoint regions. Each peak represents a single nucleotide in the DNA sequence, and each nucleotide has a different colour; A is green, T is red, C is blue and G is black. MM: Molecular Marker; A: diagnosis; B: 3 months follow-up; C: 6 months follow-up; D: 12 months follow-up; E: 18 months follow-up; F: RT negative; G: PCR negative; H: Nested-PCR negative.

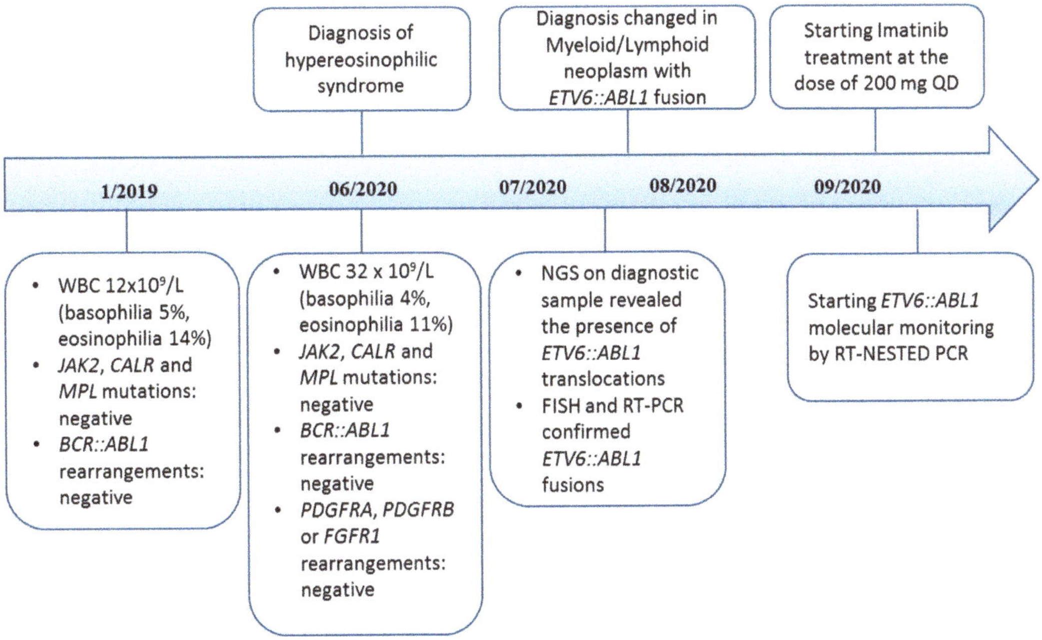

Figure 5. Timeline displaying clinical and therapy schedule (upper part) and laboratory data (bottom part).

3. Discussion

In this study, we report the case of an *ETV6::ABL1* rearranged patient with a diagnosis of Myeloid/Lymphoid neoplasm, who received imatinib mesylate treatment and achieved a durable response.

The formation of an in-frame *ETV6::ABL1* fusion gene involves complex genomic rearrangements because *ETV6* and *ABL1* genes have opposite chromosome orientations. Conventional diagnostic techniques (such as conventional cytogenetics) sometimes fail to detect this rearrangement because of its cryptic nature due to the similar G-banding pattern of the distal long arm of chromosome 9 and the distal short arm of chromosome 12. Moreover, no ready-to-use *ETV6::ABL1* FISH probes are commercially available, suggesting that the *ETV6-ABL1* fusion may remain undetected in a number of patients [5,11].

In the case we present, the use of next generation sequencing allowed us to overcome the above-mentioned limitations and to detect this fusion transcript, which changed the initial diagnosis of hypereosinophilic syndrome into the proper diagnosis of Myeloid/Lymphoid neoplasm with *ETV6::ABL1* fusion.

The patient showed the presence of both type "A" and "B" fusion transcripts, first detected by NGS and then confirmed by RT-PCR and Sanger sequencing. FISH analysis combining *ETV6::RUNX1* DCDF and BCR-ABL1 TCDF probes performed on metaphases showed a cryptic insertion of the 3′ region of *ABL1* in the *ETV6* gene on one chromosome 12, in addition to a signal consistent with trisomy 12.

ETV6::ABL1 rearrangements have been reported in different hematological malignancies and, in particular, in ALL, followed by MPNs and acute myeloid leukemia (AML) [11,12]. Eosinophilia represents a common clinical feature and a hallmark of all *ETV6::ABL1* rearranged MPNs cases reported in the literature [2], while the most frequent molecular alterations observed in ALL or in lymphoid blast crisis (LCB) patients are deletions of *CDKN2A/CDKN2B*, *IKZF1* or *PAX5* [2].

ETV6::ABL1 rearranged hematological neoplasms share many clinical features with CML. Indeed, the ETV6::ABL1 fusion protein functionally resembles the BCR::ABL1 ones, being characterized by a constitutive activation of the chimeric transcript [13], and sensitivity to both first- [14] and second-generation tyrosine kinase inhibitor (TKI) treatments [15]. For these reasons, the patient received imatinib therapy. Imatinib competitively binds the ABL1 ATP binding site in the ETV6::ABL1 fusion protein by the same mechanism of action described for the BCR::ABL1 protein.

Despite this, in the literature, few patients have received TKI treatment at first manifestation of the disease and/or at the first progression, and most of them died or relapsed/evolved [2]. Schwaab et al. presented data on *ETV6::ABL1* rearranged MPN patients that received imatinib, nilotinib or dasatinib after a prior treatment with hydroxyurea and/or cytarabine or intensive chemotherapy. Patients receiving imatinib did not achieve a complete cytogenetic (CCR) or molecular (CMR) response, which was instead obtained by patients under nilotinib or dasatinib treatment [16]. Accordingly, previous reports showed that imatinib allowed only an initial reduction of disease followed by a mild neutrophilia, basophilia and eosinophilia after 6 months, with persistent *ETV6::ABL1* positivity in FISH and nested PCR [13], or a transient response followed by transformation into ALL [17]. Moreover, most patients reported in the literature were diagnosed as atypical AML or Ph-like ALL.

Conversely, our patient presented without any blast excess at the diagnosis, and the clinical features were consistent with chronic diseases. She started TKI treatment as a frontline therapy after receiving the correct diagnosis and is still maintaining complete hematological and molecular responses after 36 months of imatinib mesylate. To our knowledge, this is the first case reporting a follow-up longer than one year without any additional [13] or previous chemotherapy treatment [18]. Our data likely rule out the co-occurrence of genomic events accounting for resistance in our patient and suggest a potential driver role for the *ETV6::ABL1* rearrangement. Studies accounting for different sensitivity profiles, gene expressions and BCR-ABL1-like signatures are warranted in this case; however, an accurate and multicenter sample collection is needed to meet this endpoint.

4. Conclusions

The detection of the *ETV6::ABL1* rearrangement remains difficult, due to its cryptic nature.

A deeper genomic characterization of patients with *ETV6::ABL1* fusion transcripts may improve our understanding of the biological complexity behind this disease. Although this could represent a limitation of our study, overall, our results underline the importance of timely and proper diagnostics, and the need to revise the current screening algorithms—for example, by recommending NGS RNA panels—in order to detect and monitor *ETV6::ABL1* rearrangements. In this case, molecular biology was instrumental in the diagnosis and, consequently, in the selection of an appropriate therapy. Notably, in the absence of molecular biology results, supportive therapies would have been the only ones administered to the patient.

Supplementary Materials: The following supporting information can be downloaded at: https://www.mdpi.com/article/10.3390/ijms25010118/s1. References [19–21] are cited in the supplementary materials.

Author Contributions: M.T.B. and G.R. drafted the manuscript and prepared figures; M.T.B., C.B., L.B., A.F., G.C., A.G.L.d.R., F.R., C.A., E.S. and A.O. conducted molecular biology, cytogenetic experiments and anatomic pathology evaluation; C.S., G.R., G.M. (Giovanni Marconi) and A.L. collected patient samples and clinical data; M.T.B., G.S., G.M. (Giovanni Marconi) and G.R. conceived, designed and interpreted the data; M.T.B. and G.R. supervised the project; G.S. provided the funding; M.T.B., G.M. (Giovanni Marconi), G.M. (Giovanni Martinelli), G.S. and G.R. revised the manuscript. All authors have read and agreed to the published version of the manuscript.

Funding: This work was partly supported by the contribution of Ricerca Corrente by the Italian Ministry of Health within the research line "Precision, gender and ethnicity-based medicine and geroscience: genetic-molecular mechanisms in the development, characterization and treatment of tumors" for IRCCS Istituto Scientifico Romagnolo per lo Studio e la Cura dei Tumori (IRST) "Dino Amadori", Meldola (FC), Italy. Part of the research activities by Carmen Baldazzi were supported by the Italian Ministry of Health, Ricerca Finalizzata GR-2018-12365278, within the expected project experimental work.

Institutional Review Board Statement: This study was approved by Comitato Etico della Romagna (protocol 5805/2019, #NCT04298892) and was carried out in accordance with the principles outlined in the 1964 Declaration of Helsinki.

Informed Consent Statement: Written informed consent was received from the patient prior to inclusion in the study. Moreover, written consent to publish the information contained in this article was also obtained from the patient.

Data Availability Statement: All data generated or analyzed during this study are included in this published article and in its Supplementary Materials.

Acknowledgments: The authors acknowledge Nicoletta Testoni and Emanuela Ottaviani from IRCCS Azienda Ospedaliero-Universitaria di Bologna, Istituto di Ematologia "Seràgnoli", Bologna (BO), Italy for their useful discussion on cytogenetics and molecular data.

Conflicts of Interest: Maria Teresa Bochicchio received honoraria as consultant from Werfen, Instrumentation Laboratory, S.p.A. Giovanni Marconi received honoraria as a consultant from/participant in a speaker bureau of Abbvie, Astellas, Immunogen, Menarini-Stemline, Pfizer, Ryvu, Servier, Syros and Takeda and received research support from Abbvie, Astellas, Astrazeneca, Jazz, Pfizer. Giovanni Martinelli has competing interests with Novartis, BMS, Roche, Pfizer, ARIAD and MSD. Gianantonio Rosti participated in a speaker bureau of Novartis, Incyte, BMD and Pfizer; and is on steering committees and advisory boards (Novartis, Pfizer, Incyte). All the other authors declare that the research was conducted in the absence of any commercial or financial relationships that could be construed as potential conflicts of interest.

References

1. De Braekeleer, E.; Douet-Guilbert, N.; Morel, F.; Le Bris, M.J.; Basinko, A.; De Braekeleer, M. ETV6 Fusion Genes in Hematological Malignancies: A Review. *Leuk. Res.* **2012**, *36*, 945–961. [CrossRef] [PubMed]
2. Zaliova, M.; Moorman, A.V.; Cazzaniga, G.; Stanulla, M.; Harvey, R.C.; Roberts, K.G.; Heatley, S.L.; Loh, M.L.; Konopleva, M.; Chen, I.M.; et al. Characterization of Leukemias with ETV6-ABL1 Fusion. *Haematologica* **2016**, *101*, 1082–1093. [CrossRef] [PubMed]
3. Cessna, M.H.; Paulraj, P.; Hilton, B.; Sadre-Bazzaz, K.; Szankasi, P.; Cluff, A.; Patel, J.L.; Hoda, D.; Toydemir, R.M. Chronic Myelomonocytic Leukemia with ETV6-ABL1 Rearrangement and SMC1A Mutation. *Cancer Genet.* **2019**, *238*, 31–36. [CrossRef] [PubMed]
4. Metzgeroth, G.; Steiner, L.; Naumann, N.; Lübke, J.; Kreil, S.; Fabarius, A.; Haferlach, C.; Haferlach, T.; Hofmann, W.K.; Cross, N.C.P.; et al. Myeloid/Lymphoid Neoplasms with Eosinophilia and Tyrosine Kinase Gene Fusions: Reevaluation of the Defining Characteristics in a Registry-Based Cohort. *Leukemia* **2023**, *37*, 1860–1867. [CrossRef] [PubMed]
5. Qi, Z.; Smith, C.; Shah, N.P.; Yu, J. Complex Genomic Rearrangements Involving ETV6::ABL1 Gene Fusion in an Individual with Myeloid Neoplasm. *Genes* **2023**, *14*, 1851. [CrossRef] [PubMed]
6. Choi, S.I.; Jang, M.A.; Jeong, W.J.; Jeon, B.R.; Lee, Y.W.; Shin, H.B.; Hong, D.S.; Lee, Y.K. A Case of Chronic Myeloid Leukemia with Rare Variant Etv6/Abl1 Rearrangement. *Ann. Lab. Med.* **2017**, *37*, 77–80. [CrossRef] [PubMed]
7. Hock, H.; Shimamura, A. ETV6 in Hematopoiesis and Leukemia Predisposition. *Semin. Hematol.* **2017**, *54*, 98–104. [CrossRef] [PubMed]
8. Amarante-Mendes, G.P.; Rana, A.; Datoguia, T.S.; Hamerschlak, N.; Brumatti, G. BCR-ABL1 Tyrosine Kinase Complex Signaling Transduction: Challenges to Overcome Resistance in Chronic Myeloid Leukemia. *Pharmaceutics* **2022**, *14*, 215. [CrossRef]
9. Xie, W.; Wang, S.A.; Hu, S.; Xu, J.; Medeiros, L.J.; Tang, G. Myeloproliferative Neoplasm with ABL1/ETV6 Rearrangement Mimics Chronic Myeloid Leukemia and Responds to Tyrosine Kinase Inhibitors. *Cancer Genet.* **2018**, *228*, 41–46. [CrossRef]
10. Okuda, K.; Golub, T.R.; Gilliland, D.G.; Griffin, J.D. P210BCR/ABL, P190BCR/ABL, and TEL/ABL Activate Similar Signal Transduction Pathways in Hematopoietic Cell Lines. *Oncogene* **1996**, *13*, 1147–1152.
11. Tirado, C.A.; Siangchin, K.; Shabsovich, D.S.; Sharifian, M.; Schiller, G. A Novel Three-Way Rearrangement Involving ETV6 (12p13) and ABL1 (9q34) with an Unknown Partner on 3p25 Resulting in a Possible ETV6-ABL1 Fusion in a Patient with Acute Myeloid Leukemia: A Case Report and a Review of the Literature. *Biomark. Res.* **2016**, *4*, 16. [CrossRef] [PubMed]

12. La Starza, R.; Trubia, M.; Testoni, N.; Ottaviani, E.; Belloni, E.; Crescenzi, B.; Martelli, M.F.; Flandrin, G.; Giuseppe Pelicci, P.; Mecucci, C. Clonal Eosinophils Are a Morphologic Hallmark of ETV6/ABL1 Positive Acute Myeloid Leukemia. *Haematologica* **2002**, *87*, 789–794. [PubMed]
13. Gancheva, K.; Virchis, A.; Howard-Reeves, J.; Cross, N.C.; Brazma, D.; Grace, C.; Kotzampaltiris, P.; Partheniou, F.; Nacheva, E. Myeloproliferative Neoplasm with ETV6-ABL1 Fusion: A Case Report and Literature Review. *Mol. Cytogenet.* **2013**, *6*, 39. [CrossRef] [PubMed]
14. Okuda, K.; Weisberg, E.; Gilliland, D.G.; Griffin, J.D. ARG Tyrosine Kinase Activity Is Inhibited by STI571. *Blood* **2001**, *97*, 2440–2448. [CrossRef] [PubMed]
15. Nand, R.; Bryke, C.; Kroft, S.H.; Divgi, A.; Bredeson, C.; Atallah, E. Myeloproliferative Disorder with Eosinophilia and ETV6-ABL Gene Rearrangement: Efficacy of Second-Generation Tyrosine Kinase Inhibitors. *Leuk. Res.* **2009**, *33*, 1144–1146. [CrossRef] [PubMed]
16. Schwaab, J.; Naumann, N.; Luebke, J.; Jawhar, M.; Somervaille, T.C.P.; Williams, M.S.; Frewin, R.; Jost, P.J.; Lichtenegger, F.S.; La Rosée, P.; et al. Response to Tyrosine Kinase Inhibitors in Myeloid Neoplasms Associated with PCM1-JAK2, BCR-JAK2 and ETV6-ABL1 Fusion Genes. *Am. J. Hematol.* **2020**, *95*, 824–833. [CrossRef] [PubMed]
17. Kakadia, P.M.; Schmidmaier, R.; Völkl, A.; Schneider, I.; Huk, N.; Schneider, S.; Panzner, G.; Neidel, U.; Fritz, B.; Spiekermann, K.; et al. An ETV6-ABL1 Fusion in a Patient with Chronic Myeloproliferative Neoplasm: Initial Response to Imatinib Followed by Rapid Transformation into ALL. *Leuk. Res. Rep.* **2016**, *6*, 50–54. [CrossRef] [PubMed]
18. Barbouti, A.; Ahlgren, T.; Johansson, B.; Höglund, M.; Lassen, C.; Turesson, I.; Mitelman, F.; Fioretos, T. Clinical and Genetic Studies of ETV6/ABL1-Positive Chronic Myeloid Leukaemia in Blast Crisis Treated with Imatinib Mesylate. *Br. J. Haematol.* **2003**, *122*, 85–93. [CrossRef]
19. Righi, S.; Novero, D.; Godio, L.; Bertuzzi, C.; Bacci, F.; Agostinelli, C.; Sagramoso, C.; Rossi, M.; Piccioli, M.; Gazzola, A.; et al. Myeloid Nuclear Differentiation Antigen: An Aid in Differentiating Lymphoplasmacytic Lymphoma and Splenic Marginal Zone Lymphoma in Bone Marrow Biopsies at Presentation. *Hum. Pathol.* **2022**, *124*, 67–75. [CrossRef]
20. Jeon, M.J.; Yu, E.S.; Kim, D.S.; Choi, C.W.; Kim, H.N.; Ah Kwon, J.; Yoon, S.Y.; Yoon, J. Performance Evaluation and Clinical Impact of the Oncomine Myeloid Research Assay for Gene Expression Analysis in Myeloid Haematologic Malignancies. *J. Clin. Pathol.* **2022**, *76*, 778–783. [CrossRef]
21. Simonetti, G.; Padella, A.; do Valle, I.F.; Fontana, M.C.; Fonzi, E.; Bruno, S.; Baldazzi, C.; Guadagnuolo, V.; Manfrini, M.; Ferrari, A.; et al. Aneuploid Acute Myeloid Leukemia Exhibits a Signature of Genomic Alterations in the Cell Cycle and Protein Degradation Machinery. *Cancer* **2019**, *125*, 712–725. [CrossRef] [PubMed]

MDPI AG
Grosspeteranlage 5
4052 Basel
Switzerland
Tel.: +41 61 683 77 34

International Journal of Molecular Sciences Editorial Office
E-mail: ijms@mdpi.com
www.mdpi.com/journal/ijms

www.ingramcontent.com/pod-product-compliance
Lightning Source LLC
Chambersburg PA
CBHW061456210926
51850CB00008B/1737